Contents

Acknowledgements

I wish to thank Miss Della Bingley of Coventry Technical College, and Ms Lyn Goldberg and Mr Alan Warren of the London College of Fashion for generous help and advice during the preparation of this book. I am also grateful for specialist advice on chapter 15 from Dr Alan Bedford of the Open University and Pamela Linforth, Principal of Sterex Academy, Coventry.

I am greatly indebted to Mrs Mary Robinson of Coventry Technical College and Mr Dick Welsh, Assistant Secretary, Northern Council for Further Education and Chief Examiner for CGLI Hairdressing and Beauty Therapy Science, for their careful reading of the manuscript and most valuable comments.

The publishers would like to thank the following for permission to reproduce photographs in this book:

Cover: Camera Press, London and The Sanctuary (see below)

Black-and-white photographs: Dr J Almeida, p 46; Dalesauna, p 256; Empire Stores Limited, p 52; John Lawrence Photography Limited, p 40; Dr D W R MacKenzie, p 44; The Sanctuary, p 273, pp 381–387; Tony Brain/Science Photo Library, p 78; NIBSC/Science Photo Library, p 261; George Solly Organisation Limited, pp 1, 49, 127, 167, 226, 295, 305, 367; John Symonds, pp 323, 341; Taylor Reeson Laboratories, pp 70, 98, 189, 245; Unilever, p 75; Walter Gardiner Photography, pp 48–49.

Every effort has been made to trace copyright holders of material reproduced in this book. Any rights not acknowledged here will be acknowledged in subsequent printings if notice is given to the publishers.

Foreword

In this book Ruth Bennett gives a full and comprehensive account of the applied science required by students for beauty therapy examinations. Students will find chapter 1 particularly useful as it gives a good insight into the basic scientific principles necessary for the understanding of the materials which follow in chapters 15 and 16.

As well as embracing all the scientific information necessary for the examinations, the science covered also concentrates on the anatomy and physiology, physical and electrical sciences and cosmetic chemistry behind the activities and treatments taking place in the beauty salon.

I congratulate Ruth on her book which has been written with great care, and the wealth of detail, coupled with her illustrations, reflect her very extensive experience. It should succeed in its aims.

Richard S Welsh
Former Chief Examiner for CGLI:
Hairdressing and Beauty Therapy Science

Preface

This book is intended for students taking courses in Beauty Therapy who are preparing for the examinations of the City and Guilds of London Institute Certificates in Beauty Therapy (304), Manicure (302), Cosmetic Make-up (303) and Electrical Epilation (305), the International Health and Beauty Council Diplomas, those of the British Association of Beauty Therapists and Cosmetologists, and of the BTEC National Diploma in Beauty Therapy. Much of the material also has relevance to courses such as the City and Guilds Science Foundation Course, CPVE modules in Beauty Care, TVEI courses and GCSE, A/S Level Human Biology.

The material in this book aims to provide a scientific explanation of the procedures carried out in a beauty salon. Chapter 1 explains the basic scientific concepts required for an understanding of the material in later chapters.

A number of self-assessment questions are included within each chapter. The answers to these will be found in the relevant chapter by careful reading of the text. Most of these questions resemble the shorter type of question which occurs in the examination papers set by the City and Guilds and the International Health and Beauty Council. Some longer questions placed at the back of the book resemble those in Section B of the examination papers mentioned above.

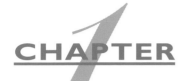

CHAPTER 1

Foundation Science

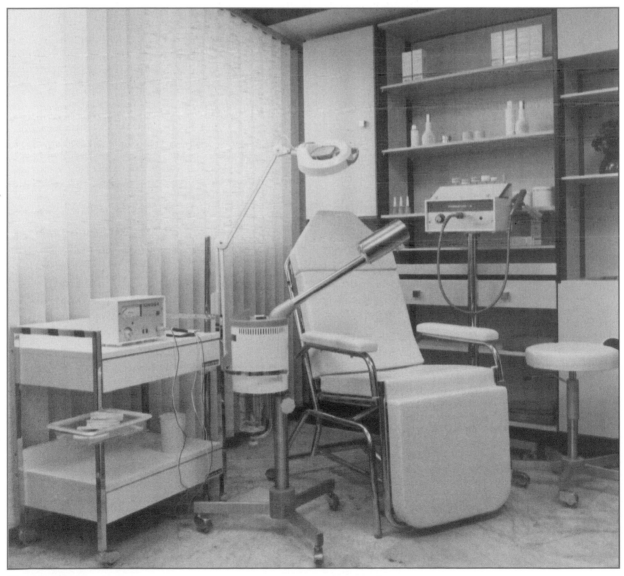

Beauty salon

PHYSICAL SCIENCE

Measurement

Both a number and a unit are needed to give a value to a particular quantity such as weight and energy. The number is obtained by measurement using a specific unit. Scientists use the metric system of measurement, and SI (international system) units. Larger or smaller quantities are derived by multiplying or dividing these units by multiples of ten.

Nature of matter

ELEMENTS AND COMPOUNDS

All substances are composed of matter, and are divided into two large groups called elements and compounds. If a substance can be split up into two or more simpler substances by a chemical change, it is a compound. If it cannot be split up by these means it is an element.

CHEMICAL AND PHYSICAL CHANGES

Chemical changes are those which are permanent and result in the formation of new substances. Changes which are easily reversed, such as ice melting or salt dissolving in water, are physical changes. New substances are not formed by physical

Table 1.1   *Units*

Name of unit	Dimension	Conversion	Subdivisions and multiples
Metre (m)	Length (distance between two points in space)	1 m = 39.37 inches	1 m = 100 centimetres (cm) 1 m = 1000 millimetres (mm) 10^{-6} m = 1 micrometre (μm) 10^{-9} m = 1 nanometre (nm)
Cubic metre (m^3)	Volume (amount of space)	16.38 cm^3 = 1 cubic inch	10^{-3} m^3 = 1 litre (l) 10^{-6} m^3 = 1 cubic centimetre (cm^3) = 1 millilitre (ml)
Kilogram (kg)	Mass (amount of matter) Weight (pull of gravity on a mass)	1 kg = 2.2 lb 28.34 g = 1 oz	1 kg = 1000 grams (g) 1 g = 1000 milligrams (mg)
Kilograms per cubic metre (kgm^{-3})	Density (mass per unit volume)		
Newton (N)	Force (a push or a pull)	4.45 N = 1 lb force	
Joule (J)	Energy (makes things happen)	4.2 J = 1 calorie 4200 J = 1 kilocalorie	1000 J = 1 kilojoule (kJ)
Degree Celsius (°C)	Temperature (hotness)	1 °C = ⅖ °Fahrenheit t °F = ⅗ (t − 32) °C	

changes. Chemical changes are often called chemical reactions, and many of them are exothermic, giving out heat.

ATOMS

Matter is composed of very small particles called atoms. An element is made up of only one kind of atom, and there are as many different kinds of atom as there are elements. As the atoms of different elements have different masses, it is useful to compare these masses to obtain the relative atomic mass. The carbon atom is chosen as the standard at 12. A hydrogen atom has only one-twelfth of the mass of a carbon atom, so its relative atomic mass is 1.

An atom is the smallest part of an element that can be involved in a chemical change. Chemical changes do not destroy or create atoms, but during them atoms will combine together to form molecules.

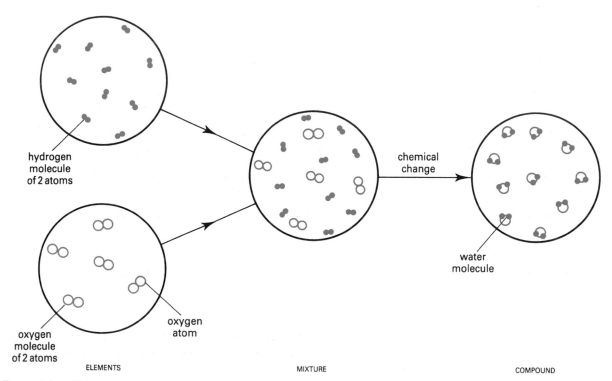

hydrogen
molecule
of 2 atoms

oxygen
molecule
of 2 atoms

oxygen
atom

ELEMENTS

MIXTURE

chemical
change

water
molecule

COMPOUND

Figure 1.1　*Elements,*
mixtures and compounds

MOLECULES

A molecule is the smallest part of an element or compound that
can exist alone. The atoms it contains may all be of the same
element, for example there are two oxygen atoms in an oxygen
molecule and three oxygen atoms in an ozone molecule. The
majority of molecules contain several different kinds of atom, for
example a water molecule contains two hydrogen atoms and one
oxygen atom.

MIXTURES

Although both mixtures and compounds contain at least two
substances, a mixture differs from a compound in that a
chemical change is not involved in its formation. Air is a mixture
of several elements (oxygen, nitrogen, neon) and compounds
(water, carbon dioxide).

SUBATOMIC PARTICLES

Atoms are made up of three smaller kinds of particle called
protons, electrons and neutrons. Protons and neutrons cluster in
the centre of the atom forming its nucleus. Electrons are much
lighter in weight and move round the nucleus at a fixed distance

Table 1.2   *Mixtures and compounds compared*

Mixtures	Compounds
Formed by a physical change (mixing)	A chemical change is involved in their formation, e.g. combustion or neutralisation
Their properties are the sum of the properties of their components	Their properties are quite different from the properties of their components
They may vary widely in their composition	Their composition is fixed, i.e. the weight of each component does not vary
Their components can be separated by physical means, e.g. filtration, evaporation or distillation	Their components cannot be separated by physical means
The atoms or molecules they contain are arranged randomly	The atoms they contain have a regular arrangement

from it in a particular orbit called an electron shell. The number of each of these subatomic particles varies in the atoms of different elements.

Figure 1.2   *Hydrogen and copper atoms*

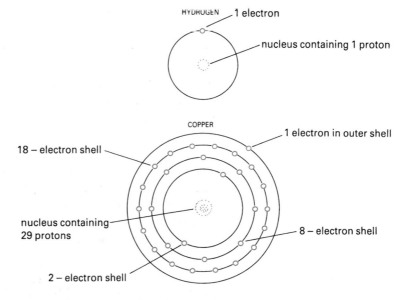

- Protons have a positive electric charge.
- Electrons have a negative electric charge.
- Neutrons have no electric charge.

As a result of their unlike charges, protons and electrons attract one another. Because each atom contains an equal number of protons and electrons, the positive and negative charges are balanced. All atoms are therefore electrically neutral.

IONS

If an atom (or molecule) loses or gains electrons, it acquires an electric charge, positive or negative respectively, and becomes an ion. Ions which have a positive electric charge are cations, and those with a negative charge are anions. Both hydrogen and copper ions are cations.

 The smallest part of a compound that can exist alone is:
(a) an electron
(b) an ion
(c) an atom
(d) a molecule

States of matter

Matter may occur in three forms, or states, known as solid, liquid or gas (vapour). If a solid becomes a liquid or a liquid becomes a

Table 1.3 *States of matter*

Gases	Liquids	Solids
Molecules move at high speeds	Molecules stick together (cohere) but can slide over one another	Molecules can move only very slightly
Exert a pressure which increases with increasing temperature	Exert a pressure which increases with temperature, but which is less than gas pressure	Molecules are often arranged in regular patterns so the solid is crystalline
Can be compressed to occupy a much smaller volume	Can be compressed very much less than gases	Cannot be compressed
As the temperature drops a liquid is formed	As the temperature drops a solid forms at freezing point. As the temperature increases a gas forms by evaporation and the liquid finally boils	As the temperature increases a liquid forms at the melting point

gas, or vice versa, this is a change of state. Melting, solidifying, evaporating, condensing, boiling and freezing are all changes of state. When they occur, latent heat is either given out or absorbed. This explains why sweat cools the body when it evaporates; it takes latent heat from the skin when changing from the liquid to the gaseous state.

Mass and weight

The mass of an object is the amount of matter contained in it. This remains constant. A person's body in air or water always has the same mass. Weight is the downward pull of gravity on that mass. A person's weight will vary if there is a force opposing the pull of gravity on their body.

Density

Density is the mass of unit volume of matter. As 1 cm^3 of water has a mass of 1 g, the density of water is 1 g/cm^3. Water has a much greater density than air, so far more muscular effort is needed for a person to move through chest high water than when surrounded by air. As the resistance of water is greater, muscles work harder and are strengthened. The heart is also made to work harder to supply the active muscles with food and oxygen.

Substances with a density less than 1 g/cm^3 will float on water while substances with a density greater than that of water will sink.

Buoyancy

Buoyancy is the tendency of water to exert a lifting effect on a body wholly or partly immersed. This is an application of Archimedes' principle that the upthrust of a body in water is equal to the weight of fluid the body displaces. The upthrust therefore counteracts the downward force of gravity. A person's body is thus supported by the water if it is wholly or partly immersed. The weight of the body on the hip, knee and ankle is thus reduced, so no damaging compression on these joints occurs. The benefits of exercise without the risk of injury to the musculo-skeletal system make exercising in water of particular value to older or less-fit individuals.

Solubility

SOLUTIONS

When some substances are added to a liquid they dissolve and form a solution. The substance which dissolves is the solute, and may be a solid, liquid or gas. The liquid in which the solute dissolves is the solvent.

Solid solutes will be left behind if the solution evaporates, for example when the water (solvent) in sweat (solution) evaporates, the salt (solute) is left behind on the skin. Liquid or gaseous solutes are separated from the solution by distillation. The solute molecules are evenly distributed throughout the solution, which is therefore a homogeneous mixture. A solution looks transparent (clear) as the dissolved particles are too small to be visible. The solute molecules cannot be removed from the solution by filtering it through a filter paper.

A concentrated solution contains a large amount of solute, while one which is dilute contains very little. A saturated solution contains as much solute as it can hold at that temperature. Concentration is usually expressed in terms of the number of moles of solute in one litre of solution (mol l^{-1}). A mole is the unit used to describe the amount of chemical substance and is calculated from the relative atomic masses of each element in the substance. The relative atomic mass (in grams) of every element contains the same number of atoms (6×10^{23}) and equals one mole of the element. Thus, since a mole of sodium chloride (salt) contains this fixed number of sodium atoms (relative atomic mass 23) and the same number of chlorine atoms (relative atomic mass 35.5), one mole of sodium chloride has a mass of:

$$23 \text{ g} + 35.5 \text{ g} = 58.5 \text{ g}$$

A solution of sodium chloride with a concentration of 1 mol l^{-1} contains 58.5 g dissolved in 1 litre of solution.

ELECTROLYTES

Some solutes ionise (split up into ions) in solution and are called electrolytes. If all the solute molecules ionise, the substance is a strong electrolyte. If only a few of the molecules ionise, the substance is a weak electrolyte. If none of the molecules ionise, the substance is a non-electrolyte.

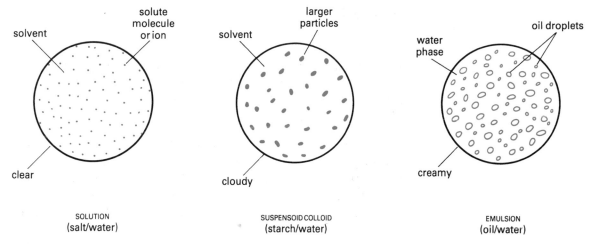

Figure 1.3   *Solutions and colloids*

SUSPENSIONS

Suspensions may form from insoluble solids which remain homogeneously mixed with a liquid. The solid particles in a suspension are usually large enough to be removed by filtering, and because they are visible the suspension looks cloudy. On standing, the solid particles slowly separate out of the liquid as a visible layer. A clay-based face pack is an example of a suspension.

COLLOIDS

In a colloid the suspended particles are smaller than those in a suspension, but larger than the individual molecules in a solution. On standing, the particles do not settle out but are kept in suspension by continuous collisions with solvent molecules. This jostling effect is known as Brownian movement. The particles in a colloid are small enough to pass through a filter paper and can be split into two classes: suspensoids where the particles are solid, and emulsoids where the particles are tiny liquid droplets. Soap and starch form suspensoids, mixing with water to form a colloid which is cloudy in appearance. If the colloid is very concentrated, a semi-solid gel is produced. Emulsoid colloids are usually called emulsions.

EMULSIONS

An emulsion is a suspension of droplets of one liquid in another liquid, where the two liquids are immiscible (one liquid does not dissolve in the other). An emulsion is known as a cream when the two liquids are oil and water, and many cosmetics are formulated as creams. The tiny droplets of the suspended liquid form the disperse phase of the emulsion, while the other liquid forms the continuous phase. Where oil droplets form the disperse phase an oil-in-water (o/w) emulsion is produced. When water droplets form the disperse phase the emulsion is of the water-in-oil (w/o) type.

A suspension of tiny droplets of one liquid in another liquid is:
(a) an emulsion
(b) a suspensoid
(c) a filtrate
(d) a solution

Figure 1.4   *Structure of an emulsion*

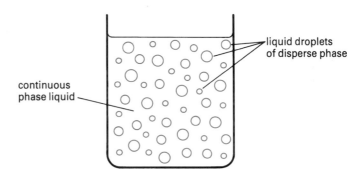

The two types of emulsion have different properties

- An o/w emulsion is less greasy and can be rinsed off the skin with water.

- A w/o emulsion is very greasy and cannot be rinsed away. It must either be wiped off the skin using a paper tissue, washed off by a detergent solution, or removed by another oil which is miscible with the continuous phase of the emulsion.

EMULSIFYING AGENTS

When preparing an emulsion, the oil and water phases must be heated separately and an emulsifying agent (emulsifier) added before stirring the two phases together.

Metal and non-metal

The elements are divided into metals and non-metals. Each element is represented by a chemical symbol which may also represent one atom of that element, for example Cu represents copper and one atom of copper. (See table 1.5.)

Table 1.4   *Metals and non-metals compared*

Metals	Non-metals
Solids, with the exception of mercury	May be gases, liquids or solids
Have lustre (shiny)	Solid non-metals are dull except carbon in the form of diamond
Dense (heavy)	Have a low density (light in weight)
Good conductors of heat and electricity	Poor conductors of heat and all except carbon are poor electrical conductors
Can be hammered into sheets and drawn out into wire	Solid non-metals are brittle
Form basic oxides	Form acidic oxides
Form positive ions (cations)	Form negative ions (anions), except hydrogen

Organic and inorganic compounds

Compounds form the majority of chemical substances and are divided into two groups:

- Organic compounds are those containing the element carbon and are usually found in, or made by, living organisms. Many have large complex molecules due to the ability of carbon atoms to link up in chains. Proteins and starches are organic compounds.

- Inorganic compounds are the rest of the compounds. They may contain any of the elements, and the majority have small molecules, for example sodium chloride (salt) and water.

Figure 1.5   *Organic and inorganic molecules*

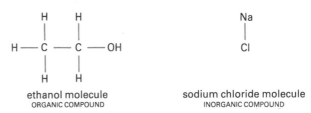

ethanol molecule
ORGANIC COMPOUND

sodium chloride molecule
INORGANIC COMPOUND

Table 1.5   *Characteristics of some important elements*

Element	State	Metal or non-metal	Protons	Symbol
Hydrogen	Gas	Non-metal	1	H
Carbon	Solid	Non-metal	6	C
Nitrogen	Gas	Non-metal	7	N
Oxygen	Gas	Non-metal	8	O
Fluorine	Gas	Non-metal	9	F
Sodium	Solid	Metal	11	Na
Aluminium	Solid	Metal	13	Al
Silicon	Solid	Non-metal	14	Si
Phosphorus	Solid	Non-metal	15	P
Sulphur	Solid	Non-metal	16	S
Chlorine	Gas	Non-metal	17	Cl
Potassium	Solid	Metal	19	K
Calcium	Solid	Metal	20	Ca
Iron	Solid	Metal	26	Fe
Cobalt	Solid	Metal	27	Co
Copper	Solid	Metal	29	Cu
Iodine	Solid	Non-metal	53	I
Tungsten	Solid	Metal	74	W
Mercury	Liquid	Metal	80	Hg
Lead	Solid	Metal	82	Pb

Compounds are arranged in a number of classes based on a study of their structure and properties.

OXIDES

Oxides are the compounds formed when elements combine with oxygen. This occurs during the chemical change of burning (combustion).

- The oxides of non-metals, for example carbon dioxide (CO_2), are acidic, turning litmus solution red.

- The oxides of metals, for example calcium oxide (CaO), are basic, turning litmus solution blue.

Litmus and other dyes which change colour in acidic and basic chemicals are called indicators.

pH

The degree of acidity or basicity (alkalinity) is measured on the pH scale. This scale goes from 0 to 14. In the range 0 to 6.9 the lower the pH value, the greater the acidity. Above 7 the greater the pH value, the more basic (alkaline) the chemical becomes. A substance which is neither acidic nor basic has a pH of 7 and is said to be neutral.

Figure 1.6   *The pH scale*

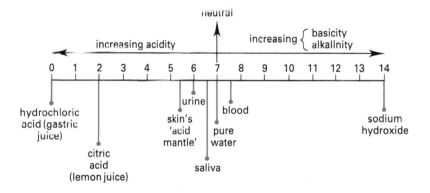

Acidity is closely related to the concentration of hydrogen ions in a solution. The pH corresponding to a hydrogen ion concentration of 1.0×10^{-3} mol l^{-1} is 3, that is the index figure 3 is used as the pH value. An increase in pH indicates a decrease in hydrogen ion concentration. A neutral solution contains 1.0×10^{-7} mol l^{-1} of hydrogen ions, so the index 7 becomes the neutral pH value. A basic solution has less than 1.0×10^{-7} mol l^{-1} of hydrogen ions, so its pH is greater than 7.

ACIDS

Acids are formed when acidic oxides react with water. They ionise in aqueous solution to give hydrogen ions.

$$CO_2 \quad + \quad H_2O \quad \rightarrow \quad H_2CO_3 \quad \rightarrow \quad H^+ \quad + \quad HCO_3^-$$

| acidic oxide | water | carbonic acid | hydrogen ion | hydrogen carbonate ion |

- Inorganic (mineral) acids in solution usually contain a high concentration of hydrogen ions as they are strong electrolytes and thus have a low pH. They are known as strong acids, examples being sulphuric acid (H_2SO_4) and hydrochloric acid (HCl). Some inorganic acids, for example carbonic and phosphoric acids, are weak electrolytes so they have a slightly higher pH and are known as weak acids.

- Organic acids are also weak electrolytes and weak acids. Examples are citric acid (in lemon juice), fatty acids and alpha hydroxy acids (AHAs) obtained from various fruits. Organic acids contain a carboxyl group (−COOH) from which hydrogen ions are produced.

Diluting an acid by dissolving it in a large volume of water increases its pH by reducing the concentration of hydrogen ions. (**Note:** it is very dangerous to add water to concentrated acid. Always add small volumes of acid to a large volume of water.)

ALKALIS

Basic oxides (bases) may react with water to form metal hydroxides. A few metal hydroxides are soluble in water, ionising to produce hydroxyl ions (OH^-), and are called alkalis. Examples of alkalis are sodium, potassium and calcium hydroxides. Although it is not a metallic hydroxide, ammonium hydroxide (NH_4OH) resembles other alkalis in its properties and is included with them.

NEUTRALISATION

A solution of an acid contains hydrogen ions and acid radical ions. A solution of an alkali contains hydroxyl ions and metal ions. When these two solutions are mixed, many of the hydrogen and hydroxyl ions disappear as they combine together to form water molecules. The acid radical and metal ions remain as an ionised salt. This chemical reaction is called neutralisation as the product, water, is neutral. It is expressed by the following equation:

$$acid + base = salt + water$$

ORGANIC BASES

Organic bases include the alcohols which contain a hydroxyl group (−OH), and the amines which contain an amine group (−NH_2). Examples of alcohols are methanol, ethanol, propanol

Table 1.6 *Properties of acids and alkalis*

Acids	Alkalis
Turn litmus red	Turn litmus blue
Dilute solutions have a sour taste	Dilute solutions have a bitter taste and feel soapy
Many are dangerous corrosive compounds causing chemical burns	Are dangerous caustic compounds causing chemical burns
Have a pH below 7	Have a pH above 7
React with alkalis to form a salt and water by the chemical change of neutralisation	React with acids to form a salt and water by the chemical change of neutralisation

and glycerol. Triethanolamine is an example of an amine. Organic bases will combine with acids to form esters and water:

organic acid + organic base = ester + water

 When an organic acid reacts with an alcohol, the products are water and:
(a) an alkali
(b) an amine
(c) an ester
(d) an alkane

SALTS

Salts are produced when the hydrogen of an acid is replaced by a metal or an ammonium group. They are also produced by the neutralisation of an acid by a base or an alkali. Salts form metal ions which are positively charged (cations) and acid radical ions which are negatively charged (anions). Soluble salts are highly ionised in water and are therefore strong electrolytes.

If a salt is formed from a strong acid and a strong base (e.g. sodium chloride), it will form a neutral solution with a pH of 7. A salt formed from a weak acid and a strong base (e.g. sodium phosphate) will form an alkaline solution with a pH above 7. This is due to a small proportion of the acid radical (e.g. phosphate) ions reacting with water to form acid molecules (e.g.

phosphoric acid) and hydroxyl ions. This reduces the number of hydrogen ions present and increases the pH.

$$\text{phosphate ions} + \text{water molecules} = \text{phosphoric acid} + \text{hydroxyl ions}$$

Table 1.7   *Salts*

Metal	Acid radical	Common name
Calcium	carbonate	Chalk
Magnesium	silicate	Talc
Potassium	palmitate	Soft soap
Sodium	chloride	Common salt
Sodium	stearate	Hard soap
Zinc	carbonate	Calamine

BUFFERS

Where it is important to keep the pH of a mixture stable, as in acid creams and chemical depilatories, a buffer is required.

A buffer can be made from a weak acid and the sodium salt of that acid, commonly phosphoric acid and sodium phosphate. As phosphoric acid is only slightly ionised but sodium phosphate is highly ionised, a mixture of the two compounds in water contains few hydrogen ions but many phosphate ions. If a small amount of acid is added to the buffer, the hydrogen ions from the acid will combine with phosphate ions to form molecules of phosphoric acid. There is thus no increase in the concentration of hydrogen ions, so the pH does not fall.

Similarly, if a small amount of alkali is added to the buffer, the hydroxyl ions from the alkali combine with hydrogen ions to form water. Further ionisation of phosphoric acid molecules then occurs to replace the lost hydrogen ions and lower the pH again.

ESTERS

Esters are produced when alcohols react with organic acids.

Ethyl, butyl and amyl acetates used as nail lacquer solvents are esters. Esters of glycerol combined with three molecules of long chain fatty acids are called triglycerides. They occur in plant and animal fats and oils. Phospholipids are more complex esters containing phosphate groups. True waxes are usually esters formed from long chain fatty acids and from alcohols such as cetyl alcohol or cholesterol.

HYDROCARBONS

Hydrocarbons (alkanes) consist of molecules containing long chains of carbon atoms to which hydrogen atoms are attached. As their name suggests, they contain the elements hydrogen and carbon only. They are present in natural gas and petroleum which are fossil fuels derived from once-living organisms. Methane (CH_4) is present in natural gas. Alkane gases, petrol, mineral oil, petroleum jelly and paraffin wax are all obtained from petroleum.

SALON WATER SUPPLY

Water authorities are required to supply tap water which is free from visible suspended particles, disease-producing organisms (pathogens) and chemical substances injurious to health (pollutants). The original source of all water supplies is rainfall, which is part of the natural water cycle on the earth.

Water is taken from lakes and rivers, and stored in reservoirs placed at a higher level than the buildings they supply. A head of water, that is the distance between the water level in the reservoir and the level of the service pipes to the buildings, produces a water pressure. Where there is no head of water available, tap water must be pumped into water towers or directly into the service pipes to achieve a water pressure.

The water must be treated in various ways to remove suspended particles (by filters), pathogens (by chlorine) and pollutants (by suitable chemical treatments) before entering the service pipes. In some areas fluoride is added as a protection against tooth decay. The service pipe must supply at least one cold tap, which should be used for drinking water, before the water enters a cold tank for storage and circulation through the salon water system.

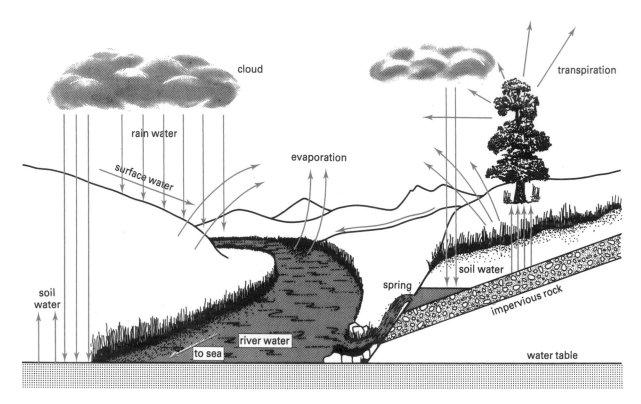

Figure 1.7   *The water cycle*

Hard and soft water

Distilled water and rainwater from clean air districts contain no dissolved solid impurities and are soft. Most tap water, however, does contain dissolved salts and is hard. Hard water forms a scum with soap, which prevents it from lathering readily. It also deposits scale when heated. Soft water, on the other hand, forms neither scale nor scum and lathers readily with soap.

The impurities which make water hard have come from the rocks over which the water source flows. They consist of the four ionised salts: calcium sulphate, calcium hydrogen carbonate (bicarbonate), magnesium sulphate and magnesium hydrogen carbonate (bicarbonate). The calcium and magnesium ions react with soap to form an insoluble calcium or magnesium soap called a scum. Thus, soapless detergents, such as sodium lauryl sulphate, have a great advantage over soap in that they do not form a scum with hard water.

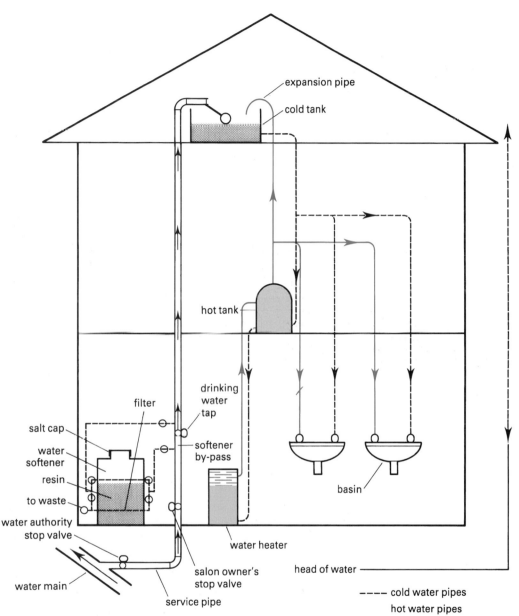

Figure 1.8   *Salon water supply*

Water softening

The natural impurities which make water hard can be removed to obtain soft water by a number of means.

BOILING

Hardness due to hydrogen carbonates will be removed by boiling the water and is said to be temporary. Boiling converts the hydrogen carbonate into insoluble metal carbonate salts and carbon dioxide is released.

$$\text{calcium ions} + \text{hydrogen carbonate ions} \xrightarrow{\text{heat}} \text{calcium carbonate molecules} + \text{carbon dioxide}$$

Hardness due to sulphates cannot be removed by boiling and is said to be permanent.

CHEMICALS

All types of hardness can be removed from tap water on a small scale by the addition of a chemical water softener such as sodium hexametaphosphate (Calgon), sodium carbonate (washing soda) or sodium borate (borax). Sodium carbonate and borate form insoluble particles by reacting with the calcium and magnesium ions in the hard water and increase its alkalinity. This method of water softening does not prevent the scaling of pipes in a hot water system.

ION EXCHANGE

For softening the entire salon water supply an ion exchange method is used. The hard water flows through a cylinder containing a column of synthetic resin (derived from polystyrene) which contains negatively charged acidic groups at the surface. These are neutralised by sodium ions to form a sodium salt of the resin. As hard water flows through the cylinder, its calcium or magnesium ions are exchanged for sodium ions from the resin. After a certain volume of hard water has passed over the resin column all its sodium ions will have been exchanged, so water softening ceases. The resin column is regenerated by passing a concentrated solution of sodium chloride through it. This washes out the calcium and magnesium ions and replaces them with sodium ions.

 When dissolved in tap water, the sulphates of calcium and magnesium produce the type of hardness called:
(a) temporary
(b) partial
(c) permanent
(d) anionic

FUNDAMENTALS OF HEATING

Heat energy

Heat is a form of energy. It is produced by burning fuels, by human bodies, and by friction when two surfaces are rubbed together, for example during massage. In a beauty salon, heat is produced by different types of appliances which convert other forms of energy into heat.

Water heating

A beauty salon requires a supply of hot water for washing and laundry all the year round. The usual temperature of a hot water supply is 60 °Celsius. This temperature will not cause much scaling of hot water pipes where tap water is hard, but is hot enough for normal salon purposes.

Space heating

A suitable air temperature must be maintained for the comfort of clients undergoing beauty treatments. The air temperature needs to be at least 20 °Celsius, with an optimum temperature two or three degrees higher for maximum comfort.

Thermometer

Temperature is measured by a thermometer, an instrument which compares the hotness of a substance (for example water or air) with that of melting ice or boiling water. A thermometer contains a liquid (mercury or coloured alcohol) in a narrow tube with a basal bulb. The liquid expands as the temperature increases, giving a reading on a scale marked in degrees Celsius (°C). The fixed points on this scale are the temperature of melting ice at 0 °C and that of boiling water at 100 °C. Body temperature is around 37 °C.

CLINICAL THERMOMETER

A special type of thermometer, called a clinical thermometer, should be used to take body temperatures. It has a strong bulb containing the mercury and a narrow temperature range from 35 °C to 45 °C. Temperatures higher than this will cause the thermometer to break due to increased expansion of the mercury, so it must always be washed in cold water. The narrow tube containing the mercury has a constriction to prevent the mercury level from falling after body temperature has been registered. The thermometer must, therefore, be shaken after use to bring the mercury level down to below 35 °C.

Figure 1.9   *Clinical thermometer*

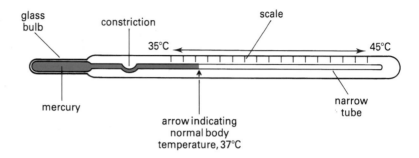

Thermostat

Temperature is regulated by a thermostat. It acts by cutting off the fuel supply to a heater once it reaches a selected temperature. When the temperature falls, the fuel reaches the heater again to bring the temperature up to its required value. Thermostats are fitted to most electrical appliances that produce heat used in a beauty salon.

BIMETALLIC STRIP

The simplest type of electrical thermostat contains a bimetallic strip. The scientific principle on which its action is based is that different metals expand by different amounts for the same temperature rise. Most metals, including brass, expand on heating and contract on cooling. The alloy invar (a mixture of steel and nickel), however, hardly expands at all on heating. Thus, if a strip of brass and a strip of invar are joined together to form a bimetallic strip which is then heated, the brass expands more than the invar, causing the bimetallic strip to bend. As the strip cools it will straighten again because the brass contracts to its original length.

In a thermostat, the electricity flows through a bimetallic strip to reach a heater. The heater warms the bimetallic strip which bends, breaking the electrical contact and preventing electricity from reaching the heating element of the appliance.

Figure 1.10   *Electric thermostat*

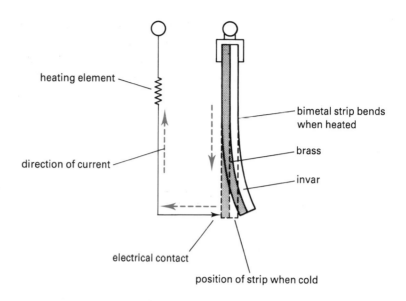

Heat transfer

Heat produced by an appliance, or by the body, can be transferred in three possible ways: by conduction, convection or radiation (see table 1.8).

Heating appliances

Water heating appliances include a central heating system, immersion heaters and instantaneous water heaters. The fuel converted is either gas or electricity. Salon space heating appliances include a central heating system, but also an air-conditioning system, electrical floor or ceiling heating systems, balanced flue heaters and infra-red wall heaters.

A bimetallic strip is part of the structure of a:
(a) thermostat
(b) heating element
(c) fuse
(d) three-pin plug

Inverse square law

All heat therapy and ultra-violet therapy treatments apply the principle of the inverse square law. This law states that the

Table 1.8   *Methods of heat transfer*

	Conduction	Convection	Radiation
How heat is transferred	Heat passes from one molecule to the next	Heat passes by the movement of heated molecules	Heat travels in straight lines as heat rays. All hot objects give out heat rays
Where the method occurs	Occurs most rapidly in solids. Metals are good thermal conductors	Occurs in liquids and gases	Occurs in gases and space
Properties of the method	Does not pass through thermal insulators such as glass, wool, plastic etc	Expansion of the heated gas or liquid increases its volume and reduces its density. The hot gas or liquid therefore rises. A stream of heated molecules forms a convection current	Dull, dark surfaces in the path of heat rays absorb them and become hotter. Shiny and light surfaces reflect heat rays and remain cool
Examples	Heat produced by friction passes by conduction through the skin to underlying muscle during massage	The movement of hot water in a hot water system and movement of warm air in a sauna are due to convection	Nichrome heating elements and infra-red heaters give out radiant heat

intensity of the radiation at the skin surface depends on the inverse square of its distance from the radiation source.

For example, if the distance of a radiant heat lamp from the skin is doubled, the intensity of the infra-red radiation on the skin is only one quarter ($\frac{1}{2}^2$) of the original intensity. Similarly, the intensity of the radiation on the skin 50 cm away from the radiant heat lamp is four times the radiation received when the lamp is placed 100 cm away.

The duration of a treatment is also determined by the inverse square law. To produce the same effect as exposure for one minute to an ultra–violet lamp placed 50 cm away from the skin, the client needs to be exposed for four minutes when the lamp is 100 cm away. The formula that can be used for calculating treatment duration is:

$$\text{new time} = \text{original time} \times \left(\frac{\text{new distance}}{\text{original distance}} \right)^2$$

Example

$$\text{new time} = 1 \text{ minute} \times \left(\frac{100 \text{ cm}}{50 \text{ cm}} \right)^2$$

$$= 1 \text{ minute} \times \left(\frac{2}{1} \right)^2$$

$$= 4 \text{ minutes}$$

FUNDAMENTALS OF LIGHTING

Light energy

Light is a form of energy which travels as waves. Light travels in straight lines, transferring energy from one place to another. A light ray is the direction of the path taken by light and is usually represented by an arrowed line. A light beam is a stream of light energy, in which the light rays may be parallel, diverging or converging.

Opacity

Objects become visible when light rays are reflected from them and reach the eye of the observer. When all the light rays falling on an object are either reflected or absorbed, the material is said to be opaque. If all the light rays pass through an object, the material is transparent. However, if some of the light rays pass through the object while the rest are reflected, the material is translucent. Thus, metal objects are opaque, clean air and clear glass are transparent, and frosted glass is translucent.

Refraction

When light passes from one transparent substance into another, the light rays are bent or refracted.

Reflection

When light rays are reflected from a shiny surface (a mirror) the angle at which the light rays strike the mirror (angle of incidence) is equal to the angle at which they bounce off (angle of reflection). These two angles are measured from a line at right angles to the mirror surface called a normal. A salon mirror usually has a flat surface and is therefore a plane mirror. The image produced in the mirror by reflection is the same size as the object and appears to be as far behind the mirror as the object is in front of it.

Figure 1.11   *Refraction and reflection of light rays*
(a) Refraction of light
(b) Reflection in a mirror

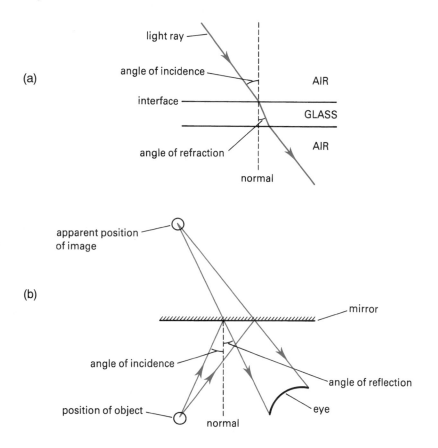

Intensity

The intensity of light is an important factor in salon lighting since clear vision depends on adequate light intensity. This is governed by the inverse square law, which states that light intensity decreases with the square of the distance from the light source. If you double the distance between yourself and a window allowing daylight to enter, only one quarter of the original light intensity will now reach your eyes. Light of low intensity causes eye strain. High light intensity without glare or deep shadows is required from a salon lighting system.

Figure 1.12   *Inverse square law*

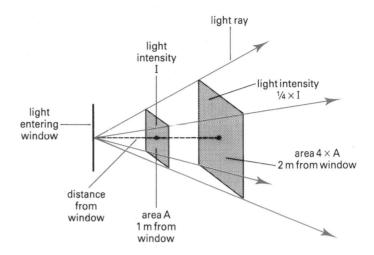

Artificial lighting

Some form of artificial lighting to increase light intensity is almost always required in a salon. Electrical energy is converted by lighting appliances into light and heat energy. The tungsten filament lamp (light bulb) converts electrical energy into 10% light and 90% heat. A fluorescent tube containing low pressure mercury vapour converts around 30% of the electrical energy into light so it is a more efficient lighting appliance.

Colour

The impression of colour is due to the nature of white light, and the way that certain molecules called pigments or dyes absorb and reflect light rays.

Figure 1.13   *Dispersion of light*

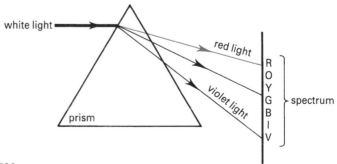

DISPERSION

White light can be split up into a number of component

coloured light rays by passing it through a prism. The process is called dispersion and the component colours of the light are a spectrum.

Figure 1.14   *Wavelength differences*

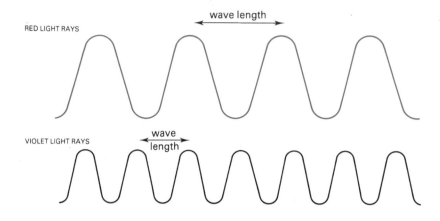

RED LIGHT RAYS

wave length

VIOLET LIGHT RAYS

wave length

WAVELENGTH

Light rays of different colours have different wavelengths. Red light, at one end of the visible spectrum, has the longest wavelength. Violet light, at the other end of the spectrum, has the shortest wavelength. The wavelength is the distance between the crest of a wave in the light ray and the crest of the following wave.

Figure 1.15   *Colour triangle*

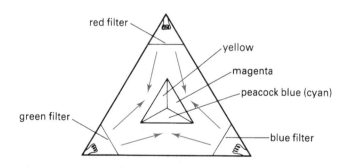

red filter

yellow

magenta

peacock blue (cyan)

green filter

blue filter

LIGHT MIXING

If red, green and blue light of equal intensity are combined, white light is obtained. Red, green and blue are therefore known as the primary colours of light. Mixing any two primary colours of light produces the secondary colours: yellow (red + green), magenta (red + blue) and cyan (green + blue). A secondary colour together with the missing primary colour will produce white light. These pairs of primary and secondary colours (for example blue + yellow), which together give white light, are said to be complementary colours. This is illustrated by the colour triangle.

PIGMENTS AND DYES

Pigments and dyes reflect light of the colour they appear to be, and absorb other colours. Viewed in white light, red pigments and dyes reflect the red light rays but absorb the green and blue rays. The colour of a pigment or dye will be affected by the colour of the light falling upon it. A pigment that looks red in white light will look more vivid in red light, but in blue light it will look black as there is no red light for it to reflect.

ARTIFICIAL LIGHT

Artificial light has a spectrum which is slightly different from that of natural daylight, so pigments and dyes look a slightly different colour in the two types of light. Tungsten filament lamps give out light containing more red and less blue light than daylight. Under this form of artificial lighting, red and orange pigments and dyes will look brighter than in daylight, magenta will look redder, and blue will look duller. Fluorescent tubes are available to produce a range of white lights (with slightly different spectra). The light produced may resemble daylight, or may contain more red light (warm white) or more blue light (cold white).

COLOUR MATCHING

The type of light is important in colour matching and in choosing coloured cosmetics suitable for day or evening make-up. Day make-up should always be applied in a salon area illuminated by natural daylight or daylight fluorescent tubes, so that the make-up will colour match day-time clothes. Evening make-up, however, should be applied in a salon area illuminated by tungsten filament lamps or warm white fluorescent tubes to obtain good colour matching of make-up with evening wear.

 Under a tungsten filament lamp, a lipstick which appears scarlet in daylight will look:
(a) paler
(b) brighter
(c) black
(d) blue

FUNDAMENTALS OF VENTILATION

Humidity

During the working day the salon air will alter in composition. As a result of evaporation the air will hold more water vapour so its humidity will increase. If air saturated with water vapour is cooled, water droplets will condense out of it at a temperature known as the dew point.

RELATIVE HUMIDITY

Air is not usually saturated with water vapour, and its humidity is expressed as % relative humidity (% RH).

$$\% \text{ RH} = \frac{\text{Actual amount of water vapour in the air}}{\text{Amount of water vapour saturating the air at the same temperature}} \times 100$$

For comfort, salon air should have a % RH between 40 and 50. If it reaches 70, sweat will not evaporate to cool the body adequately and heat fatigue will cause headache, tiredness and irritability.

Ventilation

Stale air contains an increased amount of carbon dioxide and a reduced amount of oxygen due to human breathing. The number of micro-organisms is increased and these survive well in the warm, humid, stale air, becoming a health hazard.

Ventilation is the process by which stale air is replaced by fresh air. It is needed to keep the composition of the salon air stable, and to prevent too great a rise in temperature. Over-ventilation causes draughts which reduce comfort and rapid loss of heat which is uneconomic. A balance between space heating and ventilation must be maintained for comfort.

DIFFUSION AND CONVECTION

Ventilation occurs by the physical processes of diffusion and convection, assuming that suitable entrances for fresh air and exits for stale air are provided. Diffusion is the movement of molecules to distribute themselves evenly throughout the space they occupy. Convection currents consist of the upward movement of heated molecules and the downward movement of cooling ones.

Figure 1.16 *Methods of natural ventilation*
(a) Louvred window
(b) Cooper's disc

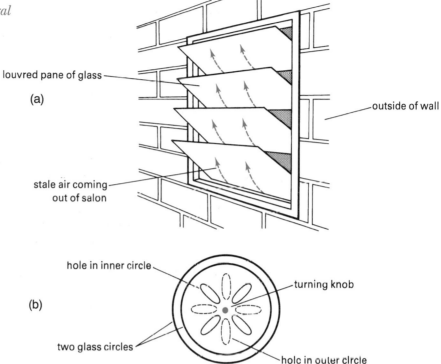

louvred pane of glass

(a)

outside of wall

stale air coming out of salon

hole in inner circle

turning knob

(b)

two glass circles

hole in outer circle

NATURAL METHODS

Natural ventilation occurs through open windows and doors, louvres, ventilating bricks and Cooper's discs placed in windows. Open windows and doors usually cause draughts, but the other three devices provide draught-free natural ventilation.

 The physical processes on which natural ventilation depends are:
(a) humidity and condensation
(b) diffusion and convection
(c) conduction and radiation
(d) evaporation and condensation

ARTIFICIAL METHODS

Extractor fans and air conditioning are methods of ventilation by artificial means. They provide controlled ventilation free from draughts.

BASIC ELECTRICITY

Conductors and insulators

STATIC ELECTRICITY

Materials such as plastic, glass, hair, nylon and ebonite produce frictional (static) electricity or electric charge when they are rubbed together. The electric charge is due to the internal structure of the atoms forming the material. Electrons from the surface atoms of one of the materials are transferred to the surface of the material rubbing against it. The surface losing the electrons becomes positively charged, while the one gaining the electrons becomes negatively charged. This happens when a plastic comb is energetically pulled through the hair. The comb gains electrons and acquires a negative charge, leaving the hair positively charged. The oppositely charged surfaces attract one another and, when they are close enough, the electrons jump back again. Energy is released as small flashes of light and crackling sounds as the electric charge is lost. Substances which develop a static electric charge are electrical insulators so an electric charge (electricity) is unable to travel through them.

ALL- AND DOUBLE-INSULATION

If the outside of an electrical appliance is made entirely of insulating material (such as plastic) it is said to be all-insulated. Double-insulated equipment may have some exposed metal, but extra insulation is fitted inside to prevent wires carrying an electric current from touching the exposed metal. The symbol

indicates that an appliance is double-insulated. All-insulated and double-insulated appliances do not need the safety device called an earth wire to prevent electric shock.

ELECTRIC CURRENT

Metals and water will allow a flow of electric charge, or current, through them. They are therefore electrical conductors, in which the outer electrons of the atoms are able to move in a random way from atom to atom. The electric current passes when the free electrons move in the same direction.

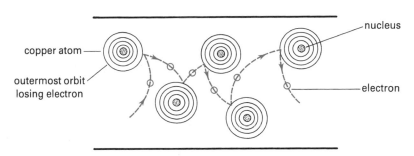

Figure 1.17 *Movement of electrons in copper wire*

ELECTRICAL RESISTANCE

In some conductors the free electrons move less readily so there is some resistance to the flow of electric current. The energy used in overcoming this resistance produces heat and light, and the material is known as a high resistance conductor. Nichrome (an alloy of nickel and chromium) used in heating elements and tungsten used in light bulb filaments are both high resistance conductors. Copper has a very low electrical resistance so it will conduct an electric current without becoming hot and is used in the conductor wires of an electric circuit.

 A radiant electric fire has a nichrome heating element to act as:
(a) an electrical insulator
(b) a source of frictional electricity
(c) a high resistance conductor

Electrical units

PRESSURE

A force is needed to drive electrons round an electric circuit, which is provided by the mains supply or a battery. This electrical force, or pressure, is called voltage, and is measured in units called volts (V).

INTENSITY

The number of electrons passing any point in the circuit in each second determines the strength or intensity of the electric current. The unit of rate of flow of electric current is the ampere (amp).

RESISTANCE

The ability of a conductor to resist the flow of electric current is measured in units called ohms. One volt of electrical pressure keeps a current of 1 amp flowing through a circuit with a resistance of 1 ohm.

$$\text{current in amps} = \frac{\text{pressure in volts}}{\text{resistance in ohms}}$$

Figure 1.18   *Relationship between electric current, pressure and resistance*

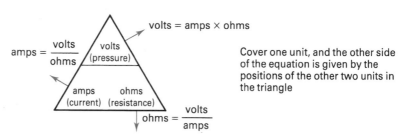

Cover one unit, and the other side of the equation is given by the positions of the other two units in the triangle

Sources of electricity

The flow of electric current from one place to another requires a potential difference between the two places. The size of the potential difference determines the electrical pressure and is measured in volts. As electrons are negatively charged, they flow through a circuit from the negative region towards a positive region where there is an electron deficit. As the direction of flow of current is usually described as being from positive to negative, this is actually in the opposite direction to the electron flow in the circuit.

Figure 1.19   *Electron flow and direction of electric current*

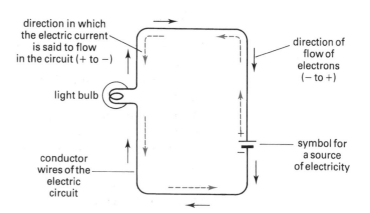

ELECTRIC CELL

An electric cell makes use of chemicals to produce a potential difference which will drive an electric current round a circuit by exerting an electrical pressure.

Figure 1.20   *Structure of a dry battery*

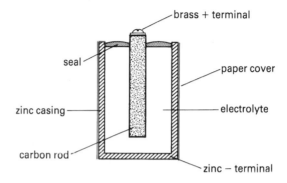

A dry battery is one type of electric cell in which there is an internal transfer of electrons from one of its terminals to the other. One terminal has a surplus of electrons, while at the other terminal there is an electron deficit. When the two terminals of a dry battery are linked by a conductor, electrons flow in one direction through the circuit. As electrons continue to be transferred inside the electric cell, the flow of current is maintained until the chemicals are used up. The chemicals used in a dry battery are known as the electrolyte, and the terminals are attached to electrodes made of conducting materials (a carbon rod and the zinc battery casing).

A direct current (DC) is produced by an electric cell, as the current always flows in the same direction.

Generator

Current electricity is provided on a large scale by electric generators. The electric current they produce is one in which the direction of flow of electrons in a circuit reverses many times a second. A complete cycle is said to have occurred when the current which is flowing one way changes and flows in the opposite direction in the circuit, and then changes again to flow in the original direction. The current therefore changes direction twice in every cycle. The number of cycles in each second is the frequency of the current and is measured in units called hertz (Hz).

An alternating current (AC), where the direction of flow reverses rapidly, is the type of electricity produced by these generators.

MAINS SUPPLY

The electricity produced in power stations has a high voltage (11,000 V). This is further increased to 132,000 V when it passes into the power lines of the National Grid. It is then reduced to 240 V for the mains supply to the salon. In the UK the mains supply is usually AC, with a frequency of 50 Hz and a pressure of 240 V. The mains supply may be different in other countries, so foreign appliances may not be suitable for UK mains. Continental mains usually provide AC of 50 Hz but 220 V, while in the USA AC of 60 Hz and 110 V is standard.

Effects of an electric current

In addition to heat and light, an electric current is able to produce mechanical movement (kinetic effects), magnetic fields, sound and chemical changes. On the body it causes muscle and nerve stimulation and electric shock. These effects are due to the conversion of one form of energy into a different one.

Table 1.9   *Energy conversions in appliances*

Appliance	Energy conversion
Fan	Electrical to kinetic
Light bulb	Electrical to heat and light
Audiosonic vibrator	Electrical to sound
Galvanic machine	Electrical to chemical effects
Faradic machine	Electrical to muscle stimulation

ELECTRIC POWER

The amount of heat, movement or other effect that the electric current can produce in 1 second is the electric power or wattage of the appliance, measured in units called watts:

$$1 \text{ watt} = 1 \text{ amp} \times 1 \text{ volt}$$

$$1,000 \text{ watts} = 1 \text{ kilowatt}$$

Q The unit of electric power is the:
(a) amp
(b) volt
(c) hertz
(d) watt

HEATING EFFECT

The heating effect of an electric current is produced when it passes through high resistance wires. A nichrome heating element becomes red hot, and a thin tungsten filament in a light bulb becomes white hot producing light as well as heat. Both AC and DC produce heating effects.

CHEMICAL EFFECTS

The chemical effects of an electric current are produced when DC flows through solutions of electrolytes, including those in the body tissues, to cause chemical changes. Water containing dissolved substances which ionise (acids, alkalis, salts) will conduct an electric current due to the movement of the electrically charged ions. Pure water contains some ionised molecules but, being a weak electrolyte, it conducts electricity less well. The process during which the chemical effects occur is called electrolysis. Two conductors called electrodes, which are connected by wires to the source of the current, are placed some distance apart in the electrolyte. The electrodes are called the anode (+), to which negatively charged anions are attracted, and the cathode (−), to which positively charged cations are attracted.

Figure 1.21 *Electrolysis of sodium chloride solution*

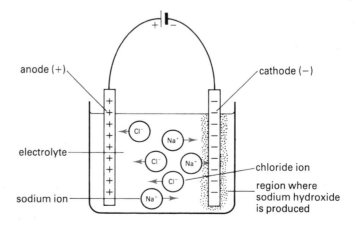

Chemical change occurs in the region of the electrodes. In human tissues, which contain salt (sodium chloride) ionised in solution, electrolysis produces sodium hydroxide at the cathode to which the sodium cations travel, so this region becomes more alkaline. Acids are produced at the anode to which the chloride anions travel.

Electric circuits

Electric circuits link electrical appliances to the mains supply, providing a path for the flow of electrons. If a number of appliances are included in the same circuit, they may be connected in series or in parallel.

CONNECTIONS IN SERIES

When connected in series the current goes through each appliance in the circuit in turn. Any break in the circuit will stop the flow of current, so all the appliances will stop working. Each additional appliance present in the circuit reduces the electric current as it increases the resistance.

Figure 1.22   *Light bulbs connected in series*

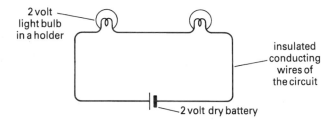

CONNECTIONS IN PARALLEL

Where the connections are in parallel, each appliance is connected directly to the source of electricity and is independent of all other appliances in the circuit. In a salon lighting circuit, each light bulb is connected in parallel so that one or several lights may be on at any one time. Provided the bulbs are of the same wattage, they will all glow equally brightly however many are in use.

RING-MAIN

The individual sockets of a ring-main circuit are connected in parallel, and any appliance may be plugged into any socket. In this type of circuit, one length of cable travels round the salon and back to the mains supply, reducing the length of cable required for power points. Extra sockets can usually be added to a ring-main relatively cheaply. The cable carries two insulated wires known as the live and neutral conductors which connect to each power socket. A third wire, called the earth, is also connected to each socket and leads into the ground, providing a path of low resistance for electric current. The earth acts as a safety device to prevent an electric shock occurring to a person using electrical equipment which has become faulty. A residual current circuit breaker (RCB) cuts off the current in the event of a fault. It is an alternative to an earth in preventing electric shock.

Figure 1.23   *Ring-main circuit*

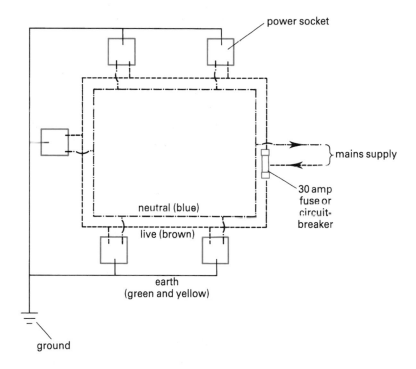

Fuses

The live conductor of a circuit passes through a fuse or a circuit breaker. These are devices to protect the wiring of a circuit from the effects of overloading, which can cause a fire as the wires become very hot. A fuse is the weakest part of a circuit as the wire it contains melts if too large a current passes through it, thus breaking the circuit. A circuit breaker (MCB) switch moves to the off position when the circuit is overloaded. A ring-main carries a 30 amp fuse or circuit breaker, while a lighting circuit is protected by one of 5 amps.

Figure 1.24   *Circuit breaker*

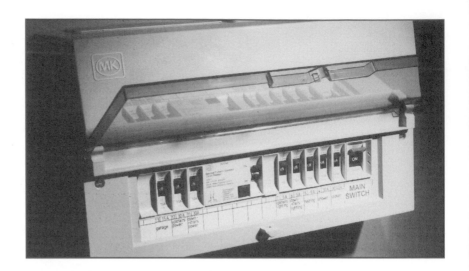

>
> **Q** A device which prevents an electric shock occurring to a person using faulty beauty therapy equipment is:
> (a) an appliance
> (b) a ring-main
> (c) a neutral conductor
> (d) an earth wire

Plugs

The appliances used in a beauty salon are connected to the sockets by means of a plug attached to a flex from the appliance. The plug should normally have three pins which enter the socket holes, unless the appliance is all- or double-insulated, when a two-pin plug is adequate requiring no earth wire.

Figure 1.25   *Connections between plug and flex*

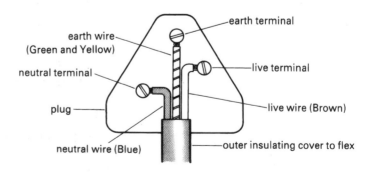

WIRING A PLUG

One pin connects with the live wire of the ring-main, one with the neutral wire and the third, longer pin connects with the earth wire. The flex must be connected to the plug so that the three wires of the flex are attached to the correct terminals inside the plug.

- The brown covered wire of the flex must be connected to the terminal marked Live or L.

- The blue covered wire must be connected to the terminal marked Neutral or N.

- The green and yellow covered wire must be connected to the terminal marked Earth or E.

All flex must conform to the international colour code described above, and all plugs to the British Standard BS/1363.

CARTRIDGE FUSE SIZE

The plug contains a cartridge fuse which lies over the live terminal. A 3 amp fuse should be placed in the plug of an appliance with a power of less than 720 watts. More powerful appliances require a 13 amp fuse. The current normally flowing through an appliance is given by the formula:

$$\frac{\text{amps}}{\text{(current)}} = \frac{\text{watts (power of appliance)}}{\text{volts (pressure of mains supply)}}$$

For an appliance with a wattage of 720 on a mains supply of 240 volts:

$$\text{current flowing} = \frac{720 \text{ watts}}{240 \text{ volts}} = 3 \text{ amps}$$

For a wattage of 720 or more, a 3 amp fuse would not allow current to flow through it as the fuse wire would become so hot that it would burn through.

Figure 1.26   *Structure of a cartridge fuse*

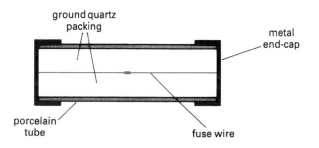

Switches

A switch allows an air gap to be introduced into an electric circuit to stop the current when the switch is in the off position. Some switches have a variable control so that different amounts of current pass through the switch to the appliance at the different numbered positions. A switch is placed in the live conductor and is a safety device. A thermal cut-out will automatically switch off the current to a heating element when an appliance begins to overheat.

Cost of electricity

KILOWATT-HOUR

The amount of electricity used by an appliance depends on its power (wattage) and the length of time it is operating. The unit of electrical energy is the kilowatt-hour, that is the electricity consumed when an appliance with a power of 1 kilowatt operates for 1 hour.

METER

The number of units of electrical energy used in a salon is measured by the Electricity Board's meter. Recently installed meters display the number of units used. Older meters record the units used on a series of four large dials. Where the pointer on the dial lies between two numbers the lower number should be read, except between 9 and 0 where 9 is the correct reading because 0 represents 10.

Figure 1.27   *Electricity meter dials*

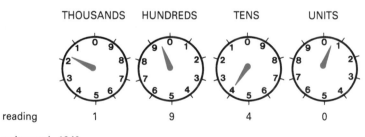

The difference between present and previous readings represents the number of units used in that time interval. The cost is obtained by multiplying the number of units by the cost per unit.

$$cost = \underbrace{kilowatts \times hours}_{units} \times cost\ per\ unit$$

MICROBIOLOGY

Micro-organisms

Micro-organisms are minute living organisms which are too small to be visible with the naked eye. Some micro-organisms become visible by using an optical microscope, but others can only be seen by using an electron microscope which has a much higher magnification. Micro-organisms are mostly either fungi (yeasts and moulds), bacteria or viruses. A few are single-celled animals called protozoans, such as Entamoeba. Micro-organisms are universally present in the natural environment and on the person.

PATHOGENS

Some micro-organisms are responsible for infectious diseases which can be passed from one individual to another. These are termed pathogens

SAPROPHYTES

Many other micro-organisms are saprophytes, feeding on dead organic material, and are non-pathogenic.

SYMBIONTS

Other micro-organisms are symbiotic, living in or on a human or animal carrier. Both the symbiont and the carrier profit by the association.

 Q Micro-organisms which cause disease are described as:
(a) pathogenic
(b) symbiotic
(c) saprophytic
(d) anaerobic

Fungi

STRUCTURE

Fungi are either unicellular organisms (e.g. yeast) or multicellular filamentous organisms (e.g. moulds). In moulds the filaments are called hyphae. They are 5–10 μm wide and of varying length. They branch to form a flat tangled mat called a mycelium. Although mycelia are visible to the naked eye, unicellular yeasts are too small to be visible.

Fungal cells and hyphae have well-defined nuclei and are surrounded by a rigid wall. They never contain the green pigment chlorophyll which is characteristic of plants.

Figure 1.28   *Fungal hyphae*

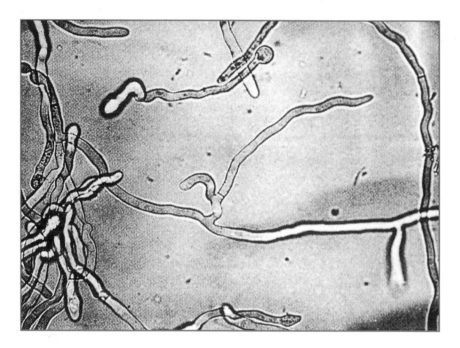

REPRODUCTION
Fungi reproduce by tiny spores or from fragments of hyphae which become detached from the mycelium.

NUTRITION
Fungi secrete enzymes which diffuse out through the cell or hyphal walls to digest surrounding organic material which is then absorbed in liquid form as food. Most fungi are saprophytic, but a few are pathogenic, feeding on the living tissues of their host (for example on human skin, causing athlete's foot and ringworm).

GROWTH
Conditions which favour fungal growth and reproduction are warmth (15–30 °C), a plentiful food supply, water and oxygen, although a few fungi (e.g. yeasts) can respire without oxygen for a short time.

Bacteria

STRUCTURE

Bacteria are unicellular organisms with no distinct nucleus. Their size varies from between 0.5 µm and 2 µm. They belong to the simplest group of living organisms.

Each bacterium is bounded by a cell wall and has a characteristic shape. It is either spherical (a coccus), rod-shaped (a bacillus), spirally coiled (a spirochaete) or comma-shaped (a vibrio). Some bacteria are surrounded by a slime capsule, and some have one or more projecting hair-like processes called flagella. Some bacteria (e.g. spirochaetes) are able to move around. Bacteria may form bunches or chains.

Figure 1.29   *Characteristic shapes of bacteria*

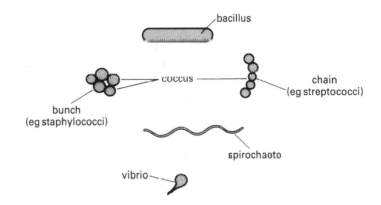

REPRODUCTION

Bacteria reproduce by dividing into two (fission). A few form thick-walled resistant spores.

NUTRITION

Bacteria secrete enzymes that digest the material they use as food. They may be parasitic or saprophytic, and some live as symbionts in the human intestine. Pathogenic bacteria produce waste products called toxins which may cause the symptoms of the bacterial disease. Large numbers of bacteria live and feed on human skin and in body cavities. Others live in water, soil and in human foods. Examples of diseases caused by bacteria are boils (by a staphylococcus) and sore throats (by a streptococcus).

GROWTH

Conditions which favour bacterial growth and reproduction are warmth (37 °C for pathogenic and symbiotic bacteria), a plentiful food supply, water and the removal of waste products. A supply of oxygenated air is needed by those bacteria which respire aerobically.

Viruses

A virus is smaller than a bacterium, for example the herpes virus is 0.1 μm in size. Viruses can grow only within the living cells of a suitable host, therefore all viruses are pathogenic and infect a specific host. A virus must pass, usually fairly directly, from an infected living cell to another cell of the same kind. Once inside the host cell, the virus takes over from the cell nucleus and programmes the cell to produce new virus material instead of the substances it would normally synthesise.

Cold sores, warts and influenza are all viral diseases.

Figure 1.30   *Wart virus*

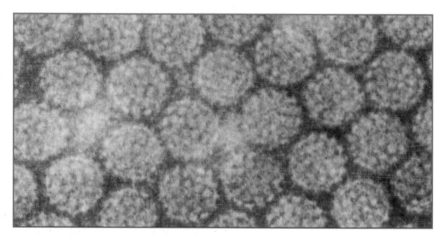

Transmission of micro-organisms

Pathogenic micro-organisms can enter the body through breaks in the skin, by being breathed in, or via the mouth, anus, urinary and vaginal openings. These pathogens are transmitted from various sources:

* air which contains suspended infected droplets, produced by the coughing, sneezing or talking of infected persons;

* equipment and towels which have become contaminated by contact with the skin of infected persons. Micro-organisms are thus transferred by indirect means from one person to another;

- contaminated food and water containing pathogens originating from sewage or insects' bodies;

- personal contact such as shaking hands, kissing and other skin contacts such as manual massage. Contagious diseases are transferred in this way;

- sexual intercourse can result in the transmission of venereal diseases;

- blood – two serious and often fatal diseases, AIDS and Hepatitis B, can be transmitted when small amounts of blood released from an infected person (the carrier) enter a small break in the skin or mucous membrane of a healthy contact. Equipment used for ear-piercing, or electrolysis needles, can transmit these viruses unless they have not been used before, or have been sterilised before re-use.

Controlling micro-organisms

Personal hygiene and disinfection provide the external methods of controlling micro-organisms. The body's natural defence mechanisms (immune system), due mainly to the white blood cells, provides internal resistance to attack by pathogenic micro-organisms.

PERSONAL HYGIENE

Personal hygiene involves the cleanliness of skin, hair and clothing. Washing frequently with soap and water removes the layer of sweat, sebum, stale make-up and dead skin cells on which skin micro-organisms feed. It is particularly important to wash the hands after using the lavatory and before preparing or eating food.

DISINFECTION

Disinfection is the process by which micro-organisms on salon surfaces or equipment are inactivated or destroyed. This is achieved using either physical processes or chemicals, some methods being more effective than others.

Physical methods of disinfection involve the use of heat or ultra-violet radiation.

- Burning will destroy all micro-organisms and is the method used to dispose of contaminated waste such as infected dressings and paper tissues.

- Glass bead sterilisers employ dry heat to destroy all micro-organisms on metal and plastic equipment such as applicators. These sterilisers take up to 30 minutes to reach the required temperature. The equipment is then put in to sterilise and immersed for around ten minutes in the case of a single piece of equipment.

Figure 1.31   *Glass bead steriliser*

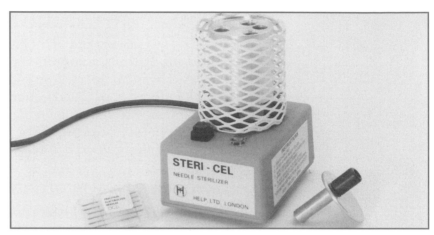

- An autoclave producing steam under pressure is a very effective means of sterilising metal and some plastic equipment, as the temperature reached is well above 100 °C and destroys all micro-organisms present.

- Boilers and steamers which reach a temperature of 100 °C are less effective than an autoclave, destroying most, but not all, micro-organisms and their spores. Natural earths used in face masks are steam-sterilised to destroy bacteria. Boilers designed for use on instruments will disinfect metal and plastic equipment reasonably well during a ten minute treatment. Infected towels and linen should also be boiled.

- Ultra-violet cabinets contain a quartz mercury vapour lamp which emits ultra-violet rays. These rays only destroy micro-organisms on the surfaces they reach. They do not sterilise the equipment placed in the cabinet, but only disinfect it.

Chemical methods of disinfection also vary in their effectiveness. The chemicals must be used at the recommended concentration and for a sufficient time. Even when used correctly, the degree of disinfection varies with the chemical involved.

Figure 1.32   *UV germicidal cabinet*

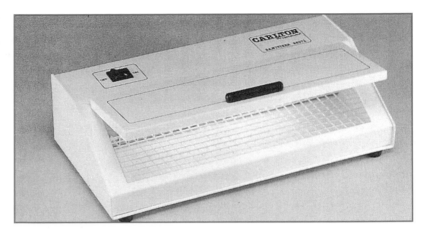

- An antiseptic will prevent micro-organisms from multiplying, but does not necessarily kill them. The simplest antiseptic is soap or detergent and hot water. This is adequate for reducing the activity of micro-organisms on salon surfaces and textiles. A 1% solution of Cetrimide (a quaternary ammonium compound) is a useful antiseptic for human skin. Antiseptics such as Nipagin are added to cosmetic preparations as preservatives to prevent the growth of micro-organisms.

- A disinfectant kills most pathogenic micro-organisms when used correctly. A 70% solution of ethanol (alcohol) or chlorhexidine in 70% ethanol are the best disinfectants for salon use. Both disinfectants are available in liquid form or as commercially prepared wipes, and may be used on metal or plastic applicators, electrodes, etc. At least 15 minutes immersion in the liquid disinfectant is necessary. Ethanol is an inflammable liquid and care must be taken to keep it away from flames or heat. Other chemical disinfectants are less suitable for salon use as they may be corrosive to the equipment, damaging to the user's health, or may deteriorate on keeping.

- Sterilising agents will destroy all micro-organisms and their spores. Neat chlorine bleach should be used as the sterilising agent on blood spills following a cut or a nose bleed. This treatment will destroy the viruses which cause the diseases AIDS and Hepatitis B. Bleach should be poured on the spilt blood and left for one minute before washing the blood away with hot water and detergent. Rubber gloves should always be worn when dealing with blood spills.

Q A sterilising agent that will destroy the viruses causing AIDS and Hepatitis B if they are present in spilt blood is:
(a) nipagin
(b) 1% Cetrimide solution
(c) chlorine bleach
(d) distilled water

Disposal of waste

Waste water from wash basins, and lavatory waste pass into pipes connecting to the drains where micro-organisms from sewage and dirty water flourish.

TRAPS

Each wash basin and lavatory bowl has a trap below it containing a water seal to prevent air-borne pathogens and unpleasant

Figure 1.33   *Waste traps*
(a) S-trap
(b) bottle trap

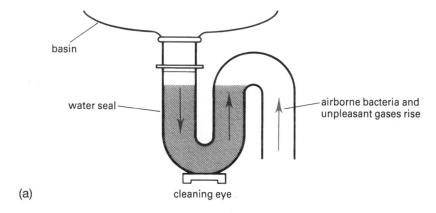

(a)

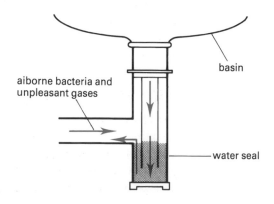

(b)

EXPLOSIVE

CORROSIVE

HARMFUL
or IRRITANT

OXIDISING

HIGHLY
FLAMMABLE

TOXIC

BIOHAZARD

Figure 1.34 *Hazard symbols for chemicals*

smelling gases from the drains entering the salon. Below the lavatory bowl and some older wash basins the trap is S-shaped. Modern wash basins usually have a bottle trap.

Below the trap the basin waste pipe runs into a waste water pipe which empties outside the building into a gulley trap (drain) just below the ground. The gulley trap also contains an S-shaped trap and water seal.

INSPECTION CHAMBER

From here the waste water enters a large underground inspection chamber covered by an air-tight drain cover. The lavatory waste passes from the trap into a soil pipe which runs down the outside of the building and opens at the bottom into the inspection chamber. The top of the soil pipe is open to allow the escape of unpleasant smelling gases at roof level. It is covered by a wire guard to prevent birds nesting in the opening. From the inspection chamber the waste water and sewage passes into the main drain which empties into the sewer in the road.

CHLORINE BLEACH

Micro-organisms in the traps of wash basins and lavatories can be destroyed by adding a small quantity of chlorine bleach, which is left in the trap for a short time before flushing it away. Chlorine bleach is a hazardous chemical as it is both acidic and an oxidising agent. It should be handled with care, kept off the skin, and disposed of with large volumes of cold water. It should not be mixed with other chemicals in case violent chemical reactions take place.

Disposal of chemicals

Bleaches, acids, alkalis and flammable solvents must all be disposed of with great care after use, and stored and handled safely. Such chemicals bear warning signs on their containers known as hazard symbols (see figure 1.34).

Disposal of 'sharps'

Used electrolysis needles and other sharp objects should be placed in a 'sharps' box or bag for disposal. This will prevent objects, which could be contaminated with blood or micro-organisms, wounding the skin of a person handling the sharp object and transmitting infection.

Body Structures

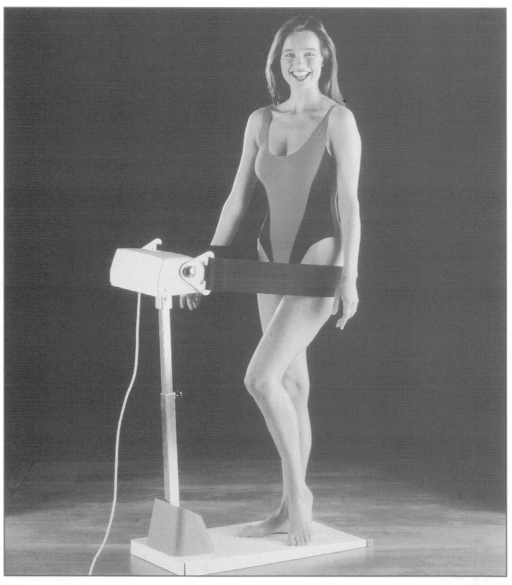

Belt massager

CELLS

A human body is composed of millions of microscopic living units called cells

Figure 2.1   *Basic structure of a cell*

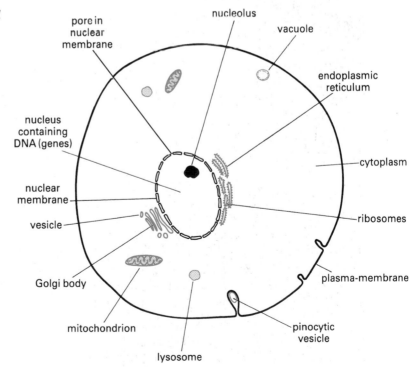

Cell structure

Cells nearly always have the same basic structure. They are bounded by a very thin living plasma membrane which encloses the cell contents, or protoplasm. This consists of a number of small structures called organelles, surrounded by a jelly-like cytoplasm.

ORGANELLES

The central organelle, called the nucleus, is round or oval and is bounded by a nuclear membrane pierced by pores which allow exchange of materials between the nucleus and the cytoplasm. The nucleus may contain one or two small nucleoli, and carries the heritable material (genes) in the form of a chemical substance called DNA.

Examining a cell under an electron microscope shows a system of membranes which divide up the cytoplasm into a network of channels. This membrane system is called the endoplasmic reticulum. Some of the membranes have small granules known as ribosomes on their outer surface. In one area, smooth membranes and associated vesicles form an organelle called the Golgi body.

Throughout the cytoplasm are rod-shaped organelles called mitochondria which are particularly numerous in very active cells. Other small membrane-surrounded bodies called lysosomes also occur in the cytoplasm. Some cells have numerous short hair-like projections from the surface called cilia which are able to move. Sperm cells have a single longer movable projection called a flagellum.

INCLUSIONS

Cell cytoplasm often contains inclusions, such as granules of chemicals being temporarily stored in the cell.

PLASMA MEMBRANE

A plasma membrane is a highly elastic structure composed of a central layer of fatty phospholipid molecules sandwiched between two layers of protein. Some of the protein molecules penetrate the phospholipid layer, and some completely span the plasma membrane. Within the plasma membrane the protein and phospholipid molecules can move around, giving the membrane some of its special properties and allowing substances to pass into and out of cells.

A plasma membrane must be able to respond to hormones, and must carry 'marker molecules' so that it is recognised as belonging to the individual.

Figure 2.2   *Portion of plasma membrane in section*

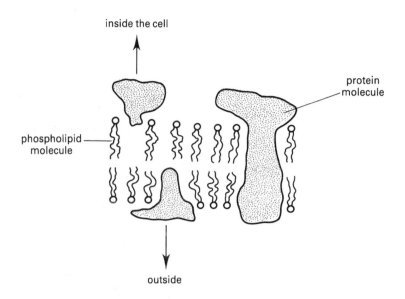

Q   In each case, name the cell structure with which each of the following is associated:
(a) ribosome
(b) DNA
(c) marker molecule

Cell function

Cells carry out a series of chemical reactions resulting in the activities which keep them alive. The chemical substances involved must move into and out of the cell through the plasma membrane.

DIFFUSION

Some of these substances pass, by the physical process of diffusion, from a region of high concentration to one of lower concentration. Oxygen is one of the substances which diffuses through the plasma membrane, which is thus permeable to oxygen.

OSMOSIS

Water will pass in and out of cells by the physical process of osmosis from an area of high water concentration (dilute solution) to an area of lower water concentration (concentrated solution). Since osmosis occurs, plasma membranes are said to be semi-permeable.

ACTIVE TRANSPORT

Some of the substances required by a cell will only pass through its plasma membrane by active processes requiring the cell to use energy for their transport. Such substances, which are already present in higher concentration inside the cell than outside, can still enter the cell by active transport. Glucose molecules enter cells by active transport, but glycogen (animal starch) molecules stored in cells are unable to pass out through the plasma membrane, which is therefore described as selectively permeable. Carrier proteins present in the plasma membrane aid active transport of some materials across the membrane.

 Explain the difference between 'semi-permeable' and 'selectively permeable' when applied to membranes.

Another form of active transport is known as pinocytosis. Droplets of liquid collect on the surface of the cell membrane which folds inwards, surrounding the liquid droplet and forming a vesicle by separating from the rest of the membrane. Fat droplets are taken up by the cells of the intestine lining by pinocytosis. Phagocytosis is a form of active transport where projections of the plasma membrane and cytoplasm surround and engulf solid particles outside the cell. The membrane closes above the particle to form a vacuole inside the cell. White blood cells engulf harmful bacteria by phagocytosis.

Each type of organelle has a particular function in the cell, shown in table 2.1.

 Give the scientific name for the cellular structures known as:
(a) suicide bags
(b) sperm tails

Table 2.1   *Functions of cell organelles*

Organelle	Functions
Plasma membrane	Protects the cell; allows substances to enter and leave the cell
Nucleus	Contains genes for inheritance; controls the cell's activities
Endoplasmic reticulum	Provides channels for moving substances round the cell; provides a large surface area for chemical reactions in the cell
Ribosomes	Provide the sites for protein synthesis
Golgi body	Region of synthesis of materials which will be secreted by the cell, e.g. mucus
Mitochondria	Involved in energy production within the cell; known as the 'power houses' of the cell
Lysosomes	Destroy worn out organelles and/or whole cells and foreign materials; known as 'suicide bags'
Cilia	Cause the movement of particles and fluid across a cell surface
Flagella	Enable cells to move about

Cell division

As cells become damaged by disease or ageing, they eventually die and must be replaced. Growth in size of the body organs also requires the production of extra cells.

MITOSIS

The process by which most cells reproduce is called mitosis. This results in a cell dividing into two daughter cells, each identical with the parent cell except in size. Each daughter cell then grows to the size of the parent cell and contains a complete set of the parental genes.

MEIOSIS

Eggs and sperms are produced from cells undergoing a different type of cell division called meiosis. Eggs and sperms contain only half the genes of the parent cells.

─────────── **SUMMARY** ───────────

Cells need chemicals to carry out the biochemical reactions involved
in living processes. The substances utilised and produced during these
reactions must be able to enter and leave the cell. The three methods
by which chemicals move through the cell's plasma membrane are
diffusion, osmosis and active transport. The cell organelles each have a
particular role in the functioning of the cell. Body growth and
reproduction occur as a result of cell division.

TISSUES

Some cells have special functions in the body and their structure
may be modified or differentiated as a result. Such differentiated
cells usually occur in groups forming a tissue, which carries out
particular activities. The body tissues are of four main types:
epithelial, connective, muscular, and nervous.

Epithelial tissue

Epithelial tissue covers the outer surface of the body and the
internal organs. It also lines body cavities and forms glands. The
cells making up the tissues have a simple shape and fit closely
together. They occur as a single, continuous layer in a simple
epithelium, or as several layers in a compound or stratified
epithelium. The bottom layer of cells always rests on a non-living
basement membrane containing a fine meshwork of collagen
protein fibres.

Epithelial tissues are further classified according to the shape of
the cells.

SQUAMOUS

Squamous epithelium consists of flat scale-like cells. It may be
simple like that forming the wall of the blood capillaries and air
sacs of the lung, or it may be stratified like that of the skin
epidermis and lining of the mouth cavity where it must survive
considerable friction.

CUBICAL

Cubical (cuboidal) epithelium with cube-shaped cells which have
a central nucleus, may be simple, as in the thyroid gland and
kidney tubules, or stratified, when lining the ducts of sweat
glands.

COLUMNAR

Columnar epithelium consists of tall cells with an elongated nucleus near the base of the cell. A simple columnar epithelium lines the stomach and intestines, and a stratified columnar epithelium lines the larger urinary ducts.

CILIATED COLUMNAR

Ciliated columnar epithelium covers wet surfaces and is often interspersed with mucus-secreting goblet cells. The hair-like cilia covering the free surface of the cell move a stream of mucus and particles along. This type of epithelium lines the air passages, where it has a filtering effect on the air breathed in.

TRANSITIONAL

Compound transitional epithelium is composed of several layers of cells when relaxed, but when stretched is reduced to one or two layers. In the bladder this type of epithelium is waterproof and allows the large changes in volume that occur.

Figure 2.3   *Types of simple epithelia*
(a)   Simple squamous
(b)   Simple cubical
(c)   Simple columnar
(d)   Simple ciliated columnar

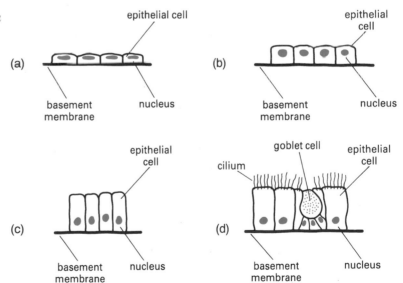

GLANDULAR

Glandular epithelium consists of cells which secrete wanted chemicals, a process requiring the use of energy. The cells may occur singly, like the goblet cells which secrete mucus, or they may be grouped to form a gland.

Figure 2.4   *Types of compound epithelia*
(a) *Stratified squamous*
(b) *Transitional*
(c) *Stratified cubical*
(d) *Stratified columnar*

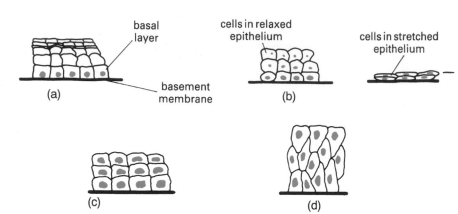

GLANDS

In glands, the substance secreted is passed into ducts in the case of exocrine glands, but into the blood from endocrine glands. The sweat and sebaceous glands of the skin are exocrine, while the hormone-producing glands are endocrine. Multicellular exocrine glands have an inner secretory part and an outer non-secretory duct. They are divided into a number of types, as shown in figure 2.5. Where the duct is unbranched the gland is simple, while compound glands have branched ducts.

> *Q* Give one important structural difference between exocrine and endocrine glands.

> *Q* Where in the body would you find the following?
> (a) stratified squamous epithelium
> (b) compound tubuloacinar glands

The exocrine glands release their secretions in one of three different ways:

- The holocrine type accumulates the secreted material and when the cells die each is discharged containing its secretion. Each cell is replaced by a new cell of the glandular epithelium, which becomes secretory. The sebaceous glands of the skin are holocrine.

- Merocrine glands, such as those producing saliva, discharge their secretions from the cells as they are produced.

Figure 2.5 *Types of exocrine glands*
(a) Simple tubular (e.g. in small intestine)
(b) Simple branched tubular (e.g. in stomach)
(c) Simple coiled tubular (e.g. sweat glands)
(d) Simple acinar (e.g. glands storing sperms)
(e) Simple branched acinar (e.g. sebaceous glands in skin)
(f) Compound tubular (e.g. glands of liver which form bile)
(g) Compound acinar (e.g. salivary glands)
(h) Compound tubuloacinar (e.g. mammary glands of breast)

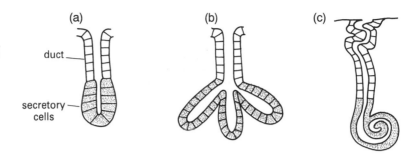
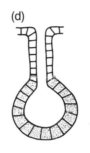
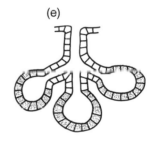
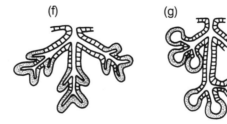
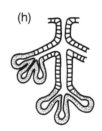

- In apocrine glands, the secreted material accumulates near the free surface of the cell, and that part is pinched off from the rest of the cell and discharged. The large sweat glands in the armpits and the milk-producing mammary glands are examples of the apocrine type.

Q Name the type of secretion release method found in:
(a) sebaceous gland cells
(b) salivary gland cells

Figure 2.6   *Secretion release
methods in exocrine glands*
(a)   *Holocrine*
(b)   *Merocrine*
(c)   *Apocrine*

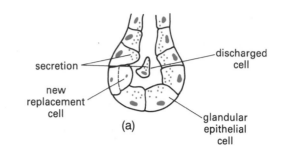

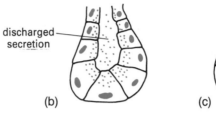
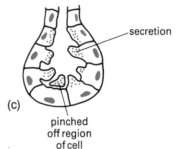

Connective tissue

The cells in these tissues lie in a matrix of non-living material
which they have secreted. Unlike epithelia, connective tissues
have a rich blood supply and the cells are not closely packed.
Fibres are always present in the matrix. The nature of the matrix
largely determines the properties of the various types of
connective tissue which are binding or supporting in function.

AREOLAR

Areolar connective tissue is smooth and moist with a semi-fluid
matrix containing hyaluronic acid which has moisturising
properties. Running through the matrix are bundles of white
fibres composed of collagen protein which strengthen the tissue,
and a network of yellow fibres composed of elastin protein to
give elasticity. The living cells of the tissue are of three types.
Large flat fibroblasts secrete the matrix and fibres. Mast cells
secrete histamine, a substance which enlarges small blood
vessels, and heparin, an anti-coagulant. Macrophages destroy
bacteria and tissue debris. This loose connective tissue binds
together the various tissues and organs, for example it attaches
the skin to the underlying muscle.

Figure 2.7   *Areolar tissue*

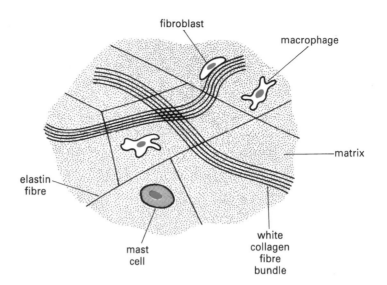

ADIPOSE

Adipose tissue is a form of loose connective tissue in which the
fibroblasts are modified for storing fat. The nucleus of each
adipose cell is flattened against the plasma membrane by the
large fat droplet, giving the cells a 'signet-ring' appearance.
Adipose tissue forms the subcutaneous layer below the skin and
occurs around the heart and kidneys. It acts as an insulating
layer, reducing heat loss from the body. It also acts as a major
food reserve.

Figure 2.8   *Adipose tissue*

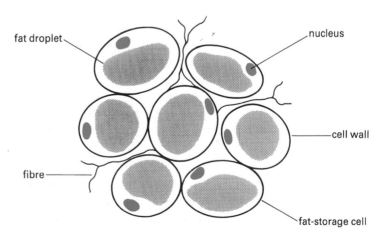

In which tissue do the following materials occur?
(a) elastin
(b) fat droplets
(c) hyaluronic acid

WHITE FIBROUS

White fibrous tissue is a dense connective tissue where many bundles of firm collagen fibres run through the matrix, pushing the fibroblasts into rows between the bundles. The tissue appears silvery-white and is very tough. It occurs in the cord-like tendons and broad aponeuroses which connect muscles to bones.

YELLOW ELASTIC

Yellow elastic tissue has a branching network of elastin fibres in the matrix which gives the tissue its yellowish colour. The fibroblasts occur in the gaps between the fibres. This elastic connective tissue occurs in the walls of arteries and lungs.

OTHER TYPES

Lymphoid tissue (see chapter 12), blood (see chapter 10), cartilage and bone (see chapter 4) are also connective tissues.

 List three characteristics of connective tissue.

Muscular tissue

This tissue brings about movement by its ability to contract and relax (see chapter 5).

Nervous tissue

This tissue transmits messages (see chapter 6).

MEMBRANES

The combination of an epithelial layer with an underlying connective tissue layer is known as a membrane. Mucous and serous membranes are of this type.

Table 2.2   *Types of tissues*

Main type	Sub-classes		Occurrence
EPITHELIAL Covers surfaces Basement membrane present	Simple: single layer of cells	Squamous Cubical Columnar Ciliated Glandular	Wall of blood capillary Thyroid gland Wall of stomach and intestine Lining windpipe Mucous membrane of nose
	Compound: several layers of cells	Transitional Stratified squamous Stratified cubical	Wall of bladder Skin epidermis Ducts of sweat glands
CONNECTIVE Binding or supporting Non-living matrix fibres present Highly vascular	Areolar – matrix semi-fluid Adipose – cells store fat White fibrous – dense collagen fibres Yellow elastic – elastin fibre network Lymphoid – fluid matrix. Fibres on clotting Blood – fluid matrix. Fibres on clotting Cartilage – matrix gel-like Bone – matrix hardened with calcium salts		Dermis of skin Subcutaneous layer Tendons and aponeuroses Lungs and artery walls Lymph in lymphatic vessels In blood vessels Ends of bones Bones and teeth
MUSCULAR Bring about movement	Cardiac Skeletal Smooth (visceral)		In heart Muscles of arms and legs In walls of food canal
NERVOUS Conduct impulses	Neurons and neuroglia		In brain, spinal cord, and nerves

Mucous

Mucous membranes line the body cavities that open to the outside, such as the food canal and air passages. Mucus is a thin slimy fluid which lubricates surfaces and prevents them from drying out. It is secreted by goblet cells in the epithelial layer.

Serous

Serous membranes line body cavities that do not open to the outside. They also cover the organs lying in those body cavities, allowing them to slide smoothly over one another. They consist of a thin layer of areolar connective tissue covered by an epithelial layer of flattened cells through which a watery fluid oozes. The pleural membranes lining the chest cavity and outer surfaces of the lungs are serous membranes.

Synovial

Synovial membranes line joint cavities and secrete a thick fluid to lubricate the movement of bones. They are composed of connective tissue with elastic fibres, but do not contain epithelium.

Q Where in the body do the following structures occur?
(a) pleural membranes
(b) goblet cells

ORGANS AND BODY SYSTEMS

Organ

In the body different kinds of tissues combine together to form organs which have one or a related group of functions. The heart, for example, is an organ with the function of pumping blood round the body. It contains muscular and nervous tissues and the connective tissue, blood.

System

Body systems consist of a group of organs which are concerned with one of the body's living processes. These living processes involve the use and supply of chemicals and energy, and the removal of waste.

METABOLISM

The living processes are collectively known as metabolism and include the activities of nutrition, respiration, excretion, movement, growth, repair and reproduction. These activities must continue in spite of changes inside and outside the body, otherwise death will eventually occur. The body must therefore be sensitive to these internal and external changes and able to respond to them.

Table 2.3   *Body systems*

System	Main organs/tissues	Functions in the body
Integumentary	Skin, hair, nails	Protection, temperature regulation, sensitivity to external changes
Skeletal	Cartilages, bones, joints	Supports, protects and gives shape to the body; forms blood cells and stores minerals
Muscular	Skeletal muscles, tendons	Causes movement, maintains posture, produces heat
	Visceral and cardiac muscles	See below
Nervous	Brain, spinal cord, nerves, sense organs	Co-ordinates the body's activities, perceives stimuli
Digestive	Alimentary canal, liver, pancreas, gall bladder	Physical and chemical breakdown of food, removal of solid waste
Respiratory	Lungs, respiratory ducts	Supplies oxygen and removes carbon dioxide
Urinary	Kidneys, urinary ducts, bladder	Regulates composition of the blood, maintains the salt/water (osmotic) balance
Vascular	Heart and cardiac muscles, blood vessels, blood	Transports materials round the body to the living cells, collects up waste products
Lymphatic	Lymphatics, lymph nodes, lymph, spleen, thymus, tonsils	Removes materials from the tissues and returns them to the blood, e.g. protein and water; protects against disease
Endocrine	Glands producing hormones	Regulates growth and development and other body processes
Reproductive	Ovaries, testes and their ducts	Produces new generations of human beings

 Distinguish between the vascular and lymphatic body systems.

BODY CAVITIES

The spaces within the body that contain internal organs are called body cavities. Inside these cavities the organs are protected.

Figure 2.9   *Body cavities (side view)*

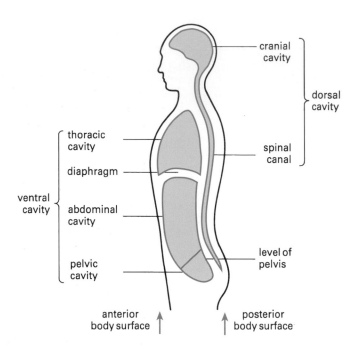

Dorsal

Close to the back, or posterior surface of the body, are the cranial cavity in the skull containing the brain, and the spinal canal formed by the vertebrae containing the spinal cord. These two cavities together form the dorsal body cavity.

Ventral

The ventral body cavity occurs nearer the front, or anterior surface of the body. It consists of the thoracic cavity in the chest and the abdominal cavity below the diaphragm. The lower part of the abdominal cavity is known as the pelvic cavity. The thoracic cavity is subdivided into two pleural cavities, one round each lung, and a pericardial cavity round the heart. The cavities are lined by serous membranes known as the pleurae and pericardium respectively. The abdominal cavity contains most of the alimentary canal below the oesophagus (gullet) and the two kidneys with their ducts. The pelvic cavity contains the bladder, the lower colon and rectum of the alimentary canal, and the reproductive organs. The serous membrane lining the cavity and binding the organs to each other is the peritoneum. The organs inside the ventral body cavities are collectively called the viscera.

ANATOMY AND PHYSIOLOGY

The anatomy of the body refers to its structure and the arrangement of the organs of the body systems. Body types have been classified into three groups, depending on the development and proportion of bone, muscle and fat in the body.

- In the endomorphic type the person has short limbs, poor bone and muscle development and much body fat. This produces a heavy physique.

- The mesomorphic individual has strong well developed bones and muscles and a healthy amount of body fat.

- Ectomorphs are tall thin individuals, less muscular and with light bones.

Definitions of anatomical terms will be found on page 400.

Physiology is the study of the way the organs function in the body.

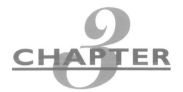

CHAPTER 3

The Skin

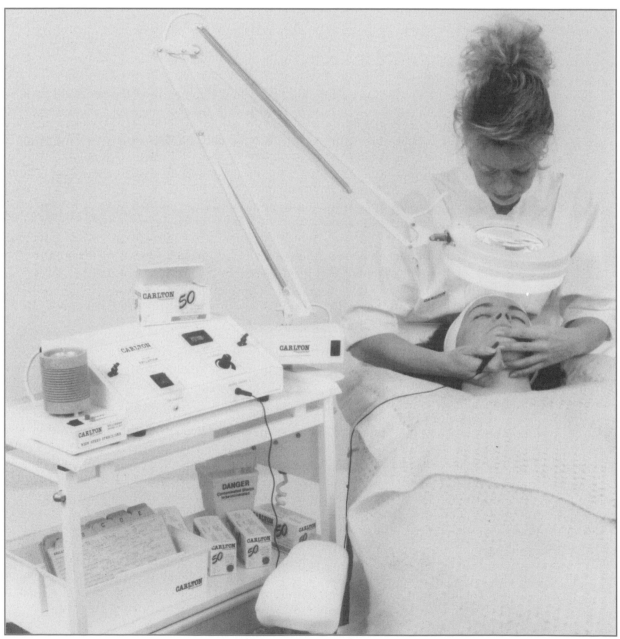

Epilation by diathermy

STRUCTURE OF THE SKIN

The skin is a large organ covering the outside of the body. Its thickness varies between 0.05 and 3 mm. Dorsal surfaces have thicker skin than ventral surfaces, except where ventral surfaces are subjected to considerable wear, as on the palms of the hands. A vertical section through the skin shows two distinct layers, an outer epidermis and an inner thicker dermis.

Epidermis

The tissue forming the epidermis is stratified squamous epithelium in which five distinct layers can be recognised. The two inner layers are composed of living cells and together form the stratum germinativum. In the three outer layers, the cells are dying or dead as a result of keratinisation. During this process the cells become filled with a horny waterproof protein called keratin.

LAYERS

- The innermost layer or stratum basale consists of a single row of columnar cells resting on a basement membrane which separates the epidermis from the dermis. The cells are capable of dividing continuously by mitosis to produce new cells and are stimulated into rapid division by friction on the skin surface. At intervals between the columnar dividing cells are large star-shaped melanocytes which form the skin pigment melanin

- Above the stratum basale, the stratum spinosum is a layer composed of eight to ten rows of rounded cells fitting closely together. Short projections emerge from these cells (prickle cells) to make contact with neighbouring cells. The living cells of this layer remain capable of dividing.

- The next layer, or stratum granulosum, consists of two or three rows of rather flattened cells that contain granules of keratohyalin produced as the first stage of keratinisation in these dying cells.

- A fourth layer, the stratum lucidum, is pronounced in the thick hairless skin on the palms of the hands and soles of the feet, but is not present in hairy skin. It consists of three or four rows of flat dead cells which look translucent as they contain eleidin droplets, produced as a further stage in keratinisation.

- The stratum corneum is the outer 25 to 30 rows of dead scaly cells which contain keratin granules. These cells flake off (desquamation).

PIGMENT

The skin melanocytes produce two types of pigment, eumelanin which is black or brown, and phaeomelanin which is yellowish-brown or red. The amount and distribution of these melanin pigments is responsible for the variation in skin colour. In the Caucasian (white) races, eumelanin is present in relatively small amounts in the basale, spinosum, and granulosum strata. In the *Negroid* (black) races much more eumelanin is present, and it occurs in all the epidermal layers.

 In which layers of the skin epidermis do the following processes occur?
(a) keratinisation
(b) mitosis
(c) desquamation

Dermis

The dermis is composed of connective tissue, containing cells and both collagen and elastin fibres in the matrix.

LAYERS

- The outer region of the dermis is called the papillary layer and its outer ridged surface pushes up into the epidermis as the dermal papillae. The papillary layer is continued round the hair follicles as a connective tissue sheath.

- The inner region of the dermis is the reticular layer. It contains more collagen fibres, making the tissue both strong and flexible. Hyaluronic acid in the matrix of the dermis has excellent moisturising properties.

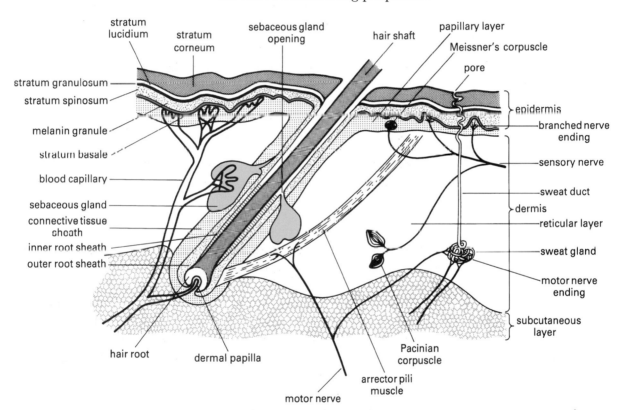

Figure 3.1   *Vertical section through the skin*

The dermis contains a number of structures which have grown down into it from the epidermis. These are the pilosebaceous units, consisting of a hair follicle and its associated sebaceous glands, and the sweat glands. Blood vessels, nerves, and muscles are all dermal structures.

Q   List the structures which together form a pilosebaceous unit.

BLOOD VESSELS

Unlike the epidermis, the dermis is highly vascular. Arterioles (small arteries) enter the dermis from below and branch into networks of blood capillaries round active or growing structures. Such networks occur in the dermal papillae to provide the stratum basale of the epidermis with food and oxygen. A network forms the dermal hair papilla at the growing root of each hair. Similar networks surround the sweat glands and the arrector pili muscles which pull the hairs upright. The capillary networks drain into venules (small veins) which carry the blood away from the skin.

NERVES

Nerves run through the dermis, terminating in nerve endings of various types. Branched nerve endings which are sensory occur in the papillary layer and hair root, and respond to touch and temperature changes. More complex nerve endings also occur such as Meissner's corpuscles in the dermal papillae, sensitive to gentle pressure, and Pacinian corpuscles in the reticular layer, responsive to deep pressure. The nerve endings in the sweat glands and arrector pili muscles are motor, affecting the rate of secretion and state of contraction respectively. Motor nerve endings in the walls of the dermal blood vessels cause them to contract or dilate.

MUSCLES

The arrector pili muscles are attached to hair follicle walls at one end and to the papillary layer just below the epidermis at the other end. When these muscles contract they pull the hair follicles vertical and pinch up the surrounding skin to produce 'gooseflesh'.

 Q | What is the function of Meissner's and Pacinian corpuscles?

SWEAT GLANDS

Eccrine or sudoriferous glands are simple coiled exocrine glands. The glandular region is deeply embedded in the reticular layer and the long duct passes to the skin surface, opening at a pore. In the dermis the duct is straight, but becomes coiled where it passes through the epidermis, as an adaptation to skin stretching. The pores occur on the top of the epidermal ridges to aid the evaporation of sweat. Very large numbers of pores occur on the palms of the hands, soles of the feet, armpits, and forehead.

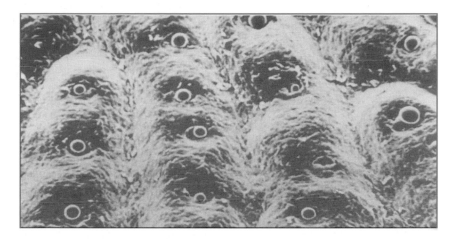

Figure 3.2 *Pores in skin indicated by sweat droplets*

The blood capillaries supply the water and solutes which are secreted as sweat. Sweat contains water and sodium chloride as its main components, together with small amounts of urea, uric acid, ammonia and lactic acid, which are waste products. There are also traces of amino acids, sugar, and ascorbic acid (Vitamin C) in sweat, which provide materials for bacterial growth on the skin surface. The activity of sweat secretion is under nervous control.

Apocrine sweat glands (odoriferous glands) are slightly larger than eccrine sweat glands, and produce a milky fluid containing small amounts of organic substances, such as fats, sugars, proteins and pheromones (sexual attractants). They occur in the axillae (armpits) and pubic region associated with hair follicles into which they usually open. Bacterial breakdown of apocrine sweat produces an unpleasant smell. The activity of these glands begins at puberty and is under both nervous and hormonal control.

SEBACEOUS GLANDS

Sebaceous glands are simple branched acinar exocrine glands which lie on the outside of the hair follicles and open into them. The sebaceous glands are particularly large in the skin of the face, neck, breasts, and upper part of the back. The fatty sebum secreted by these glands contains fats, cholesterol, proteins and some salts, providing material for bacterial and fungal growth on the skin and hair. The activity of the sebaceous glands is controlled by hormones brought by the blood. Secretion of sebum is increased at puberty by male sex hormones, and reduced during pregnancy by the higher level of female sex hormones.

 What controls the rate of secretion in the following?
(a) eccrine sweat glands
(b) sebaceous glands

Figure 3.3   *Pilosebaceous unit*

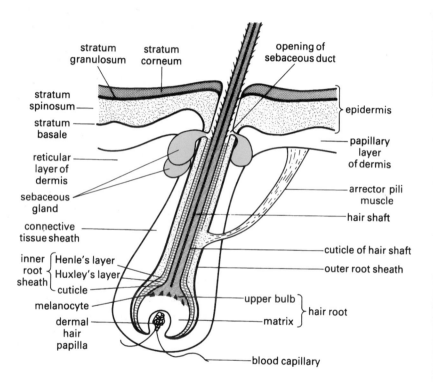

HAIR FOLLICLES

Hair follicles have a two-layered wall formed by the outer and inner root sheaths.

• The outer root sheath is formed from, and continuous with, the epidermis, and narrows down to the single stratum basale layer at the hair root.

• The inner root sheath is three-layered and extends only two-thirds of the way up the follicle, being absent above the sebaceous gland opening. On its outer edge, where it is in contact with the outer root sheath, is Henle's layer, a single row of cuboid cells with flattened nuclei. In the middle is Huxley's layer, consisting of one or two rows of flattened cells. On the inside and pressed against the hair is the cuticle, a single layer of flattened cells. The inner root sheath is formed from the matrix of the hair root. The inner root sheath interlocks with the cuticle of the hair shaft, so that hair and sheath grow up together.

- At its base the follicle is enlarged to form the bulb or hair root. The bulb is pushed in from below, the space formed being occupied by the capillary network of the dermal hair papilla. The hair root consists of two regions, the matrix and the upper bulb. The matrix is the lower region where the unpigmented cells are all alike and dividing rapidly. The matrix lies over the dermal hair papilla, whose blood capillaries supply the food and oxygen needed for hair growth. Above the matrix is the upper bulb where the cells formed by the matrix are differentiating into cells of the inner root sheath, and cuticle, cortex, and medulla of the hair shaft.

- Between the matrix and the upper bulb is a layer of melanocytes, which secrete the hair pigment granules and pass them into the developing cortex cells of the hair shaft.

SUMMARY

Skin is composed of two layers of tissues, the epidermis and the dermis. The outer epidermis has five layers and contains the skin pigment. The inner dermis contains a number of structures; some are epidermal in origin (hair follicles and glands), while the others are dermal structures (blood vessels, nerves and muscles).

Q Explain the difference in origin of the inner and outer root sheaths of the hair follicle.

Hair

TYPES

Two types of hair occur on the body. Short fair vellus hair covers most of the body, except the palms of the hands, soles of the feet, lips, nipples, terminal joints of the fingers and regions occupied by the second type or terminal hair. Terminal hair occurs on the scalp, face (eyebrows, eyelashes, moustache and beard), axillae, pubic region, chest (in men), and round the nipples (in women).

STRUCTURE

The hair shaft is a dead structure composed of keratin. The first centimetre of the hair emerging from the scalp is not fully keratinised and hardened. The diameter of the hair shaft in terminal hairs varies with the individual, and there are racial differences also. Coarse terminal hairs may have a diameter eight times that of the finest hairs. The Caucasoid races have hair which is oval in cross-section, while that of Negroid races is much more flattened. The yellow skinned Mongoloid races have hair which is round in cross-section.

The cells making up the hair shaft are arranged in three layers in coarse terminal hair, but fine terminal and vellus hair have only two layers, the central medulla being absent.

- The outer protective cuticle consists of seven to ten layers of irregular scaly bands composed of colourless transparent keratin. These bands are short and overlapping, and each one extends sideways about one-third of the distance round the hair shaft. The cuticle bands have their free edge towards the tip of the hair.

Figure 3.4   *Hair showing cuticle bands*

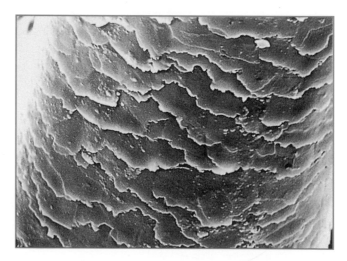

- The cortex is originally composed of long interlacing spindle-shaped cells full of keratin. The walls of the cells soon break down leaving the long parallel keratin fibres which give the cortex its strength. Between the fibres are pigment granules of eumelanin and phaeomelanin, which give the hair its natural colour.

- The medulla, when present, contains large air spaces and loosely packed cells containing eleidin granules. It forms a soft spongy tissue in the centre of the hair shaft.

SUBCUTANEOUS LAYER

Beneath the dermis is a layer of areolar and fat-storing adipose tissues called the superficial fascia. The boundary between the dermis and superficial fascia is irregular in outline, the two layers being held together by collagen fibres. Small blood vessels and lymphatic vessels occur in the subcutaneous tissue, and hair follicles project down into it from the dermis.

The superficial fascia is attached to underlying muscle or bone by its areolar connective tissue. The adipose tissue reduces heat loss through the skin. Below the waist in the region of the hips and buttocks, the subcutaneous layer may contain regions of lumpy dimpled fat called cellulite. The presence of cellulite indicates lack of exercise and a poor diet.

GROWTH OF SKIN AND HAIR

Skin growth

MITOSIS
Skin growth is due to mitosis in the cells of the stratum basale of the epidermis. New cells are produced towards the outside and are continuously pushed upwards by subsequent cell divisions in the stratum basale. Ultra-violet radiation increases the rate of skin growth and thickens the stratum corneum.

MIGRATION
It takes between 40 and 56 days for a new cell to complete its migration to the skin surface, where it forms part of a skin scale and is finally removed by friction.

NUTRITION

Blood capillary networks in the dermal papillae provide the food and oxygen for skin growth.

Hair growth

MITOSIS

Growth at the hair root is initiated by mitosis in the cells of the matrix. As the cells are pushed outwards by further divisions, differentiation occurs. The cells in the upper bulb therefore become altered structurally according to the region of the hair or inner root sheath in which they will ultimately occur. Apart from changes in shape, the differentiating cells undergo keratinisation and die. On the scalp the average rate of hair growth is 0.35 mm per day.

GROWTH CYCLE

A hair-growth cycle occurs in each hair follicle. A period of hair growth is followed by a resting period after which the hair is shed as a new hair develops in the follicle. The life span of a scalp hair is between one and a quarter and seven years, with three years being an average growing period. Eyelashes and eyebrows are replaced every four to five months, while vellus hairs have a life span of around six months. A hair loss of between 50 and 100 hairs daily is normal for the scalp. Pregnancy reduces hair loss temporarily, but after the birth the drop in sex hormone level causes many more hairs to fall out at once.

- The growing phase of a hair is known as anagen. During this phase the cells of the hair matrix are dividing rapidly. Anagen is followed by a short transition period lasting two weeks called catagen.

- During catagen the bulb and lower part of the hair follicle break down, except for a column of epithelial cells which remain in contact with the dermal papilla. The hair has now become a club hair in the shortened follicle, and remains in this condition throughout the resting phase or telogen.

- Telogen lasts for three to four months in terminal hairs and two and a half months in vellus hairs. At the end of telogen the epithelial column becomes active, forming a new hair root at its lower end and lengthening the follicle at its upper end. The club hair is shed as a new hair develops below it and a new anagen phase begins. Plucking a hair out of the follicle starts the growth of a new hair from a resting follicle. It takes 61 days for a plucked eyebrow hair to be replaced.

GROWTH RATE

The rate of hair growth is slowed down by illness and malnutrition, and by pregnancy and using the oral contraceptive pill.

FUNCTIONS OF THE SKIN

Protection

The skin protects the body against mechanical damage due to friction, as cells lost from the stratum corneum are replaced by the stratum basale.

MOISTURISER

As the stratum corneum is waterproof and the dermis contains natural moisturising factors such as hyaluronic acid which binds water, the skin protects the body against water loss.

'ACID MANTLE'

The slightly acid and salty film known as the 'acid mantle' which coats the skin surface has a pH of between 5.6 and 5.8 and prevents micro-organisms from multiplying rapidly on the skin surface. The horny stratum corneum prevents micro-organisms becoming established on, or penetrating, the skin to cause disease. Macrophages in the dermis connective tissue will also destroy micro-organisms by phagocytosis.

MELANIN

The melanin in the epidermis protects underlying tissues from radiation damage by the ultra-violet (UV) rays, and from burning by the infra-red rays in sunlight. UVA (wavelength 320–400 nm) and UVB (wavelength 290–320 nm) rays reach the skin. UVC (wavelength shorter than 290 nm) rays, however, are unable to penetrate the earth's atmosphere to reach the skin. In the UK, the skin's sensitivity to UV damage is greatest in early spring when the skin's melanin level is reduced.

Only a small amount of UVB reaches the earth's surface as it is absorbed by the ozone layer. However, due to depletion of the ozone layer by atmospheric pollution, more UVB is getting through to the earth's surface than in the past. UVA reaches the earth's surface during the hours of daylight, all the year round.

UVA penetrates more deeply into the skin than UVB. UVA affects the dermis, causing premature ageing of the skin. UVB is absorbed in the outer layers of the skin, stimulating the production of melanin and increasing the growth rate of the cells of the stratum basale, which thickens the epidermis. UVB is also the cause of most of the radiation damage to the DNA of the growing cells, resulting in skin cancer, particularly in pale-skinned people.

Figure 3.5   *The part of the electromagnetic spectrum which affects the skin*

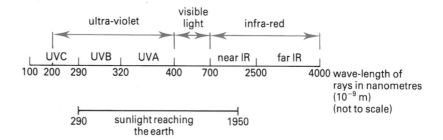

SKIN CANCER

There are two main types of skin cancer caused by ultra-violet rays.

- **Malignant melanoma** causes over 1,200 deaths each year in the UK and occurs more commonly in women than in men. People who have been severely sunburnt in childhood are particularly at risk. Approximately 3,500 new cases develop each year, which is double the number of cases reported in 1974, so the increase is causing concern. The tumour arises from the pigmented cells of moles, which enlarge and darken.

- **Non-melanoma** forms of skin cancer are less dangerous and are usually curable. Although there are around 30,000 new cases each year, only 500 deaths result. Men and women are equally vulnerable. This type of cancer is more common in the elderly, particularly in people who have worked out of doors.

Q State the wavelength limits of the following types of radiation:
(a) UVB
(b) near IR
(c) visible light

Regulating body temperature

The skin has a major role in regulating the body temperature so that it is maintained around 37 °C.

INSULATION

The adipose tissue in the dermis and subcutaneous layer insulates the body against heat loss.

SWEATING

The evaporation of sweat from the skin surface lowers the skin temperature by removing the latent heat required for evaporation, and so cools the body. The removal of latent heat is also the cause of the cold sensation when perfume or toilet water on the skin evaporate rapidly.

BLOOD VESSELS

Variations in blood flow due to changes in diameter of the skin blood vessels regulate the heat lost by radiation from the skin surface.

Sensitivity

The skin is sensitive to changes in the body's external environment. Nerve endings detect temperature changes and indicate the nature of objects in contact with the skin (see chapter 6).

Nutrient supply

Vitamin D is formed in the skin by the action of UVB rays on a substance derived from cholesterol present in the adipose layer. The stored fat in the dermis and subcutaneous layer acts as an energy source. It is continually released from storage and transported by the blood to be used in cell metabolism.

Excretion

The skin also functions as a minor excretory organ. Sweat contains small amounts of waste products (urea, uric acid, ammonia and lactic acid) which are therefore removed from the body.

SUMMARY

The skin protects the body from damage by friction, chemicals and micro-organisms. It reduces water loss from the internal organs and protects them from damage by UV rays. It regulates body temperature, is sensitive to environmental changes and excretes small amounts of waste products. It stores fat and allows Vitamin D formation within it.

SPECIAL FEATURES OF BLACK SKIN

Epidermis

The stratum corneum of the epidermis is much thicker in black skins and the surface tends to desquamate, giving a greyish scaly appearance. The scales contain melanin granules, as melanin is present in all five epidermal layers.

Figure 3.6   *Epidermis in black and white skins*
(a)   Black skin
(b)   White skin

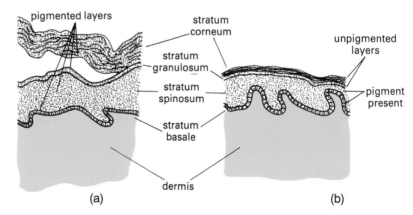

(a)   (b)

Melanin

The number of melanocytes in black skin is approximately the same as in white skin, but the melanin granules secreted are four times larger.

Collagen

There are more collagen fibres in the dermis of black skin, making it very tough. Degeneration of collagen due to ageing is much slower in black skins, which retain their elasticity for a longer time.

Sweat glands

Black skin contains many more apocrine and eccrine sweat glands and they are larger than those of white skin. The glands and ducts of eccrine sweat glands are pigmented and have large pores.

Sebaceous glands

Sebaceous glands are also more numerous and a greater proportion open directly onto the skin surface instead of into a hair follicle. Although the sebum secreted is richer in fats, black skins are not greasy even though the surface is shiny.

Hair

Woolly hair is flattened in cross-section and a medulla is absent.

Reaction to UV

The epidermis of black skin absorbs 70% of the ultra-violet radiation reaching it, while white skin absorbs only 25%. However, the heavy pigmentation allows only 5% to pass through it to reach the dermis. In white skins 15% reaches the dermis. The damaging effect of ultra-violet radiation on the deeper tissues is thus much less in black skins and skin cancers occur less frequently. The melanic pigment increases the absorption of near infra-red heating rays from sunlight (wavelength 700–2,500 nm), but the greater sweat secretion of black skin reduces the heating effect. The reduced ultra-violet penetration in a less sunny climate causes lower Vitamin D production, and this can cause a dietary problem in immigrants with black skins.

—— SUMMARY ——

A black skin has pigment throughout the epidermis, which is thick and scaly. Black skin retains its elasticity longer than white skin. It contains more glands, and is shiny but not greasy. It absorbs more UV rays, but they penetrate less deeply into black skin and cause less damage.

 State three ways in which the epidermis of black and white skins differ.

DISEASES AND DISORDERS OF THE SKIN

A damaged area of skin is known as a lesion, and is a symptom of a disease or disorder. Diseases of the skin arise because there is both a causal agent known as a pathogen, and a predisposition in the person to succumb to the disease due to lowered skin resistance.

Infectious

The diseases caused by pathogenic living organisms can be passed from one person to another, and are said to be infectious. Where a disease is passed on by contact with the lesion, or with infected material, it is said to be contagious. Where the causal agent is a small animal parasite, the disease is known as an infestation. Infectious diseases are often acute, having a rapid onset but lasting for a short time only. When an infectious skin disease is present, beauty therapy treatments are contra-indicated (not advisable).

Table 3.1   *Infectious skin diseases and infestations*

Name	Pathogen	Effects on the skin
Carbuncle	Staphylococcus aureus (bacterium)	Forms large red painful lumps involving a group of hair follicles and discharges pus
Conjunctivitis	Staphylococcus (bacterium)	Inflammation of the mucous membrane covering the eye and lining the eyelids
Face mites	Demodex folliculorum (animal parasite)	Infestation of hair follicles of eyelashes, nose, and chin; usually harmless; may cause irritation
Favus (honeycomb ringworm)	Trichophyton (fungus)	Forms saucer-shaped yellow crusts 1 cm in diameter; causes hairs to break off
Fleas	Pulex irritans (insect parasite)	Sucks blood; bites appear as groups of small red spots which itch intensely
Folliculitis	Staphylococcus aureus (bacterium)	Pustules develop at the opening of the hair follicles; whole scalp may be affected
Furuncle (boil)	Staphylococcus aureus (bacterium)	Forms an inflamed lump round a hair follicle and discharges pus
Herpes simplex (cold sore)	A virus living in the skin of the lips	Red itchy spots form round the mouth which blister, ooze and then form crusts

Table 3.1 *continued*

Name	Pathogen	Effects on the skin
Herpes zoster (shingles)	Modified chickenpox virus	Vesicles develop along the pathway of a nerve, often on face, neck, or waist; pain persists after lesions heal
Impetigo contagiosa	Streptococcus pyogenes Staphylococcus aureus (bacteria)	Blisters develop where skin is damaged, then dry to form yellow crusts; often occurs round the mouth and ears
Pediculosis capitis (head lice)	Pediculus capitis (insect parasite)	Infestation of the scalp starts behind the ears; blood sucking causes irritation leading to scratching and secondary infections, e.g. impetigo
Pediculosis corporis (body lice)	Pediculus humanus (insect parasite)	Lives in the underclothing and sucks blood; bites are small red spots with dried blood in the centre
Pediculosis pubis (crab lice)	Phthirus pubis (insect parasite)	Infests the pubic area, sucking blood; it clings to the pubic hair
Scabies (itch mites)	Sarcoptes scabiei (animal parasite)	An infestation where the mite burrows into loose skin at joints, e.g. wrist; a very irritant disease
Stye	Staphylococcus (bacterium)	Infection of the sebaceous gland of an eyelash follicle, which discharges pus
Sycosis barbae (barber's itch)	Staphylococcus aureus (bacterium)	Infection of the hair follicles of the beard, forming pustules; a form of folliculitis
Tinea capitis (scalp ringworm)	Microsporum (fungus)	Infects the epidermis and hair shafts of the scalp, forming grey scaly areas with short broken hairs
Tinea corporis (body ringworm)	Microsporum or Trichophyton fungi	Infects the epidermis, forming red scaly patches which heal at the centre and spread outwards
Tinea pedis (Athlete's foot)	Epidermophyton (fungus)	Infects the skin between the toes, forming red patches which blister and scale; itchy or sore
Verrucae (warts)	Papova virus	Infects the skin, causing rapid cell division in the epidermis, forming a small raised papilloma; plantar warts on the feet grow inwards and are painful

Non-infectious

Non-infectious diseases are not caused by pathogens and cannot be transmitted to other people. They are often chronic (long-term) disorders, which are difficult to treat effectively. Among their causes are physiological and growth disorders, external skin irritation by chemicals and climatic conditions, and abnormalities of pigmentation. Only some of these conditions contra-indicate beauty therapy treatments.

Table 3.2   *Non-infectious skin disorders*

Name	Cause	Effects on the skin
Achrochordon (skin tag)	Localised hypertrophy (excessive growth)	Small, greyish, projecting fibrous growth usually on the neck or eyelids
Acne vulgaris	Overactivity of the sebaceous glands	Inflammation of the sebaceous glands due to blocking of hair follicles by sebum; infected sebum plugs form pustules (spots)
Bromidrosis (body odour)	Overactive sweat glands	Very unpleasant smell, particularly from the feet, due to bacterial breakdown of copious sweat
Callosity (callus)	Hypertrophied area of skin	Thickened and hardened skin on hands, feet, knees and elbows due to external pressure
*Cancer of skin (tumour)	Excessive exposure to strong sunlight – UVB is the most damaging	It may begin as a small pearly lump or an ulcer that does not heal; melanoma is a cancer due to the growth of a dark mole
Chilblains (Erythema pernio)	Abnormal vascular response to cold	Reddish-blue swellings on exposed skin which itch intensely
Comedo (blackhead)	Blocked hair follicle	A plug of sebum oxidises at the skin surface forming a small black spot
Corn	Localised hypertrophy of skin of the foot	A cone of hard skin pointing inwards on the foot which is painful under pressure
*Dermatitis (contact dermatitis)	External skin irritant	Reddening, blistering, oozing or swelling of the skin soon after contact with the irritant
*Eczema	Allergy with a genetic cause	Red patches which itch, blister, ooze and form crusts or become scaly; no form of water therapy (sauna, jacuzzi) should be undertaken
Erythema	Vascular disorder usually due to UV or infra-red rays	Blood capillaries dilate making the skin red; it occurs with any skin injury or inflammation
Freckles	Hyperactive scattered melanocytes in the skin	Small darker-coloured areas of the skin, level with its surface (macules)

Table 3.2   *Non-infectious skin disorders*

Name	Cause	Effects on the skin
Hyperidrosis	Overactive sweat glands	Localised excessive sweating of hands, feet and axillae
Keratosis	Skin hypertrophy, one cause being excessive exposure to sunlight	Thick stratum corneum forms firm dry adherent scales; surrounding skin is red and pigmentation is patchy
Milia (whiteheads)	Blocked hair follicle	A plug of sebum is covered by stratum corneum so no oxidation occurs; small spots are pearly-white
Naevus (birthmark)	Abnormal skin pigmentation often present at birth	Flat or raised areas of skin varying in colour; red (strawberry mark), purple (portwine stain) or brown (mole)
*Psoriasis	General skin hypertrophy; may be inherited	Reddish slightly raised patches, on any part of the body, which are covered with silvery scales
*Sunburn	Prolonged exposure to sunlight or UV lamps	Painful erythema with blistering; rapid growth of stratum corneum, followed by desquamation (peeling)
Vitiligo	Groups of melanocytes in skin stop functioning	Absence of any pigment in small defined skin areas

Those contra-indicating beauty therapy treatments are marked *

HAIR AND SCALP DISORDERS

Non-infectious diseases of the head and scalp are due to physiological or growth anomalies, or to mechanical and chemical damage caused by unskilled practitioners.

 Distinguish between the terms 'vitiligo' and 'alopecia'.

Table 3.3   *Hair and scalp disorders*

Name	Cause	Effect on the hair and scalp
Alopecia areata (patchy hair loss)	Nervous disorder	Round bald patches on the scalp with smooth glossy skin and no broken hairs
Alopecia totalis	Nervous disorder	Total baldness of the scalp
Fragilitas crinium (split ends)	Mechanical or chemical damage to hair shaft	Loss of cuticle on ends of hairs allows splitting of the cortex layer
Hypertrichosis or Hirsuties (superfluous hair)	Terminal hair grows in follicles normally producing vellus hair	Facial hair in women in beard and moustache regions; it is often related to hormone imbalance
Male patterned baldness	Male sex hormones and increasing age in men; an inherited condition	Baldness starting at the temples and crown on the scalp
Monilethrix (beaded hair)	Uneven rate of hair growth in a follicle	Hair shafts are constricted at intervals along their length and break easily
Pityriasis simplex (dry dandruff or scurf)	Normal skin growth of scalp, where scales are small and dry	Itchy scalp, with the accumulation of dry powdery scales which are trapped by the hairs
Pityriasis steatoides or Seborrhoeic dermatitis	Overactive sebaceous glands on the scalp	Scalp scales have a greasy covering of sebum and stick together; the underlying skin is erythematous
Seborrhoea	Overactive sebaceous glands	Very greasy hair and scalp
Sebaceous cyst (wen)	Blocked sebaceous gland	Sebum is held in a sac under the skin and may become a large projection devoid of hair on the scalp
Trichonodosis (knotted hair)	Hair follicle damage often after unskilled electrolysis treatment	Hairs become looped or knotted just above the skin
Trichorrhexis nodosa	Chemical or mechanical damage to the hair shaft	Rough swellings on the hair shaft where cuticle damage leaves the cortex exposed
Trichotillomania	Nervous disorder	Tugging at the hair causes irregular bald patches with a few short hairs

ALLERGIES

Allergens

An allergy is a condition of sensitivity to a substance, the allergen, to which most other people do not react. Allergens are usually proteins, and when taken internally, or touching the skin, cause tissue damage in hypersensitive people. A hypersensitive skin prone to allergic reaction contra-indicates facial massage.

External allergens (primary irritants) cause contact dermatitis or eczema in the skin. Cosmetics and essential oils may produce an allergic reaction on the skin. Allergens present in certain foods such as shellfish, strawberries, eggs and cheese cause rashes. Some drugs, particularly penicillin and aspirin, may produce the allergic reaction called urticaria.

Sensitisation

On first contact with an allergen, defence cells of the body's immune system produce antibodies which remain attached to the cell. These antibodies attach themselves to the allergen molecules and destroy them, therefore tissue damage does not occur. The antibodies remain in the blood, leaving the body sensitised to the allergen.

HISTAMINE

Later contact with the same allergen stimulates a massive production of the antibody and causes the dermal mast cells to release histamine. This chemical causes inflammation, the skin becoming hot and red due to dilation of the blood capillaries. Histamine also increases the permeability of the blood vessel walls, so that more fluid enters the tissue causing oedema (swelling). Tissue damage results, often not confined to the area of contact.

CROSS-SENSITISATION

Cross-sensitisation may occur where a person has previously been in contact with another allergen (e.g. an azo-dye food colourant) to which they have become sensitised. A later first contact with the new allergen (e.g. a para-dye used to tint eyelashes) produces a strong immune response, which immediately results in tissue damage (dermatitis) due to the cross-sensitisation.

PHOTOSENSITISATION

Certain chemicals become activated in the body by sunlight and become allergens. Typically, a rash appears on skin areas exposed to the sun, and the condition is called photosensitisation. Some drugs (e.g. tetracycline), food constituents (e.g. Vitamin B2) and perfume oils (e.g. oil of bergamot) are photosensitisers. Foods which can cause photosensitivity if eaten in large amounts are lemons, figs, fennel, parsley, celery and carrots.

 Describe how body tissues respond to the presence of an allergen.

EFFECTS OF AGEING ON THE SKIN

Wrinkling

Wrinkling of the skin is due to loss of elasticity, so that stretched skin does not immediately return to its original area when stretching stops. This effect is due to changes in the collagen and elastin fibres of the dermal connective tissue, and to progressive dehydration of the skin, as water is required to keep the collagen pliable. UVA penetrates into the dermis causing premature ageing of collagen.

Collagen synthesis starts in the dermal fibroblast cells with the formation of procollagen molecules. These consist of three chains of amino acids (polypeptide chains) coiled round each other, and known as a triple helix. The amino acids in these chains are mainly glycine, proline and hydroxyproline. The three polypeptide chains are held together by hydrogen bonds, giving considerable tensile strength to the procollagen.

The procollagen molecules pass out of the fibroblast cells into the matrix of the dermal connective tissue. Groups of five procollagen molecules become arranged lengthways to form microfibrils in which the procollagen molecules are staggered, but held together by firm cross-links. There are gaps between adjacent ends of the procollagen molecules, which give a banded appearance when collagen is seen under an electron microscope. Microfibrils are themselves coiled, and combined into larger fibrils.

Figure 3.7   *Structure of collagen*
(a)   Procollagen molecule
(b)   Collagen microfibril
(c)   Collagen fibril

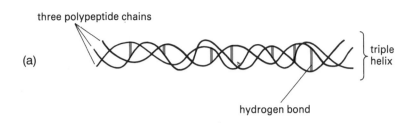

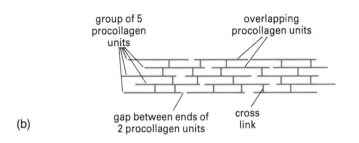

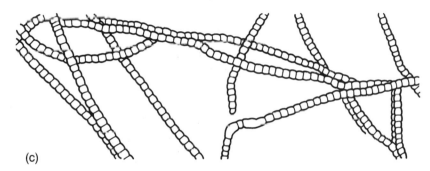

An increase in the number of cross-links in collagen with increasing age is thought to be the cause of its reduced solubility, increased hardness and loss of flexibility which reduces skin elasticity. Degeneration of collagen is considerably slower in black skin.

Drying

The amount of hyaluronic acid in the dermis declines with increasing age, so the skin is less able to bind water and prevent its loss to the atmosphere.

Pigmentation

The number of functioning melanocytes decreases in skin and hair, so the skin colour becomes lighter and white terminal hairs develop. The mixture of white and coloured hairs on the scalp is called canities. Localised groups of melanocytes in the skin may become more active causing pigmented areas known as 'liver spots', which occur commonly on the back of the hand.

Thinning

With ageing, the blood flow to the skin is reduced, and the rate of mitosis in the stratum basale slows down. The stratum corneum is therefore thinner, making the skin more fragile. The skin looks thinner, especially on the backs of the hands. The basement membrane below the stratum basale becomes flattened and broken. Sebaceous and sweat glands are less active and loss of subcutaneous fat often occurs.

NAILS

Nails are protective structures on the end joints of fingers and toes which have developed from the skin epidermis.

Structure

Each nail is a curved sheet of the protein keratin called the nail plate. This has a root which is buried in the epidermis and a body with a distal free edge, forming the visible part of the nail. The horizontal insertion of the nail root splits the epidermis, so

Figure 3.8   *Nail structure*
(a)   Cross section of finger nail
(b)   Longitudinal section of finger nail

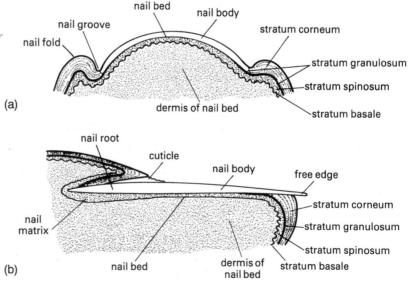

part is above the nail plate and part is below it. The upper part, representing the stratum corneum, forms the cuticle and nail fold around the base and sides of the nail. The furrow between the nail body and the nail fold is the nail groove. The lower part, representing the strata basale and spinosum, forms the matrix which extends below the lunula (half-moon). The nail plate is a thickening of the stratum lucidum. Below the body of the nail the epidermis is called the nail bed. The dermis below the nail is very strongly ridged, which holds the nail plate firmly to the nail bed. The colour of the blood in the dermal capillaries below the nail bed shows through the nail plate producing its pink colour.

 Q Which layers of the skin epidermis form the following nail structures?
(a) cuticle
(b) nail plate
(c) nail matrix

Growth

The matrix is the region from which the nail grows. The lateral walls of the nail fold and the nail bed also contribute to the growth of the nail. The cuticle prevents infection of the nail matrix by closing the space between the nail plate and the roof of the nail fold.

The average weekly growth in length of finger nails is 1 mm, while that of toe nails is only 0.5 mm. The dermis below the nail bed and matrix contains the blood capillaries supplying the food and oxygen needed for nail growth.

Diseases and disorders

The three main causes of nail defects are mechanical damage, physiological disorders and infections. During manicure, hygienic working practices and the use of sterilised implements are important in preventing nail diseases and disorders. Where manicure is contra-indicated, the following diseases and disorders are marked with an *.

• **Agnail** (hang nails) occur when narrow strips of horny epidermis split away from the lateral nail fold. They should be cut away with sharp scissors. They may be the result of damage during a manicure and are common in nail-biters.

- **Atrophy** may occur in nails which were normal at birth but become progressively ridged and deformed and the whole nail plate decreases in size. Ultimate loss of the nail, with scarring, often occurs.

- **Beau's lines** are single transverse furrows running across the nail plates of all the fingers. They are a growth disorder due to a damaged matrix, possibly resulting from an illness such as measles or from trapping the fingers in a door.

- **Blueish coloration** of the nail plate is due to circulatory defects where the blood contains insufficient oxygen (cyanosis). It can also be due to a bruise below the nail.

- **Clubbing**, where the nails are strongly curved downwards over the top of the fingers, is an indication of chronic chest disorder.

- ***Eczema** of the nails is shown by irregular ridges and coarse pitting, and part of the nail may be shed.

- **Fragilitas unguium** (brittle nails) is the effect of dehydration of the nail plate causing the free edge to break or split. Frequent use of detergents and non-oily nail varnish remover are common causes of this disorder. It does not respond to dietary supplements.

- **Hypertrophy** is the thickening and lengthening of the nail plate, usually as a result of physical damage (trauma).

- ***Ingrowing nails** occur only on the toes and are the effect of pressure by badly fitting shoes, or by cutting away the corners of the toe nails. The skin below the free edge of the nail becomes inflamed and painful, requiring medical attention. Toe nails should be cut straight across to prevent this disorder.

- **Koilonychia** is a condition where the nails are concave (spoon-shaped) due to abnormal growth of the nail matrix. It may be a symptom of anaemia.

- **Leuconychia** is the presence of white spots on the nail plate. These are the result of injury to the nail matrix, separating small areas of the nail plate from the nail bed. Refraction of light from abnormal keratin in these areas may cause the white colour.

- ***Onycholysis** is the gradual separation of the nail plate from the nail bed beginning from the free edge. It can be caused by accidental tearing or by using sharp metal implements for cleaning below the nail. Psoriasis or ringworm infections may also cause this disorder.

- ***Onychomycosis** (nail ringworm) is due to the Trichophyton fungus infecting the nail plate. White patches may form, and the free edge of the nail crumbles as it becomes brittle. Yellow streaks develop in the nail plate and Onycholysis may occur. Medical treatment for several months is required.

- ***Paronychia** is an acute infection round the sides and base of the nail plate. Pain, redness and swelling occur with pus oozing below the cuticle. The condition requires medical treatment. It can be due to nail biting injury.

- **Psoriasis** of the nails may result in the nail plate becoming pitted, resembling the surface of a thimble. Alternatively the nail may become roughened and the free edge begin to crumble. Onycholysis often occurs, with a yellow margin between the pink nail and the white separated region.

- **Pterygium unguis** results when the cuticle grows forward over the nail plate, splitting it into two side pieces, and continuing to grow until the nail is eventually lost. The epidermis of the nail fold fuses to the matrix and nail bed. It may result from poor circulation in the hands.

- **Traumatic nail dystrophy** is seen as a depression about 2 mm wide down the centre of the thumb nail, bearing a series of parallel cross ridges. It may occur on one or both of the thumb nails. It is due to overactive pushing back of the cuticle during manicuring or repeated pressure on the nail plate by rubbing with another finger.

- ***Whitlow** is an abscess which develops following infection of the nail fold and causes the terminal joint of the finger to be hot, swollen and inflamed. This condition is very painful and requires medical treatment.

Figure 3.9   *Examples of diseases and disorders of the nail*
(a)   Nail showing onychomycosis
(b)   Nail showing psoriasis
(c)   Traumatic nail dystrophy
(d)   Nail showing pterygium

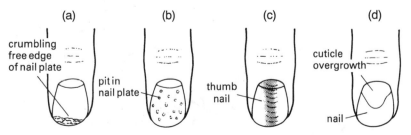

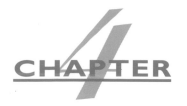

CHAPTER 4

The Skeletal System

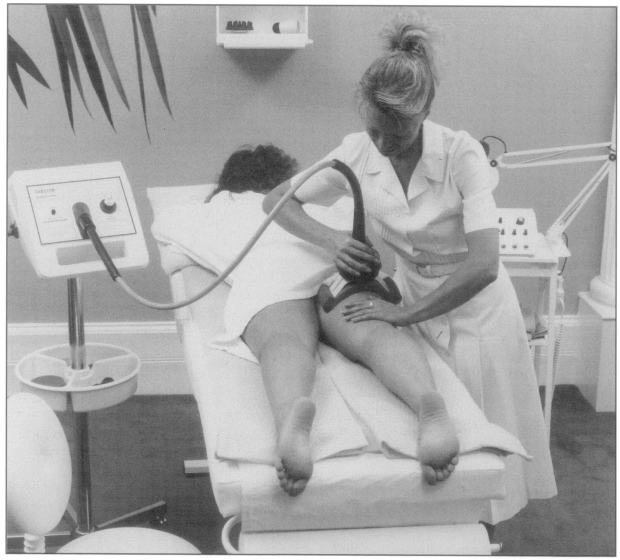

Body massage (mechanical)

SKELETON

The body has an endoskeleton, which is under the skin, covered and moved by the muscles. The skeleton is made of the connective tissues, bone and cartilage and consists of a large number of separate structures (the bones) which articulate (meet at a joint) with one another.

Functions

The functions of the skeletal system include support, protection, and movement. In its supportive role, the skeleton raises the body from the ground, maintains body shape and suspends some of the internal organs. It protects delicate organs by surrounding them with a hard covering. Bones act as levers, and when muscles pull on bones, parts of the body undergo movement. Locomotion, or movement from place to place, is the result of the co-ordinated action of muscles on the bones. Movements of the skeleton require a system of joints and muscle attachments. Muscles are usually attached to bones by tendons composed of tough fibrous non-elastic connective tissue.

 Give four functions of the human skeletal system.

BONE TISSUE

Bone is a porous connective tissue containing living cells, nerves and blood vessels. It has a matrix hardened by the minerals calcium phosphate and calcium carbonate. Collagen fibres in the matrix form a scaffolding on which the minerals are deposited. The collagen makes bone tissue less brittle.

Compact

In compact bone the osteocytes (bone cells) are arranged in concentric rings called Haversian systems, round a branching system of Haversian canals which contain the nerves and blood vessels. The osteocytes secrete the hard matrix, which fills the spaces between the rings of bone cells. Narrow canals called canaliculi pass through the layers of matrix, allowing tissue fluid to pass between the rings of bone cells. The layers of hard matrix between the rings of osteocytes are called lamellae. A small space or lacuna surrounds each osteocyte.

Figure 4.1   *Compact bone tissue*

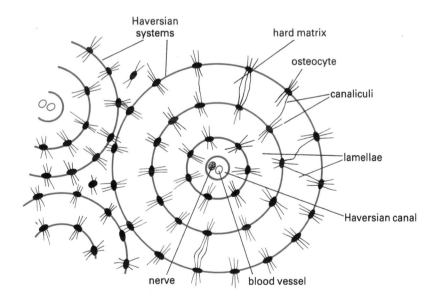

Cancellate

Cancellate (spongy) bone tissue does not have the concentric ring structure of compact bone. It consists of a meshwork of thin plates of bone called trabeculae containing the osteocytes. The large spaces between the trabeculae are filled with bone marrow. Red bone marrow consists of cells which make new red blood cells. Yellow bone marrow contains fat cells and makes certain types of white blood cells.

CARTILAGE TISSUE

Structure

Cartilage is a more flexible connective tissue than bone. Single cells, or groups of two or four cells, are embedded in a tough matrix containing a dense network of collagen and elastic fibres. The cells are surrounded by a small space or lacuna.

Types

There are three types of cartilage, hyaline, fibro and elastic, which have different properties.

HYALINE

Hyaline cartilage (gristle) is a blueish glossy tissue which covers the ends of bones. Separate cartilages of this tissue occur in the nose and trachea (windpipe) and join the ribs to the sternum (breast bone).

FIBROCARTILAGE

Fibrocartilage contains many bundles of collagen fibres, making it strong and rigid. It occurs in the discs between the vertebrae and in the knee (menisci).

Figure 4.2   *Hyaline cartilage*

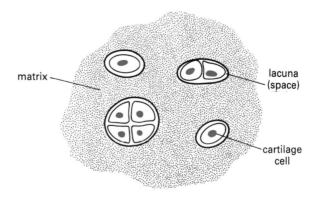

ELASTIC

Elastic cartilage contains more elastic fibres, making it more flexible. It occurs in the larynx (voice box) and the external part of the ear. It also forms the epiglottis which closes the trachea when swallowing.

CLASSIFICATION OF BONES

Types

Bones are divided into types according to their shape or position.

LONG

Long bones have a long, slightly curved shaft or diaphysis, and two wider ends or epiphyses. They have more compact than cancellate bone, which makes them stronger. Red bone marrow occurs in their ends, and yellow bone marrow in their hollow shafts. The thigh and upper arm bones are long bones.

SHORT

Short bones are roughly cube-shaped and are mainly composed of cancellate bone, with only a thin surface layer of compact bone. The bones of the wrist and ankle are short bones.

FLAT

Flat bones consist of two thin surface layers of compact bone, surrounding a central layer of cancellate bone in which red bone marrow occurs. Most of the skull bones, and the scapulae (shoulder blades) are flat bones.

IRREGULAR

Irregular bones have a more complicated shape and do not fit into any of the other three groups. The vertebrae and the zygomatic (cheek bone) are irregular bones.

SESAMOID

Sesamoid bones are a special type which develop in tendons. The patella (knee cap) is of this type.

Where in the body would you find the following structures?
(a) Haversian systems
(b) a flat bone
(c) hyaline cartilage

BONES OF THE SKELETON

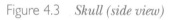

The adult human skeleton usually consists of 206 bones arranged in two groups known as the axial and appendicular skeletons. The axial skeleton of 80 bones comprises the skull, hyoid, vertebral column, sternum, ribs and the auditory ossicles in the ears. The appendicular skeleton of 126 bones comprises the shoulder and hip girdles and the limb bones. For the terms used in describing bones, see Appendix II.

The skull

The skull encloses and protects the brain and sense organs. It consists of two regions, the cranium and the face.

Figure 4.3   *Skull (side view)*

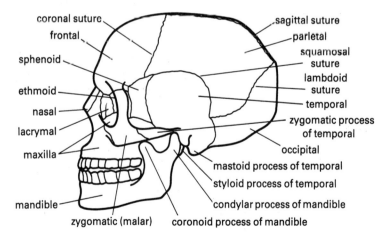

CRANIUM

There are eight flat bones forming the cranium, which articulate at interlocking joints called sutures and surround the brain.

- The frontal bone forms the forehead and upper wall of the orbits (eye sockets). It contains two frontal sinuses above the nose, which are air chambers giving resonance to the voice.

- The two parietal bones form the sides and roof of the cranium.

- Two temporal bones form the lower part of the sides of the cranium. Each temporal bone has a projection behind the ear called the mastoid process, and an anterior zygomatic process which forms part of the zygomatic arch (cheek bone).

- The occipital bone forms the back and base of the cranium. It contains a large hole, the foramen magnum, through which the spinal cord, blood vessels and nerves pass. On each side of the foramen are the occipital condyles which articulate with the first vertebra (Atlas).

- The single sphenoid bone forms the anterior part of the base of the cranium. It binds the cranial bones together, articulating with the frontal, temporal, occipital and ethmoid bones. It is bat-shaped, with a central body, greater and lesser wings and two pterygoid processes. It forms part of the floor and sides of the orbits. The optic foramen for the optic nerve from the eye occurs between the body and lesser wing of the sphenoid bone.

- The single ethmoid bone is anterior to the sphenoid, forming part of the cranial floor and the medial wall of the orbits. It roofs the nasal cavities and forms part of the nasal septum. The region of the ethmoid bone between the nasal cavity and the orbits contains several air spaces known as the ethmoidal sinuses. On either side of the nasal septum, the ethmoid bone has two thin scroll-like conchae which project into the nasal cavity.

The four main sutures of the cranium are the coronal (frontal/parietal), the sagittal (parietal/parietal), the lambdoidal (parietal/occipital) and the squamosal (parietal/temporal).

FACE

The face consists of 14 bones, most of which are irregular in type.

- The paired nasal bones are small and oblong and form the upper part of the bridge of the nose. The lower portion of the nose is supported by more flexible cartilage. The nasal bones articulate with the frontal bone and the maxillae.

Figure 4.4 *Skull from below (mandible removed)*

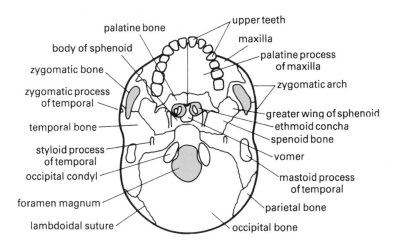

palatine bone

upper teeth

body of sphenoid

maxilla

zygomatic bone

palatine process of maxilla

zygomatic process of temporal

zygomatic arch

temporal bone

greater wing of sphenoid

ethmoid concha

spenoid bone

styloid process of temporal

vomer

occipital condyl

mastoid process of temporal

foramen magnum

parietal bone

lambdoidal suture

occipital bone

- The two maxillae unite to form the upper jaw and carry the upper teeth. They articulate with all the other bones of the face except the mandible. They also form part of the floor of the orbits and nasal cavities. A horizontal projection, the palatine process, forms part of the roof of the mouth (hard palate).

- Two irregular zygomatic or malar bones occur on the outside of the orbits, forming their outer rim and walls and part of their floor. Each zygomatic bone has a temporal process which articulates with the zygomatic process of the temporal bone to form the zygomatic arch of the cheek.

- The single mandible is the only movable facial bone and forms the lower jaw and chin. Its condylar process articulates with the temporal bone, forming a condyloid joint below the ear. Its coronoid process provides the attachment for the temporalis muscle which moves the lower jaw. The mandible carries the lower teeth. The movements of the mandible include raising and lowering, protrusion and retraction (forwards and backwards) and slight side-to-side movements.

- The paired lacrymal bones, which are only the size of a finger nail, form the inner walls of the orbits. They each have a vertical groove for the tear duct.

- Two palatine bones, which are L-shaped, form the back part of the hard palate and walls of the nasal cavities.

- Two turbinate bones occur in the lateral wall of the nasal cavities below the ethmoid conchi. They are scroll-like bones and, like the conchi, are covered with mucous membrane to filter and warm the air before it passes into the lungs.

- The single triangular vomer forms part of the nasal septum, articulating with the ethmoid bone and cartilage which form the rest of the nasal septum.

 In each case, name the bone on which the particular feature occurs:
(a) sockets for the upper teeth
(b) coronoid process
(c) mastoid process

SUMMARY

The skull is the bony protection of the brain and sense organs in the head. It consists of the cranium, with eight bones, and the face, with fourteen bones. The cranium is composed of flat bones with immovable interlocking joints called sutures. The mandible (lower jaw) in the face is the only movable bone.

The hyoid bone

This single U-shaped bone is unique as it does not articulate with any other bone. It is suspended from the styloid process of the temporal bone of the skull by ligaments. It occurs in the neck between the mandible and the larynx, and supports the tongue.

The vertebral column

A series of 26 bones in the posterior wall of the trunk forms a strong flexible vertebral column. Between successive vertebrae are intervertebral discs of fibrocartilage which have a cushioning effect. If one of these discs is ruptured, the condition known as 'slipped disc' occurs.

FUNCTIONS

Its functions are to protect the spinal cord while allowing nerves to pass out between the vertebrae, to support the head, and to provide attachment for the ribs and muscles of the back.

REGIONS

The vertebral column has five distinct regions in which the vertebrae show small structural differences. There are:

- seven cervical vertebrae in the neck;

- twelve thoracic vertebrae articulating with the ribs in the thorax;

- five strong lumbar vertebrae in the lower back;

- five sacral vertebrae fused into one sacrum in the pelvic region;

- four bones fused into one coccyx at the base of the vertebral column.

CURVES

Viewed laterally, the vertebral column has four curves which are alternately concave and convex in the posterior view. The upper concave cervical curve develops as a baby learns to hold its head up. The concave lumbar curve develops as a baby learns to walk. The thoracic and sacral curves retain the foetal convexity. These curves increase the strength of the vertebral column, help to maintain balance in the upright position, and absorb mechanical shocks when walking or running.

Postural defects may occur due to abnormal spine curvatures. Where the spine curves outwards markedly in the thoracic region, the condition is known as kyphosis. A marked inward curvature in the lumbar region is lordosis. A sideways (lateral) curvature of the spine in any region is scoliosis.

 State the functions of the vertebral column.

STRUCTURE OF A TYPICAL VERTEBRA

All vertebrae have a basically similar structure. They are irregular bones consisting of a ventral body and a dorsal vertebral (neural) arch. This arch has a dorsal spinous process, two transverse processes and four articulating processes that form joints with the two adjacent vertebrae. The body comprises a centrum and the ventral ends of the vertebral arch. A vertebral foramen for the spinal cord occurs between the body and the vertebral arch.

Figure 4.5 *Typical vertebrae (from above)*

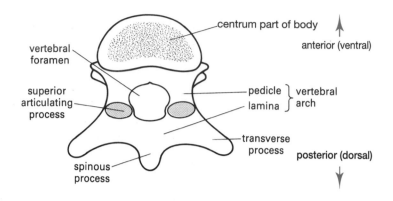

REGIONAL DIFFERENCES IN STRUCTURE

In the different regions of the vertebral column, the vertebrae have special features.

- Cervical vertebrae have a small body and a large arch with a forked spinous process. Each transverse process has a foramen for the vertebral blood vessels. The first cervical vertebra or atlas is ring-shaped, without a centrum or spinous process. Its superior surface has two concave articular surfaces to receive the occipital condyles of the skull, which allows the nodding movement of the head. The second cervical vertebra or axis has a body from which an odontoid process projects up through the ring-shaped atlas to allow the small rotary head movements.

Figure 4.6 *Thoracic vertebra (side view)*

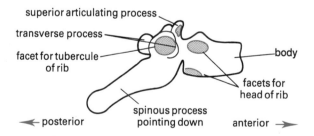

- Thoracic vertebrae have long spinous processes directed downwards, and their transverse processes have facets for articulating with the tubercles of the ribs. Facets on the body articulate with the heads of the ribs.

- Lumbar vertebrae are large and strong with short, thick processes for the attachment of the large back muscles. A considerable amount of bending (flexion) occurs in the lumbar region of the vertebral column, but almost no rotation.

- The sacrum is triangular, articulating on both sides with the pelvic girdle which it supports. The anterior surface has four pairs of pelvic foramina, and the posterior surface has four pairs of dorsal foramina. Nerves and blood vessels pass through the foramina.

- The coccyx is a very small, triangular bone at the apex of the sacrum, which represents the vestige of a tail. It is easily displaced by falling heavily onto the buttocks.

— SUMMARY —

The vertebral column is a curved chain of bones which forms the spine in the dorsal body wall. It supports the head and helps to maintain the body's upright posture. Each vertebra has a basic shape, consisting of a body which is anterior (ventral) and a posterior (dorsal) arch. The arch surrounds and protects the spinal cord. It has projecting articulating processes for adjacent vertebrae and ribs. Between the bodies of adjacent vertebrae are cushioning intervertebral discs. There are five distinct regions in the vertebral column, known as cervical (neck), thoracic (chest), lumbar (lower back), sacral (pelvic) and coccyx ('tail').

Thoracic cage

The skeleton supporting the thorax is cone-shaped, narrowing towards the neck. It comprises the bodies of the thoracic vertebrae, the ribs and costal cartilages, and the sternum (breast bone).

FUNCTIONS

Its functions are to protect the heart and lungs, and to support the pectoral (shoulder) girdle. It is essential for breathing and provides attachment for many of the muscles moving the arm.

RIBS

There are 12 pairs of ribs, each pair articulating with a thoracic vertebra by synovial gliding joints at the head and tubercle. The first seven pairs of ribs are connected to the sternum by costal cartilages and are called true ribs. The remaining five pairs are false ribs. In the eighth to tenth pairs of ribs, the costal cartilages connect with those of the seventh pair. The short eleventh and twelfth pairs are called floating ribs, as they have no attachment to the sternum.

Figure 4.7   *Typical rib*

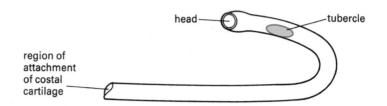

> *Q*   State the functions of:
> (a) an odontoid process
> (b) foramina
> (c) costal cartilage

STERNUM

The sternum is a flat bone lying medially in the anterior wall of the thorax. It consists of three parts: an upper wider manubrium articulates with the first two pairs of ribs; a body articulates with the second to tenth pairs of ribs; and it terminates in a xiphoid process. The manubrium also articulates superiorly with the two clavicles (collar bones) of the pectoral girdle.

Figure 4.8   *Sternum (anterior view)*

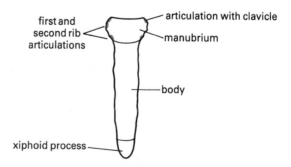

Shoulder (pectoral) girdle

The pectoral girdle connects the arm bones to the axial skeleton and is formed by two clavicles and two scapulae (shoulder blades). It is incomplete posteriorly as the scapulae do not

articulate with the vertebral column. Anteriorly the clavicles
articulate with the sternum.

CLAVICLE

The clavicles are long bones with a slight S-shaped curvature and
are placed horizontally at the top of the anterior thoracic wall.
Their medial end is rounded where it articulates with the
manubrium. Their lateral end is flattened and articulates with
the acromion process of the scapula. Both lateral and medial
articulations are gliding joints. The coracoid tuberosity on the
inferior surface of the clavicle is for attachment of ligaments
from the coracoid process of the scapula. The clavicles provide
the only attachment of the pectoral girdle to the axial skeleton
and are the most frequently fractured bones in the body.

Figure 4.9   *Clavicle (anterior view)*

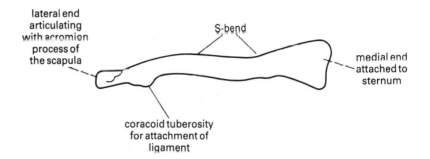

SCAPULA

The scapulae are two large, triangular, flat bones in the upper
part of the posterior thoracic wall between the second and
seventh ribs. A ridge, the scapular spine, runs diagonally across
the posterior face of the bone. The end of the spine projects as
the acromion process at the shoulder, and the scapula has a

Figure 4.10   *Scapula (posterior view)*

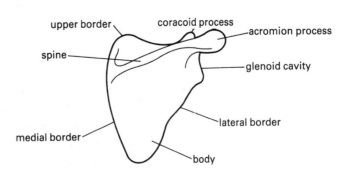

coracoid process just anterior to it. Just below these two processes the scapula has a depression, the glenoid cavity, which articulates with the humerus of the upper arm. The acromion process articulates with the clavicle.

Pelvis (hip or pelvic girdle)

STRUCTURE

The pelvis is basin-shaped and consists of two pelvic bones joined anteriorly at the symphysis pubis. Posteriorly, the bones articulate with the sacrum at a gliding joint where movement only occurs during childbirth.

Each pelvic bone has three regions, a superior ilium, an inferior posterior ischium and an inferior anterior pubis. The three regions meet at the acetabulum, where the femur (thigh bone) articulates with the pelvis at a hip joint. The ischium has a posterior ischial tuberosity for muscle attachment. The ischium and pubis surround the obturator foramen, a large gap in the pelvic bone occupied by a fibrous membrane. Nerves and blood vessels supplying the legs pierce this fibrous membrane.

Figure 4.11   *Pelvis (anterior view)*

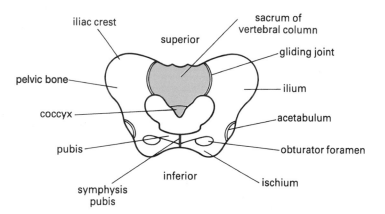

FUNCTIONS

The functions of the pelvis are to provide a strong support for the legs which carry the weight of the body, to protect the organs in the pelvic cavity, and to provide a surface for attachment of the muscles of locomotion.

 List the functions of the pelvis.

Arm (fore limb)

The arm contains 30 bones arranged on a pentadactyl (five-fingered) plan. Most are long bones. (For the nature of the joints, see later section.)

HUMERUS

The humerus is the bone of the upper arm between the shoulder and the elbow. At the proximal end is the head, a lateral greater tubercle and an anterior lesser tubercle. Between the tubercles is a sulcus, the bicipital groove. The distal end of the humerus at the elbow has a capitulum articulating with the radius of the forearm, and a trochlea articulating with the ulna of the forearm. The medial and lateral epicondyles are rough projections on either side of the distal end of the humerus.

Figure 4.12   *Right humerus (anterior view)*

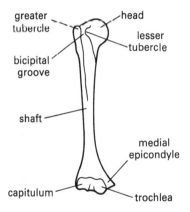

ULNA

The ulna is the medial bone of the forearm, on the little finger side. Its proximal end has a projecting olecranon process forming the elbow.

RADIUS

The radius is the lateral bone of the forearm, on the thumb side. Its distal end has a lateral styloid process and articulates with the proximal carpals. Its proximal end articulates with the humerus and the ulna. The radial tuberosity below the head is a roughened area where the biceps muscle is attached.

Figure 4.13   *Right radius and ulna (anterior view)*

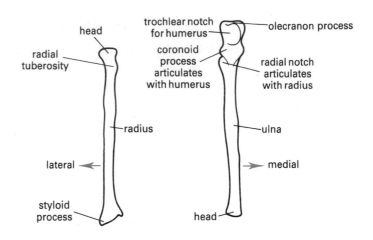

WRIST

The wrist is composed of eight small carpal bones arranged in two rows of four. The carpals are of the short bone type. The proximal row of carpals comprise the scaphoid (on the thumb side), lunate, triquetral and pisiform. The distal carpals comprise the trapezium (on the thumb side), trapezoid, capitate and hamate. The bones are joined together by ligaments.

HAND

The hand has five metacarpal bones in the palm and 14 phalanges in the digits. The pollex (thumb) has two phalanges, while each finger has a proximal, middle, and distal phalanx.

Figure 4.14   *Bones of right wrist and hand (palmar surface)*

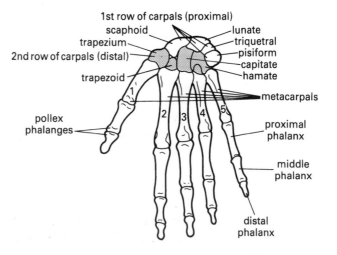

Leg (hind limb)

The leg is built on the same plan as the arm, and it also contains 30 bones. (For the nature of the joints, see later section.)

FEMUR

The femur (thigh bone) is the largest and strongest of the long bones of the limb. Its shaft inclines medially towards the knee, particularly in women, who have wider hips than men. This line brings the knee joint closer to the mid-line. Although it gives a narrower base to support the body's weight, making the body less stable, it allows easier body movements. The proximal head of the femur articulates with the acetabulum of the pelvic bone at the hip joint. Proximally, there is a lateral greater trochanter and a medial lesser trochanter for attachment of buttock and thigh muscles. There is a narrow neck between the head and the trochanters, which may fracture in elderly people. The distal end of the femur has medial and lateral condyles which articulate with the tibia (shin bone) and patella (knee cap). The patellar surface is a triangular area between the condyles.

Figure 4.15   *Right femur (anterior view)*

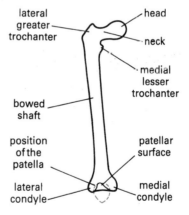

lateral greater trochanter

head

neck

medial lesser trochanter

bowed shaft

position of the patella

patellar surface

lateral condyle

medial condyle

PATELLA

The patella is a sesamoid bone which develops in the tendon of the quadriceps femoris muscle and lies anterior to the knee joint.

TIBIA

The tibia (shin bone) is the larger medial bone of the lower leg and bears the body weight. Its proximal end has lateral and medial condyles articulating with the femur. The tibial tuberosity on its anterior surface is where the patellar ligament is attached. The distal end of the tibia has a medial malleolus forming the projection on the inner side of the ankle. A fibular notch articulates with the end of the fibula.

FIBULA

The fibula bone lies parallel to the tibia in the lower leg. It is lateral to the tibia, and does not articulate with the femur. At its proximal end, the head of the fibula articulates with the lateral condyle of the tibia. Its distal end has a lateral malleolus forming the projection on the outside of the ankle.

 In each case, name the bone on which the particular feature occurs:
(a) lesser tubercle
(b) greater trochanter
(c) olecranon process
(d) patellar surface

Figure 4.16   *Right tibia and fibula (anterior view)*

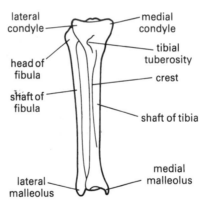

ANKLE

The ankle consists of seven tarsal bones. The talus and calcaneum are posterior, the cuboid, navicular and three cuneiform bones are anterior. The talus is the only tarsal that articulates with the tibia and fibula, and thus bears the weight of the leg. The calcaneum forms the heel.

FOOT

The foot has five metatarsal bones which, with the tarsals, support the arches of the foot. The metatarsals articulate

Figure 4.17 *Bones of right ankle and foot (side view)*

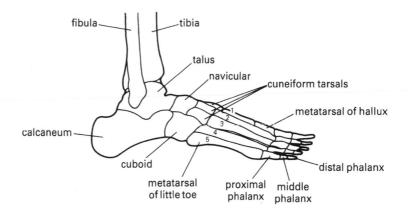

proximally with the three cuneiform tarsals and the cuboid, and distally with the phalanges. There are 14 phalanges in the toes, two in the hallux (big toe) and three in each of the other toes.

ARCHES OF THE FOOT

The bones of the foot form arches to support the body weight and provide leverage when walking. They yield slightly when weight is applied and spring back when the weight is lifted. Two of the arches run longitudinally along the foot, while the other two are transverse.

- The medial longitudinal arch on the big toe side is the highest of the arches and is formed by the calcaneum, navicular, three cuneiform and first three metatarsal bones. Only the calcaneum and metatarsal bones should make contact with the ground.

- The lateral longitudinal arch is formed by the calcaneum, cuboid and last two metatarsal bones. The cuboid is the 'keystone' of the arch.

- The posterior transverse arch is formed by the calcaneum, navicular and cuboid tarsals.

- The anterior transverse arch is formed by the posterior parts of the five metatarsals.

 Q Name the bones forming:
(a) the median longitudinal arch of the foot
(b) the ankle

MOVEMENTS OF BONES

All movements that change the position of the bones occur at joints. Several different kinds of movement may occur.

- **Flexion** is a movement which bends a limb, for example at the elbow when the forearm and hand moves towards the face, or when bending the head forward onto the chest.

- **Extension** is a movement which straightens a limb or the spine, and is the reverse of flexion.

- **Hyperextension** involves bending further back than the vertical position, for example bending the head backwards to look up at the ceiling.

- **Abduction** is a movement away from the mid-line of the body, for example when the arms are raised horizontally sideways.

- **Adduction** is a movement towards the mid-line of the body, for example lowering the arms to the sides.

- **Circumduction** is a circular movement in which the moving bone describes a cone in the air, for example circling the extended arm at the shoulder.

- **Dorsiflexion** is the upward movement of the top of the foot towards the tibia at the ankle joint.

- **Plantar flexion** is the movement of the sole of the foot downwards, extending the foot at the ankle joint, for example when standing on tip-toe.

- **'Eversion'** is turning the sole of the foot outwards at the ankle, so that the body weight is on the inner edge of the foot.

- **'Inversion'** is turning the sole of the foot inwards at the ankle so that the body weight is on the outer edge of the foot.

- **Pronation** is a movement of the flexed forearm, turning the palm to face downwards by rotating the radius on the ulna; also 'eversion' of the foot when feet planted far apart.

- **Supination** is a movement of the flexed forearm, turning the palm of the hand upwards; also 'inversion' of the foot when feet are close together or crossed.

- **Rotation** is the movement of a bone turning about its long axis, either towards or away from the mid-line of the body. For example, the atlas is rotated on the odontoid process of the axis when shaking the head, producing rotation on a horizontal plane.

 | Distinguish between plantar flexion and dorsiflexion.

JOINTS

Joints occur where bones articulate, and are classified according to the amount and type of movement between them.

Fibrous

Fibrous joints are immovable, as the bones are held together by fibrous connective tissue and there is no joint cavity. The sutures between the bones of the skull and the joints between the teeth and jawbones are examples of fibrous joints.

Cartilaginous

Cartilaginous joints are only slightly movable. The articulating bones are held together by a pad of cartilage and there is no joint cavity. The joints between the centra of successive vertebrae are cartilaginous.

SYMPHYSIS

A symphysis, such as the joint between the two pubic bones of the pelvis, has a broad flat disc of fibrocartilage between the bones.

Figure 4.18 *Synovial joint (vertical section)*

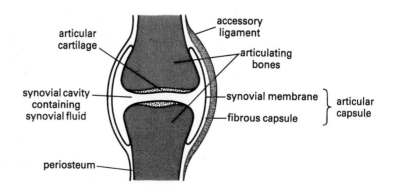

Synovial

Synovial joints are freely movable, and a joint cavity is present as there is a space between the articulating bones. The articulating surfaces at the ends of the bones are covered with a thin layer of smooth hyaline cartilage to reduce friction. In the space between the bones is the lubricating synovial fluid, secreted by a synovial membrane lining the joint cavity. Outside the synovial membrane is a fibrous capsule continuous with the periosteum of each bone. The synovial membrane and fibrous capsule together make up the articular capsule, which is strong and flexible and retains the synovial fluid. Fluid filled sacs called bursae occur around joints to reduce friction. The sacs are lined by a synovial membrane which secretes the fluid. A bursa may become inflamed, a condition called bursitis.

LIGAMENTS

The bones are held in position at the joint by additional accessory elastic ligaments, which prevent dislocation during normal movement. Ligaments are fibrous or fibroelastic bands of dense connective tissue which are silvery in appearance.

MENISCI

Inside some synovial joints, discs of fibrocartilage (menisci) lie between the articular surfaces of the bones. They help to stabilise the joint and are found in the knee joint. A 'torn cartilage' in the knee is due to damage to the menisci.

Synovial joints are divided into several types according to the kind of movement which occurs.

BALL-AND-SOCKET

Ball-and-socket joints allow rotation and movement in all three planes (one horizontal and two vertical at right angles). The rounded head of one bone fits into a cup-shaped socket in another bone. The head of the humerus fits into the glenoid socket in the scapula at the shoulder, and the head of the femur fits into the acetabulum of the pelvis at the hip. Thus there is great freedom of movement at the shoulder and hip joints.

HINGE

Hinge joints allow flexion and extension, which are movements in one plane only. The cylindrical end of one bone fits into a notch in another bone. The elbow is a hinge joint, where the lower end of the humerus fits into the trochlear notch in the ulna. Hinge joints also occur at the knee and between the phalanges of the fingers and toes.

GLIDING

Gliding (sliding) joints only allow side-to-side and back-and-forth movements in two planes. The articulating surfaces of the bones are flat. The joints between the carpals in the wrist and between the tarsals in the ankle are gliding joints. These intertarsal joints allow changes in the foot's contact with the ground during 'inversion' and 'eversion'.

CONDYLOID

Condyloid joints occur where an oval condyle projecting from one bone fits into an oval cavity on another bone, allowing side-to-side and back-and-forth movements. The occipital condyles of the skull fit into concavities on the atlas vertebra. Condyloid joints occur between the metacarpals and proximal phalanges in the hands, and at the wrist between the ulna and radius and the proximal row of carpals. A condyloid joint occurs between the skull and the lower jaw.

SADDLE

Saddle joints allow movements which are slightly freer than those of condyloid joints. The articular surfaces of the bones are saddle-shaped, concave on one side and convex on the other. The convexity on one bone fits the concavity in the other. In the thumb joint the trapezium articulates with the first metacarpal by a saddle joint.

PIVOT

Pivot joints allow rotation only. The radius and ulna rotate round one another at the elbow, and the odontoid peg of the axis vertebra rotates in a ring-shaped socket in the atlas vertebra.

Structure of major joints

Table 4.1 summarises the type and structure of each major joint and lists the movements which occur there.

Table 4.1   *Major joints of the body*

Name	Type	Structure	Movements
Shoulder	Synovial: ball-and-socket	Head of the humerus fits into the glenoid cavity of the scapula. The acromion process of the scapular spine articulates with the clavicle. The tendon of the biceps runs through the articular capsule; ligaments and deep shoulder muscles strengthen the joint	Flexion/extension; abduction and adduction; rotation outwards; rotation inwards; circum-duction
Elbow	Synovial: hinge	The capitulum of the humerus articulates with the head of the radius. The trochlea of the humerus fits into the trochlear notch of the ulna, behind which is the olecranon forming the elbow (funny bone)	Flexion/extension
	pivot	The radius articulates with the radial notch of the ulna	Pronation and supination
Wrist	Synovial: condyloid	The radius articulates with the scaphoid lunate and triquetral carpals. It is strengthened by ligaments and surrounded by a capsule	Flexion/extension; abduction and adduction; circumduction
	gliding	Joints between the carpals	Flexion/extension; abduction and adduction
Hip (bears 66% of the body weight)	Synovial: ball-and-socket	The head of the femur articulates with the acetabulum of the pelvic bone. The articular capsule is very strong and there are ligaments and muscles which strengthen the joint	Flexion/extension; abduction and adduction; rotation outwards; rotation inwards; circum-duction
Knee (bears 88% of the body weight)	Synovial: hinge	Between the femur and tibia. Cruciate ligaments hold the bones together. Menisci occur between tibial and femoral condyles	Flexion/extension; some rotation

Table 4.1   *continued*

Name	Type	Structure	Movements
	gliding	Between femur and patella. The patella is supported by the patellar ligament and the tendon of the quadriceps femoris. There is no complete articular capsule but a large number of ligaments strengthen the joint	Abduction and adduction
Ankle (bears whole weight of the body)	Synovial: hinge	The talus articulates with the malleoli of the tibia and fibula. A very strong deltoid ligament passes from the tibial malleolus to the talus, navicular and calcaneum, binding the leg to the foot. Several smaller ligaments also occur	Dorsiflexion; plantar flexion
Intervertebral	Cartilaginous: symphysis	A broad, flat intervertebral disc of fibrocartilage occurs between the centra of adjacent vertebrae. All movements are very small, but are additive	Flexion/extension; lateral flexion; rotation; circum-duction

 List four body regions where a hinge joint occurs.

Figure 4.19   *Shoulder joint*

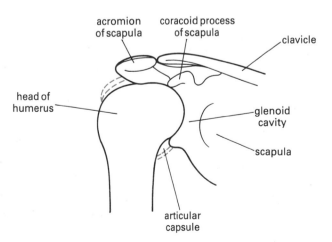

Figure 4.20   *Elbow joint*

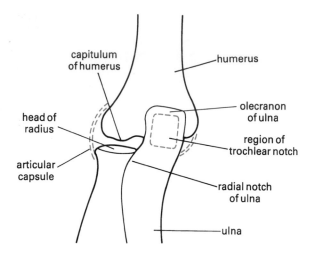

Figure 4.21   *Hip joint (vertical section)*

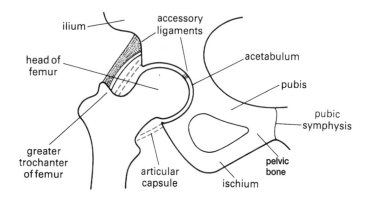

Figure 4.22   *Knee joint (vertical section)*

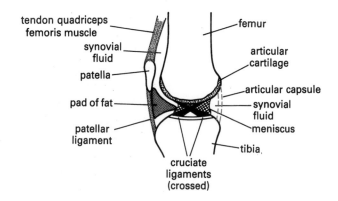

Figure 4.23   *Intervertebral joint (side view)*

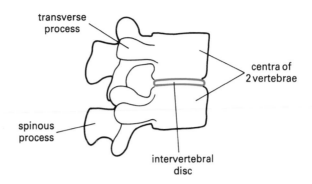

EFFECTS OF AGEING ON THE SKELETAL SYSTEM

Osteoporosis

With increasing age, especially menopausally, osteoporosis, a decrease in bone mass, occurs and there is a shortening of the legs due to compression of the softened bone. An average height loss of 1.5 cm occurs between the ages of 30 and 60 years in women.

Arthritis

Arthritis is a degenerative inflammatory condition of the joints. There are several types of arthritis; osteoarthrosis and rheumatoid arthritis commonly affect women. In osteoarthrosis the ends of the bones slowly degenerate, starting with the crumbling of the articular cartilage. It commonly affects hip, knee, shoulder and terminal finger joints, and is found in many women over 60 years of age. Rheumatoid arthritis is an autoimmune disease (where the defence mechanism attacks the body's own normal tissues) which usually starts between the ages of 35 and 40 years. There is a thickening of the synovial membrane of the joint, crumbling of the articular cartilage and over-production of connective tissue. The joint eventually becomes fixed.

EFFECTS OF INJURY ON JOINTS

Tendinitis

Tendinitis is the result of inflammation of the synovial membrane and tendon sheaths in a joint. It is caused by excessive or unusual physical activity and is painful and disabling. Repetitive strain injury caused by constant use of a keyboard is due to tendinitis in the arms and hands.

Sprain

A sprain is an injury in or around a joint, where twisting or wrenching has occurred. Ligaments and tendons may be torn and blood vessels damaged, leading to swelling and discolouration. Movement at the joint becomes restricted.

Hallux valgus

Hallux valgus is a condition where the base of the big toe is pushed outwards at the joint and a bunion occurs. The condition is due to the pressure of badly fitting footwear on the joint.

CHAPTER 5

The Muscular System

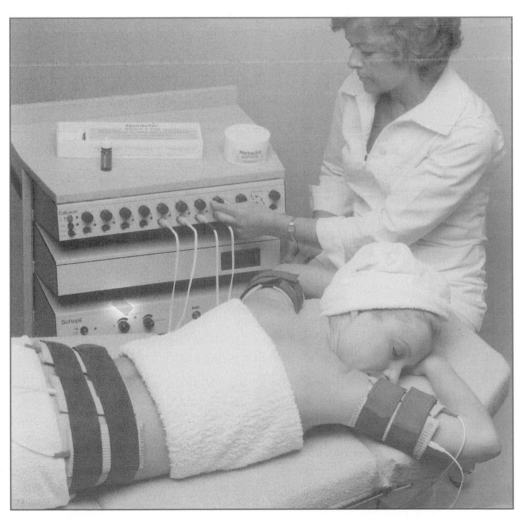

Electrical muscle stimulation

The muscular system consists of the skeletal muscle tissue and connective tissue that make up the individual muscles which are attached to the bones of the skeleton. These muscles form the flesh, covering the bones on the outside and helping to give the body its shape.

FUNCTIONS OF THE MUSCULAR SYSTEM

The muscular system has three main functions, those of causing movement (see below), maintaining posture (see page 133) and producing heat (see page 165). It brings about movement by exerting a pull on tendons which move bones at joints. The pulling force is due to the contraction or shortening of the muscle. Parts of the body, such as the limbs, are moved in this way. When the entire body moves from one place to another, locomotion is said to occur.

Usually muscles are attached by their tendons to two articulating bones on either side of the joint. When a joint is moved, one of the two articulating bones remains stationary while the other one moves. The attachment of the muscle to the stationary bone is the muscle origin, that is the anchorage end of the muscle. The attachment to the bone that moves is the insertion, that is the pulling end of the muscle. In the limb muscles the origin is usually proximal, while the insertion is distal.

Lever action

During movement, bones act as levers, hinged at the joint which acts as the fulcrum (F). The muscle provides the effort (E), while the weight of the part being moved is the load (L). The positions of the fulcrum, effort and load determine the type of lever action.

FIRST-CLASS LEVER

In a first-class lever, the fulcrum is placed between the effort and the load. The movement of the head on the vertebral column is an example of first-class lever action. When the head is lifted, the muscles at the back of the neck provide the effort, while the weight of the facial region of the skull is the load. The joint between the skull and atlas vertebra is the fulcrum.

THIRD-CLASS LEVER

In a third-class lever, the fulcrum is at one end, the load is at the other end of the lever, and the effort is between them. Flexing the arm at the elbow is an example of third-class lever action. The elbow joint is the fulcrum, the biceps muscle provides the effort, and the weight of the forearm and hand is the load.

Body movements usually involve lever action of these two types.

SECOND-CLASS LEVER

In a second-class lever, the fulcrum is at one end and the effort at the other, with the load in between. An example of this type of lever action is raising the body onto the toes. The weight of the body is the load, the ball of the foot is the fulcrum, and the contraction of the calf muscles provides the effort which lifts the heel off the ground.

MECHANICAL ADVANTAGE

The mechanical advantage which lever action provides is greatest when a large weight (load) can be moved by a small muscular effort. This occurs in the second-class lever action where the body is raised onto the toes. In the third-class lever action at the elbow joint, great muscular power develops in the biceps muscle to move the small weight of the hand, so the mechanical advantage is small.

Figure 5.1   *Lever action in body movements*
(a)   *First-class lever*
(b)   *Second-class lever*
(c)   *Third-class lever*

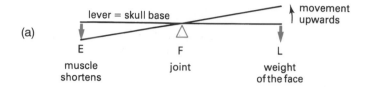

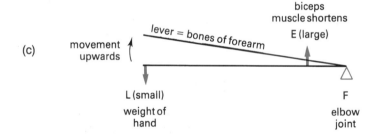

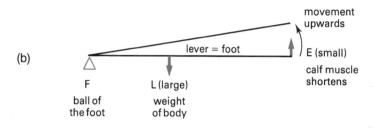

Antagonistic pairs

In most cases movements are brought about by several muscles acting in groups. Many muscles work in antagonistic pairs, where one contracts to move the bone one way and the other contracts to move the bone back. The calf and shin muscles form an antagonistic pair which lower and raise the foot.

Types of contraction

Isotonic contractions develop tension and the muscle shortens (for example the raising of the arm at the elbow by the biceps muscle, which bulges outwards as it shortens). Isometric contractions develop tension, but the muscle does not shorten (for example carrying a weight on the hand with the arm extended, when the biceps muscle does not bulge).

Define, in relation to muscular movement, the terms:
(a) insertion
(b) tendon
(c) origin
(d) antagonistic pair

MUSCLE TISSUE

Characteristics

Muscle tissue has four main characteristics.

- It has the ability to shorten or contract.

- It can be stretched when it is relaxed, so it is extensible.

- After contraction or extension it can return to its original shape, so it has elasticity.

- Muscle tissue responds to stimuli provided by nerve impulses.

Functions

By contracting, muscle tissue performs the functions of causing movements, maintaining posture, and producing heat which helps to maintain normal body temperature. Muscular movements aid the flow of blood and lymph through the veins and lymphatics respectively.

Types

There are three types of muscle tissue: skeletal, cardiac and smooth.

SKELETAL

Skeletal muscle is attached to the bones of the skeleton and is under voluntary conscious control by the brain and nerves. Viewed under a microscope, transverse stripes are visible, so the muscle is said to be striated. It is red in colour due to the presence of an oxygen-storing pigment called myoglobin. Skeletal muscle tissue consists of bundles of parallel muscle fibres. Each fibre has an outer membrane enclosing cytoplasm containing contractile protein fibrils and many nuclei. Skeletal muscle can do a great deal of work, but will tire easily. Postural muscles contain more slow-acting fibres (red), while primary movers contain more fast-acting fibres (pale).

Figure 5.2   *Muscle tissue*
(a)   Skeletal muscle
(b)   Cardiac muscle
(c)   Smooth muscle

(a)

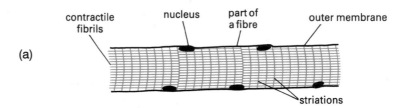

(b)

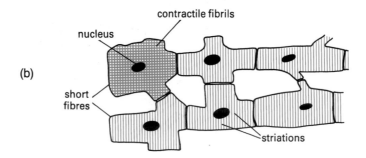

(c)

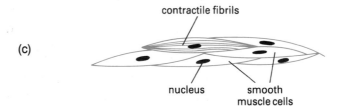

CARDIAC

Cardiac muscle is found only in the wall of the heart. The muscle fibres are striated, but short, and have a single nucleus. Cardiac muscle contracts automatically and rhythmically without any nervous stimulation, but its rate of contraction can be regulated by the autonomic nervous system and the hormone adrenalin. It does not tire readily, but works continuously throughout life.

SMOOTH

Smooth muscle is found in the walls of the food canal, blood vessels and urinary system. It consists of spindle-shaped cells which interlock. Each cell has one nucleus, contains contractile fibres, but is unstriated. Smooth muscle is regulated by the autonomic nervous system and adrenalin but exhibits rhythmic contraction in the absence of nervous stimulation. Smooth muscle is capable of slow but sustained contraction, and does not tire readily.

 Give two similarities and two differences between skeletal and smooth muscle.

Nerve supply

All muscle tissue must be well supplied with nerves in order to contract. In skeletal muscle, nerves bring the impulses which stimulate the muscle tissue to contract according to the all-or-none principle, where the muscle fibre either contracts fully or not at all.

Blood supply

Blood vessels bring glucose and oxygen to supply energy and the calcium ions necessary for normal contraction. They also remove waste products such as carbon dioxide and lactic acid (see chapter 8). Blood also brings adrenalin, which causes some muscle tissue to contract.

Adenosine triphosphate (ATP)

Muscle tissue contains molecules of ATP which store energy produced from food and release it to the tissue as it contracts.

Muscle tone

If all the skeletal muscles relaxed at once, the body would crumple. All the muscles must be slightly contracted for the body to remain upright. At any one time some of the muscle fibres in skeletal muscle tissue are contracted, while the rest are relaxed. This small amount of contraction will tense a muscle without causing movement. Different groups of fibres contract at different times to spread the work load. This continuous slight tension of the muscle tissue is involuntary and is known as muscle tone. It is essential for maintaining posture.

Effect of temperature

When muscle tissue is warmer, the process of contraction occurs faster due to the speeding up of the chemical reactions involved. However, muscle tone is reduced as the body temperature rises, so more of the skeletal muscle fibres are relaxed. Massage is more easily carried out when the muscle tissue is warm and relaxed. Heat cramps will occur in muscles which are active at high temperature. Increased sweating causes loss of salt, resulting in a lower concentration of sodium ions in the blood supplying the muscle. Cramp is a sudden involuntary contraction of the muscle which is painful.

As muscle tissue is cooled the chemical reactions slow, so the contraction takes longer to occur. There is an involuntary increase in muscle tone, eventually resulting in shivering. Hypothermia finally occurs, when the muscles become rigid and shivering stops as the reflex actions slow down. Once this stage is reached, the person is unable to move and survival is unlikely without external warming.

Muscle fatigue

When skeletal muscle is continuously stimulated, its contraction becomes progressively weaker and eventually ceases. This condition is muscle fatigue and is due both to the accumulation of the toxic waste products lactic acid and carbon dioxide, and the shortage of ATP (adenosine triphosphate, an energy-rich compound), glucose, and oxygen, which provide the energy for contraction. When all the skeletal muscles are fatigued, the muscles exert very little balancing effect, so the ligaments and tendons must support the body and may become strained.

Mechanism of muscle contraction

PROTEIN FILAMENTS

The longitudinal fibrils in skeletal muscle consist of two kinds of protein filaments, one type being thicker than the other. The thinner filaments are composed of actin and the thicker ones of myosin, and the two types of filaments are arranged in alternating bands, which gives the fibre its striated appearance. As contraction of the muscle fibre proceeds, the thinner actin filaments slide further and further in-between the myosin

Figure 5.3   *Relaxed and contracted muscle fibres*

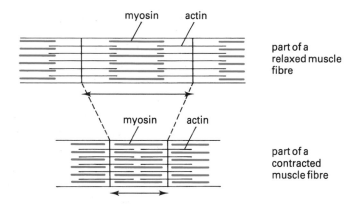

filaments. The energy for this sliding movement comes from ATP in the muscle fibre.

MOTOR POINT

A skeletal muscle fibre will only contract if a stimulus is applied to it by a motor nerve cell or neuron. A long fibre of the neuron called the axon carries the stimulus to the muscle fibre and transmits it at a neuro-muscular junction. Here the axon ends in fine knobbed branches resting on the muscle fibre membrane, which are known as motor end plates. A single motor neuron may transmit stimuli to one or two muscle fibres, or to as many as 150. The point at which a motor nerve enters a muscle is called the motor point.

MUSCLES

Structure

Within a muscle, the skeletal muscle fibres are arranged in bundles called fasiculi. Each bundle of fibres is surrounded by a sheath of connective tissue (perimysium). The entire muscle is surrounded by a layer of fibrous connective tissue (epimysium) which is an extension of the deep fascia. The deep fascia is a layer of dense, inelastic connective tissue lining the body wall and limbs, which holds the muscles together and divides them into functioning groups. It contains no fat (unlike the superficial fascia) but carries nerves and blood vessels. The fascia lata is the deep fascia of the thigh thickened laterally as the iliotibial tract.

The epimysium and perimysium continue into the tendons which attach the muscle to bones. Skeletal muscles are well supplied with nerves and blood vessels, and blood capillaries occur between the muscle fibres in each fasiculus.

Position

Some of the muscles are superficial, lying just below the skin and superficial fascia. Others lie beneath the superficial muscles and are said to be deep muscles.

Muscles of the head

The muscles of the head fall into two groups. One group comprises the muscles of mastication, used in chewing. The muscles of the other group are responsible for facial expression and may be attached to skin instead of bone. The wrinkling of the skin which occurs when they contract results in the various facial expressions.

Table 5.1   *Muscles of mastication*

Name	Position	Origin	Insertion	Action
Masseter	Lateral region of cheek between the cheek bone and angle of the jaw	Zygomatic arch	Mandible	Raises the lower jaw and clenches the teeth
Temporalis	On the side of the head, above and in front of the ear, to the lower jaw	Temporal bone	Mandible	Raises the lower jaw and retracts it if it is protruding
Lateral and medial ptergyoids	On the lateral region of the cheek beneath the masseter muscle	Sphenoid and maxilla	Mandible	Open the mouth and protrude the lower jaw. Move the jaw from side to side

All these muscles of mastication are supplied by the mandibular branch of the fifth (trigeminal) cranial nerve

Q | Which muscles move the mandible? Give the origin of each muscle and the name of the nerve which supplies them all.

Figure 5.4   *Muscles of mastication (side view)*

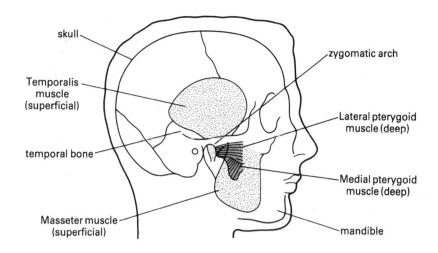

Table 5.2   *Muscles of facial expression*

Name	Position	Origin	Insertion	Nerve supply	Action
Occipitalis	Back of skull	Occipital	Epicranial aponeurosis	Auricular VII	Moves scalp backwards
Frontalis	Forehead	Epicranial aponeurosis	Skin above orbits	Temporal VII	Moves scalp forwards, raises eyebrows and wrinkles forehead; expresses fright
Corrugator	Below eyebrow	Orbit and inner edge of eyebrow ridge	Skin of eyebrow	Temporal VII	Forms vertical wrinkles between the eyebrows when frowning
Orbicularis oculi	Surrounding the eye	Rim of the orbit	Skin of the eyelid	Temporal and zygomatic VII	Closes the eyelids. Used in blinking and winking. Forms 'crows feet' folds from outer angle of the eyes
Nasalis	At the side of the nose	Maxilla	Nasal bone	Buccal VII	Compresses and dilates the nostril. Expresses anger

Table 5.2   *Muscles of facial expression*

Name	Position	Origin	Insertion	Nerve supply	Action
Procerus	At the top of the nose between the eyes	Nasal bone	Skin between the eyebrows	Buccal VII	Forms transverse wrinkles over the bridge of the nose. Also expresses distaste
Quadratus (Levator) labii	Radiates from the upper lip	Lower rim of orbit	Skin of upper lip and nose	Buccal VII	Raises the lip and flares the nostril; forms the nasolabial furrow, giving a sad expression
Orbicularis oris	Surrounding the mouth	Skin and other muscles round the mouth	Skin at the corners of the mouth	Buccal VII	Closes and puckers the lips; shapes the lips during speech
Buccinator	At the side of the face	Maxilla and mandible	Skin at the angle of the mouth and orbicularis oris	Buccal VII	Compresses the cheek; keeps food between the teeth when chewing; used in sucking and blowing
Zygomaticus, major and minor	Radiates from the upper lip	Zygomatic arch	Skin at the angle of the mouth and orbicularis oris	Buccal VII	Draws the angle of the mouth upwards when smiling and laughing
Risorius	Radiates laterally from the corner of the mouth	In fascia over the masseter muscle	Skin at the angle of the mouth	Buccal VII	Draws the mouth sideways and outwards in the 'grin of death'
Triangularis (depressor angulioris)	Radiates from the lower lip over the chin	Lower margin of the mandible	Skin at the angle of the mouth	Mandibular VII	Draws the angle of the mouth down, giving a sad expression
Depressor labii inferioris	Radiates from the lower lip over the chin	Base of mandible	Skin of the lower lip	Mandibular VII	Pulls down the lower lip, giving a sulky expression

Table 5.2   *Muscles of facial expression*

Name	Position	Origin	Insertion	Nerve supply	Action
Mentalis	Radiates from lower lip over centre of the chin	Mandible	Skin of chin and lower lip	Mandibular VII	Lifts and protrudes the lower lip and wrinkles the chin when expressing doubt
Platysma	Side of the neck and chin	Skin and fascia of pectoral and deltoid muscles	Skin of the lower face	Cervical VII	Depresses the mandible and draws the lip up when annoyed; loss of muscle tone causes crepey neck

Figure 5.5   *Muscles of facial expression (side view)*

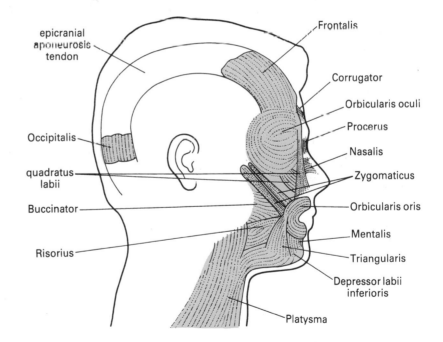

epicranial aponeurosis tendon

Frontalis

Corrugator

Orbicularis oculi

Procerus

Nasalis

Zygomaticus

Occipitalis

quadratus labii

Buccinator

Orbicularis oris

Mentalis

Triangularis

Risorius

Depressor labii inferioris

Platysma

Q   Which muscle is used in the following facial movements?
  (a) sucking
  (b) frowning
  (c) smiling
  (d) blinking

Muscles of the neck

The muscles of the neck are responsible for moving the head. The platysma muscle of facial expression rises obliquely from the side of the neck to below the centre of the chin and up onto the lower jaw. It is superficial to the muscles moving the head.

Table 5.3 *Muscles of the neck*

Name	Position	Origin	Insertion	Nerve supply	Action
Sternocleido-mastoid	Obliquely down the side of the neck from below the ear to the breastbone	Sternum clavicle	Mastoid region of the temporal bone	XI cranial	When both contract together, the chin is pulled down onto the chest; when only one contracts, the head turns to the opposite side
Trapezius	Down the back of the neck onto the shoulders	Occipital and seventh cervical, and all the thoracic vertebrae	Clavicle and scapula	XI cranial	Lifts the clavicle and rotates the scapula upwards; it extends the head (hyperextension)
Splenius capitis	Up the back of the neck beneath the trapezius to just behind the ear	Spines of seventh cervical and first four thoracic vertebrae	Occipital, and mastoid process of the temporal	Cervical spinal	When both contract together the neck is lengthened to hold the head upright; contraction of one muscle rotates the head to the same side

Figure 5.6 *Muscles of the neck (side view)*

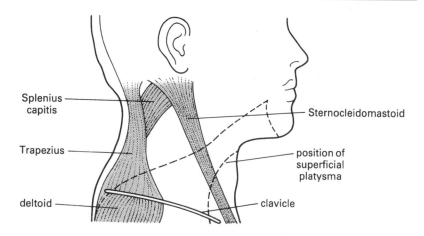

Muscles of the shoulder and chest

MOVING THE SCAPULA

Pectoralis minor

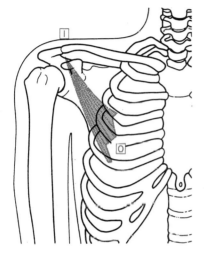

Position:
across front of upper part of
thorax beneath pectoralis
major
Origin:
third to fifth ribs
Insertion:
coracoid process of scapula
Nerve supply:
pectoral nerves of brachial
plexus
Action:
draws shoulder down and
forwards

Serratus anterior

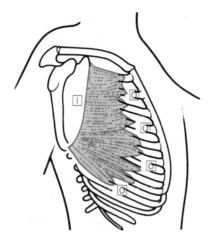

Position:
sides of ribcage below
armpits
Origin:
upper ribs
Insertion:
medial edge of scapula
Nerve supply:
cervical spinal nerves
Action:
draws scapula forwards and
rotates it upwards; used in
pushing movements

Levator scapulae

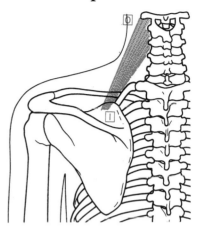

Position:
at back and sides of neck,
onto shoulder
Origin:
upper four cervical vertebrae
Insertion:
upper edge of scapula
Nerve supply:
cervical spinal nerves
Action:
lifts scapula and shoulder

Key: ☐ Origin
      ☐ Insertion

Rhomboids

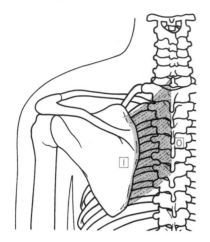

Position:
on back of thorax between
shoulders
Origin:
thoracic vertebrae
Insertion:
medial edge of scapula
Nerve supply:
cervical spinal nerves
Action:
abducts and braces shoulder,
and rotates scapula upwards

MOVING THE ARM

Pectoralis major

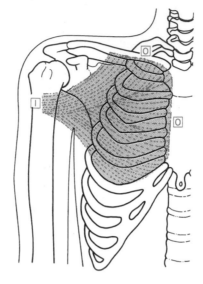

Position:
across front of upper part of
thorax, beneath breasts
Origin:
clavicle, sternum and rib
cartilages
Insertion:
shaft of humerus below its
head (greater tubercle)
Nerve supply:
pectoral nerves of brachial
plexus
Action:
flexes and adducts arm, and
rotates it inwards (throwing
action)

Coracobrachialis

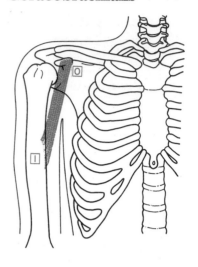

Position:
at the upper medial part of
arm, beneath deltoid
Origin:
coracoid process of scapula
Insertion:
middle of shaft of humerus
on medial side
Nerve supply:
from brachial plexus
(musculocutaneous branch)
Action:
flexes arm and adducts it,
drawing it forward and
towards mid-line of body

Latissimus dorsi

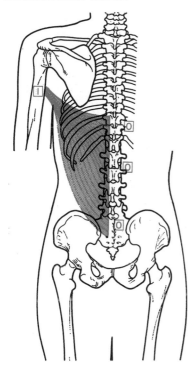

Teres major

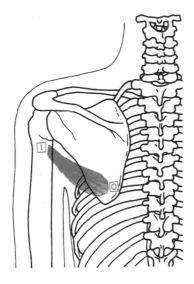

Deltoid

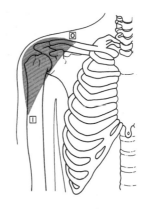

Position:
a large sheet of muscle down
back of lower thorax and
lumbar region
Origin:
lower thoracic vertebrae,
lumbar vertebrae, sacrum and
rim of pelvis
Insertion:
shaft of humerus below its
head
Nerve supply:
from brachial plexus
(thoracodorsal branch)
Action:
draws shoulder downwards
and backwards; adducts and
rotates arm; with both arms
fixed when climbing, helps
pull body upwards

Position:
across back of shoulders; a
deep muscle
Origin:
lateral edge of the scapula
Insertion:
shaft of humerus just below
lesser tubercle
Nerve supply:
lower subscapular nerves of
brachial plexus
Action:
extends, adducts and rotates
humerus inwards (medially)
in its socket, and assists in
drawing arm downwards

Position:
caps top of shoulder and
upper arm
Origin:
clavicle, scapula spine, and
acromion process
Insertion:
shaft of humerus on lateral
side, below its head
Nerve supply:
axillary nerves of brachial
plexus
Action:
abducts arm, and draws it
backwards and forwards

Supraspinatus

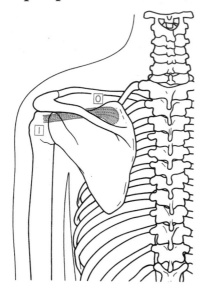

Position:
across back of shoulders; a deep muscle
Origin:
upper edge of the spine of scapula
Insertion:
greater tubercle of humerus
Nerve supply:
suprascapular nerve of brachial plexus
Action:
abducts humerus, assisting deltoid muscle

Infraspinatus

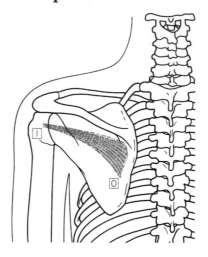

Position:
across back of shoulders; a deep muscle
Origin:
lower edge of spine of scapula
Insertion:
greater tubercle of humerus
Nerve supply:
suprascapular nerve of brachial plexus
Action:
rotates humerus outwards (laterally)

Teres minor

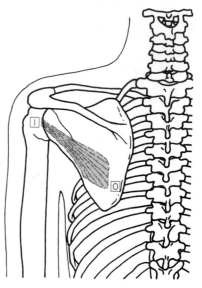

Position:
across back of shoulders; a deep muscle
Origin:
lateral edge of scapula
Insertion:
greater tubercle of humerus
Nerve supply:
axillary nerve of brachial plexus
Action:
rotates humerus outwards (laterally) in its socket

Q List the names of three muscles which lower the arms to the side.

Muscles of respiration

Diaphragm

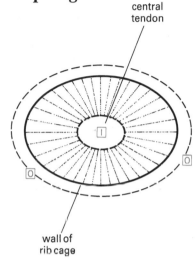

central tendon

wall of rib cage

Position:
separating thoracic and abdominal cavities
Origin:
xiphoid, cartilages of last six ribs and lumbar vertebrae
Insertion:
central tendon forming membranous part of diaphragm
Nerve supply:
phrenic nerves of cervical plexus
Action:
flattens diaphragm to increase thoracic cavity for inspiration

External intercostals

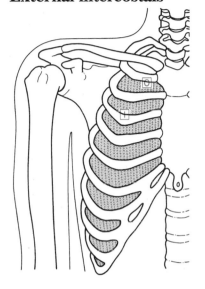

Position:
between ribs, running obliquely downwards
Origin:
lower edge of rib above
Insertion:
upper edge of rib immediately below
Nerve supply:
intercostal nerves
Action:
raise ribs to increase thoracic cavity for normal inspiration

Internal intercostals

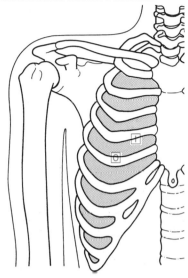

Position:
between ribs, beneath external intercostals
Origin:
upper edge of rib below
Insertion:
lower edge of rib immediately above
Nerve supply:
intercostal nerves
Action:
pull ribs down during forced expiration

Q List the muscles involved in breathing. What actions do they have when they contract?

Muscles of the abdominal wall

ANTERIOR

External oblique

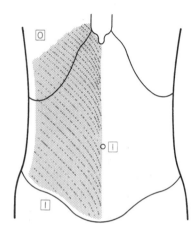

Position:
extends laterally down the front of the abdomen
Origin:
lower eight ribs
Insertion:
linea alba (tendon from xiphoid process to pubic symphysis) and iliac crest of pelvis
Nerve supply:
intercostal nerves (eight to twelfth) and upper nerves of lumbar plexus
Action:
both acting together compress abdomen; one acting alone twists trunk, turning front of abdomen towards opposite side

Internal oblique

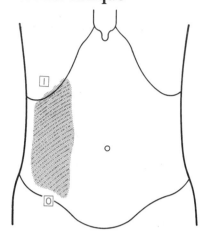

Position:
laterally on front of abdomen, deep to external oblique muscle, running diagonally in the opposite direction to it
Origin:
iliac crest of the pelvis
Insertion:
cartilages of the last four ribs
Nerve supply:
intercostal nerves (eighth to twelfth) and upper nerves of the lumbar plexus
Action:
both acting together compress abdomen; one acting alone twists trunk turning front of abdomen towards same side; works with external oblique muscle of opposite side

Rectus abdominis

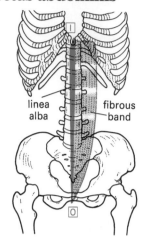

linea alba   fibrous band

Position:
extends whole length of front of abdomen and is divided into four sections by three fibrous bands
Origin:
pubic bone of pelvis
Insertion:
cartilages of fifth to seventh ribs and xiphoid
Nerve supply:
intercostal nerves (seventh to twelfth)
Action:
both acting together bend trunk forwards, flexing spine; one acting alone compresses abdomen, pushing internal organs towards spine to keep centre of gravity over arches of feet; this is therefore an important muscle in maintaining posture; draws front of pelvis upwards

Transversus abdominis

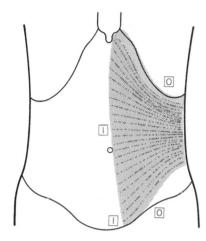

Position:
laterally on front of
abdomen, deep to internal
oblique muscle
Origin:
ilium of pelvis, lumbar fascia
and last six ribs
Insertion:
xiphoid, linea alba and pubis
of the pelvis
Nerve supply:
intercostal nerves (seventh to
twelfth) and upper nerves of
lumbar plexus
Action:
compresses abdomen

POSTERIOR

Quadratus lumborum

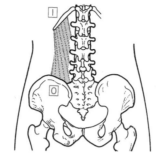

Position:
medially, on the lower part of
back
Origin:
iliac crest of pelvis
Insertion:
twelfth rib and upper four
lumbar vertebrae
Nerve supply:
last thoracic and first lumbar
nerves
Action:
flexes spine laterally

Erector spinae (three groups of muscles)

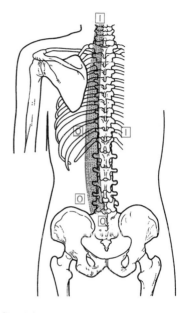

Position:
medially on posterior surface
of neck, thorax and abdomen
Origin:
iliac crest, lumbar vertebrae,
ribs and thoracic vertebrae
Insertion:
ribs, cervical and lumbar
vertebrae
Nerve supply:
cervical, thoracic and lumbar
nerves
Action:
extends spine; the main
postural muscle holds the
body upright

 List the muscles of the anterior abdominal wall and describe their positions in relation to one another.

Psoas (part of iliopsoas)

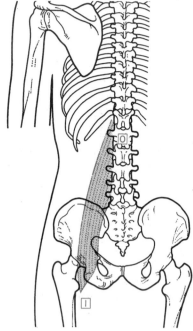

Position:
in lumbar region from spine to rim of pelvis and across hip joint
Origin:
transverse processes of lumbar vertebrae
Insertion:
lesser trochanter of femur
Nerve supply:
second and third lumbar nerves
Action:
flexes and rotates thigh laterally and flexes spine when rising from a lying to a sitting position

Iliacus (part of iliopsoas)

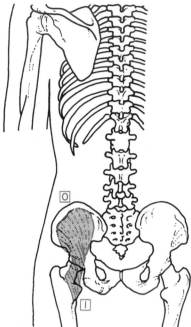

Position:
laterally, inside the pelvis and across the hip joint
Origin:
iliac bone of pelvis
Insertion:
lesser trochanter of femur, with tendon of the psoas
Nerve supply:
femoral nerve of lumbar plexus
Action:
flexes and rotates thigh laterally; acts as a postural muscle, helping to keep body erect at hip joint

Muscles of the buttocks

Gluteus maximus

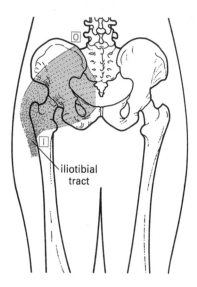

iliotibial tract

Position:
lower part of back, forming buttocks
Origin:
ilium of pelvis, sacrum and coccyx
Insertion:
posterior surface of shaft of femur iliotibial tract
Nerve supply:
gluteal nerve of sacral plexus
Action:
extends and rotates thigh laterally; used in running and jumping, and raises body after stooping; through the iliotibial tract it steadies the femur on the tibia during standing

Gluteus medius

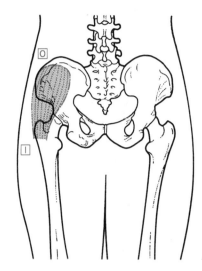

Position:
lateral area of the buttocks,
posterior part covered by
gluteus maximus
Origin:
ilium of pelvis
Insertion:
greater trochanter of femur
Nerve supply:
gluteal nerve of sacral plexus
Action:
abducts and rotates thigh
medially; used in walking and
running; maintains the
balance when standing on
one leg

Gluteus minimus

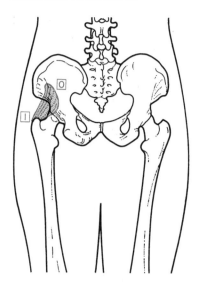

Position:
immediately deep to gluteus
medius, on lateral area of the
buttocks
Origin:
ilium of pelvis
Insertion:
greater trochanter of femur
Nerve supply:
gluteal nerve of sacral plexus
Action:
abducts and rotates thigh
laterally; used in walking and
running; maintains the
balance when standing on
one leg

Muscles of the pelvic floor

The muscles of the pelvic
floor, together with their
fasciae, are known as the
pelvic diaphragm. They
support the organs in the
pelvic cavity, including the
bladder. Damage to these
muscles during childbirth can
result in prolapse of the uterus
or stress incontinence. The
muscles can also be damaged
by inappropriate exercise.

Levator ani

Position:
forms funnel-shaped floor of
pelvic cavity; contains
openings through which the
anal canal, urethra and
vagina pass
Action:
supports and slightly raises
the floor of the pelvis,
resisting any downward
pressure in the abdomen;
constricts lower end of vagina
and rectum

Coccygeus

Position:
behind levator ani muscle
Action:
supports and slightly raises
floor of pelvis, resisting any
downward pressure in
abdomen; pulls coccyx
forward after it has been
pushed back during
defaecation or childbirth

Muscles moving the forearm

Biceps brachii

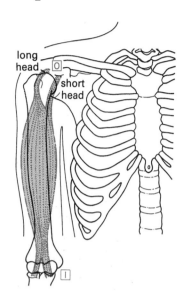

Position:
down anterior surface of the humerus; has two heads
Origin:
on scapula: long head – above glenoid cavity; short head – on coracoid process
Insertion:
on radius, just below elbow
Nerve supply:
from brachial plexus (musculocutaneous nerve)
Action:
flexes and supinates (turns palm upwards) forearm

Brachialis

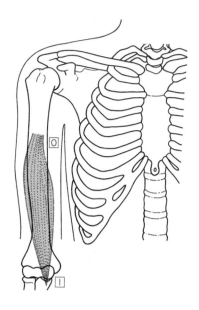

Position:
anterior surface of lower part of humerus, deep to biceps and across elbow joint
Origin:
halfway down shaft on the anterior surface of humerus
Insertion:
coronoid process of ulna
Nerve supply:
from brachial plexus (musculocutaneous and radial nerves)
Action:
flexes the forearm

Brachioradialis

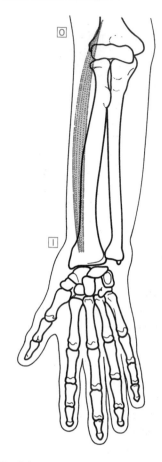

Position:
on radial (thumb) side of forearm
Origin:
shaft of humerus above lateral condyle
Insertion:
distal end of radius above styloid process
Nerve supply:
from brachial plexus (radial nerve)
Action:
flexes forearm

Triceps brachii

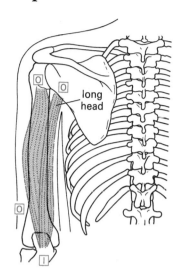

Position:
posterior surface of humerus;
has three heads
Origin:
long head on scapula; other
two heads on humerus
Insertion:
olecranon process of the ulna
Nerve supply:
from brachial plexus (radial
nerve)
Action:
extends the forearm

Pronator teres

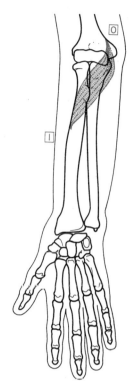

Position:
on anterior side of forearm
across elbow joint
Origin:
distal end of humerus and
coronoid process of ulna
Insertion:
lateral surface of radius
Nerve supply:
from brachial plexus (median
nerve)
Action:
pronates (turns palm
downwards) forearm, and
flexes it at the elbow

Supinator

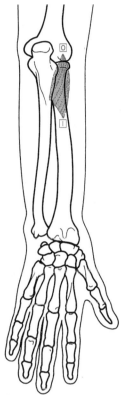

Position:
surrounds upper part of
radius
Origin:
lateral epicondyle of humerus
and ridge on ulna
Insertion:
lateral surface of radius
Nerve supply:
from brachial plexus (radial
nerve)
Action:
supinates the forearm

Muscles moving the wrist and fingers

ANTERIOR

Pronator quadratus

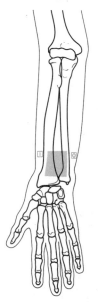

Position:
crosses lower part of front of forearm
Origin:
lower part of ulna just above wrist
Insertion:
lower part of radius just above wrist
Nerve supply:
from brachial plexus (median nerve)
Action:
pronates forearm and prevents separation of lower ends of radius and ulna when falling on wrist

Palmaris longus

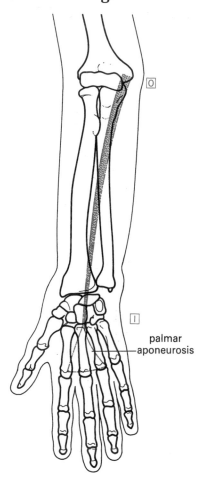

palmar aponeurosis

Position:
down anterior medial side of forearm
Origin:
medial epicondyle of humerus
Insertion:
palmar aponeurosis in palm of hand
Nerve supply:
from brachial plexus (median nerve)
Action:
flexes wrist

Flexor carpi radialis

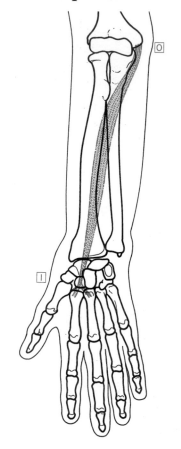

Position:
down anterior side of forearm from inside elbow joint towards thumb
Origin:
medial epicondyle of humerus
Insertion:
second and third metacarpals
Nerve supply:
from brachial plexus (median nerve)
Action:
flexes and abducts wrist (moving hand away from the body)

Flexor carpi ulnaris

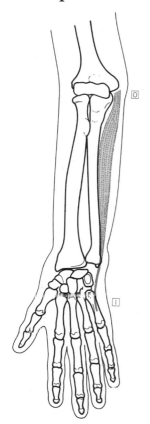

Position:
along ulnar (little finger) side
of forearm
Origin:
medial epicondyle of
humerus
Insertion:
fifth metacarpal and pisiform
and hamate carpals
Nerve supply:
from brachial plexus (ulnar
nerve)
Action:
flexes and adducts wrist
(moving the hand in towards
body)

Flexor digitorum sublimis (superficialis)

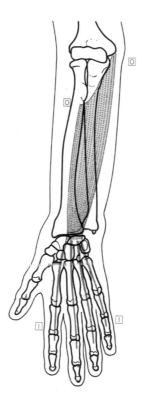

Position:
down medial side of forearm,
deep to palmaris longus
Origin:
medial epicondyle of the
humerus, coronoid process of
ulna, and shaft of the radius
Insertion:
the middle phalanx of each
finger
Nerve supply:
from brachial plexus (median
nerve)
Action:
flexes middle phalanx of each
finger

Flexor digitorum profundus

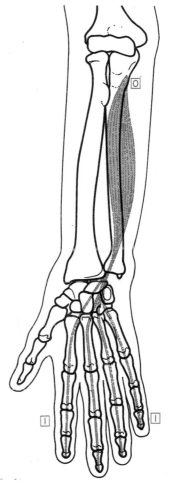

along ulnar side of forearm; a
deep muscle
Origin:
upper part of ulna
Insertion:
bases of distal phalanges
Nerve supply:
from brachial plexus (median
and ulnar nerves)
Action:
flexes distal phalanx of each
finger

POSTERIOR

Extensor carpi radialis longus

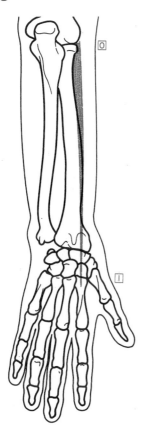

Extensor carpi radialis brevis

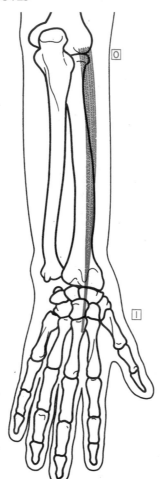

Extensor carpi ulnaris

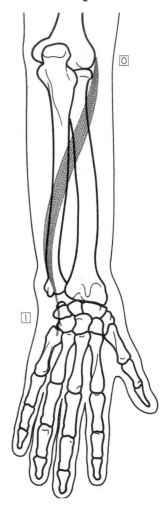

Position:
along radial (thumb) side of forearm
Origin:
lateral epicondyle of humerus
Insertion:
second metacarpal
Nerve supply:
from brachial plexus (radial nerve)
Action:
extends and abducts wrist

Position:
along radial side of forearm; a deep muscle
Origin:
lateral epicondyle of humerus
Insertion:
base of third metacarpal
Nerve supply:
from brachial plexus (radial nerve)
Action:
extends and abducts wrist

Position:
along back of forearm on ulnar side
Origin:
lateral epicondyle of humerus
Insertion:
fifth metacarpal
Nerve supply:
from brachial plexus (radial nerve)
Action:
extends and adducts wrist

Extensor digitorum

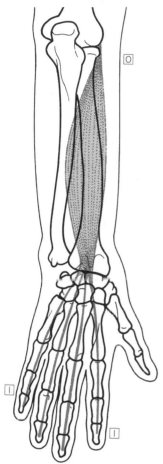

Muscles of the thigh

ACTING AT THE HIP JOINT
ONLY

Adductors brevis, longus and magnus

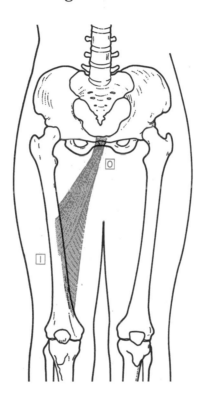

Pectineus

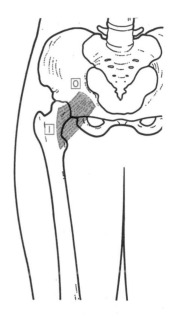

Extensor digitorum

Position:
along back of forearm on
radial side
Origin:
lateral epicondyle of humerus
Insertion:
middle and distal phalanges
of each finger
Nerve supply:
from brachial plexus (radial
nerve)
Action:
extends fingers

Adductors brevis, longus and magnus

Position:
on medial side of thigh;
longus is the most superficial
Origin:
pubis of pelvis
Insertion:
shaft of femur
Nerve supply:
from lumbar plexus
(obturator nerve)
Action:
adduct, rotate and flex thigh
at hip

Pectineus

Position:
crosses front of thigh at top,
from the medial to lateral
side
Origin:
front of pubis
Insertion:
lesser trochanter of femur
Nerve supply:
femoral nerve of lumbar
plexus
Action:
flexes, adducts, and rotates
thigh laterally

Piriformis

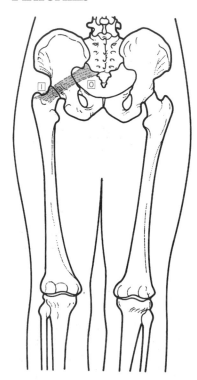

Obturator internus

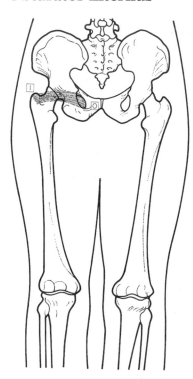

Tensor fasciae latae

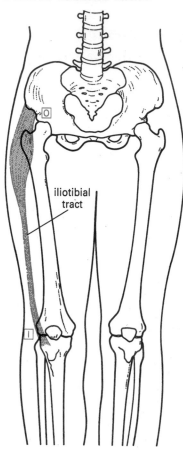

iliotibial tract

Piriformis

Position:
crossing top of thigh below buttocks; a deep muscle
Origin:
sacrum
Insertion:
greater trochanter of the femur
Nerve supply:
from the sacral plexus (1 and 2 sacral nerves)
Action:
rotates the thigh laterally and abducts it. It is a postural muscle controlling the position of the neck of the femur

Obturator internus

Position:
crosses top of thigh below buttocks; occurs partly within pelvis and partly at back of hip joint
Origin:
margin of obturator foramen of pelvis
Insertion:
greater trochanter of femur
Nerve supply:
from sacral plexus (obturator nerve)
Action:
rotates thigh laterally and abducts it; a postural muscle assisting piriformis and other lateral rotators

Tensor fasciae latae

Position:
along lateral side of thigh
Origin:
iliac crest of pelvis
Insertion:
tibia, by iliotibial tract
Nerve supply:
from sacral plexus (gluteal nerve)
Action:
flexes and abducts thigh

ACTING AT BOTH HIP AND
KNEE
Biceps femoris
(one of the hamstrings)

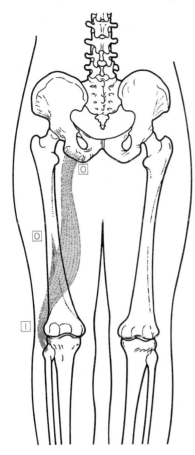

Position:
down back of thigh
Origin:
femur and ischium of pelvis
Insertion:
head of fibula and lateral
condyle of tibia
Nerve supply:
sciatic nerve of sacral plexus
Action:
extend thigh and flex leg at
knee

Semitendinosus and
semimembranosus
(hamstrings)

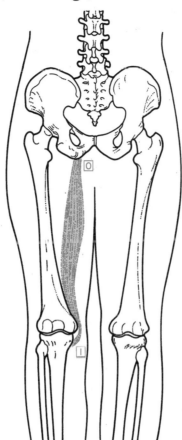

Position:
down posterior medial side of
thigh
Origin:
ischium of pelvis
Insertion:
tibia
Nerve supply:
sciatic nerve of sacral plexus
Action:
extends thigh, flexes leg at
knee

Sartorius

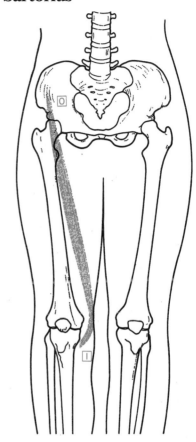

Position:
crosses front of thigh from
lateral to medial side
Origin:
ilium of pelvis
Insertion:
medial side of tibia
Nerve supply:
femoral nerve of lumbar
plexus
Action:
flexes hip and knee as when
sitting cross-legged

Gracilis

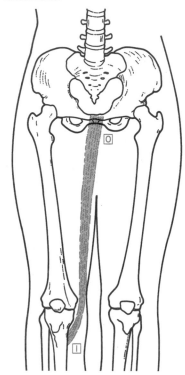

Position:
down medial side of thigh
Origin:
pubis of pelvis
Insertion:
medial side of tibia
Nerve supply:
from lumbar plexus
(obturator nerve)
Action:
adducts thigh and flexes leg
at knee

Rectus femoris (part of the quadriceps femoris)

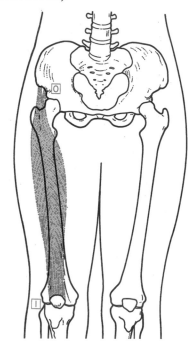

Position:
down front of thigh
Origin:
ilium of pelvis
Insertion:
upper border of patella, and
head of tibia via patellar
ligament
Nerve supply:
femoral nerve of lumbar
plexus
Action:
flexes thigh and extends leg
at knee

ACTING AT THE KNEE ONLY
Vastus (part of the quadriceps femoris)

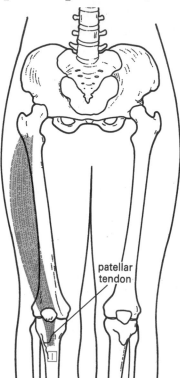

patellar
tendon

Position:
    down front of thigh
Origin:
femur
Insertion:
patella, and tibia via patellar
tendon
Nerve supply:
femoral nerve of lumbar
plexus
Action:
extends leg at knee

 List the muscles which cause movement at both the hip and knee joints. For each muscle, name the type of movement they perform at each joint.

Muscles moving the foot and toes

ANTERIOR

Tibialis anterior

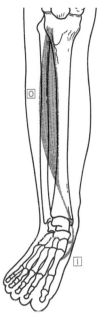

Position:
down shin, on lateral side of tibia

Origin:
lateral condyle and upper half of shaft of tibia

Insertion:
first cuneiform tarsal and first metatarsal

Nerve supply:
from sciatic nerve (deep peroneal branch)

Action:
dorsiflexes (bends ankle to pull foot up) and inverts foot (soles facing one another)

Peroneus tertius

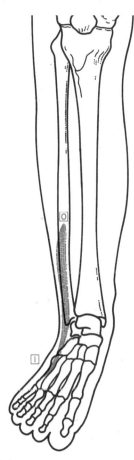

Position:
lower lateral part of shin

Origin:
lower part of shaft of fibula

Insertion:
fifth metatarsal

Nerve supply:
from sciatic nerve (deep peroneal branch)

Action:
dorsiflexes and everts (soles facing outwards) foot

Extensor digitorum longus

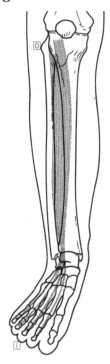

Position:
lateral part of shin

Origin:
lateral condyle of tibia and shaft of fibula

Insertion:
middle and distal phalanges of four outer toes

Nerve supply:
from sciatic nerve (deep peroneal branch)

Action:
dorsiflexes and everts foot and extends toes

 Q List the muscles which bend the ankle to pull the foot upwards towards the tibia.

Extensor hallucis longus

Gastrocnemius

Soleus

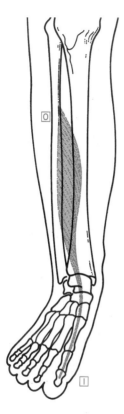

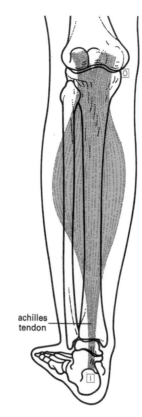

achilles
tendon

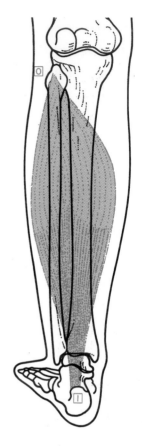

Position:
down shin, partly beneath
tibialis muscle
Origin:
middle region of shaft of
fibula
Insertion:
base of distal phalanx of big
toe
Nerve supply:
from sciatic nerve (deep
peroneal branch)
Action:
extends big toe

Position:
at back of lower leg, forming
calf
Origin:
lateral and medial condyles of
femur
Insertion:
calcaneum, via Achilles
tendon
Nerve supply:
from sciatic nerve (tibial
branch)
Action:
plantar flexes foot (pointing
the toes) and propels the
body in walking and running

Position:
at back of lower leg, deep to
gastrocnemius
Origin:
head of fibula and upper part
of tibia shaft
Insertion:
calcaneum, via Achilles
tendon
Nerve supply:
from sciatic nerve (tibial
branch)
Action:
plantar flexes foot; has
postural function, steadying
leg

Plantaris

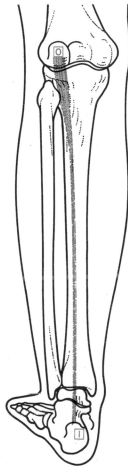

Position:
down back of lower leg, beneath gastrocnemius
Origin:
above lateral condyle of femur
Insertion:
calcaneum
Nerve supply:
from sciatic nerve (tibial branch)
Action:
plantar flexes foot

Tibialis posterior

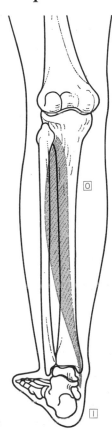

Position:
deepest muscle on back of lower leg
Origin:
shafts of tibia and fibula
Insertion:
second, third and fourth metatarsals, navicular, third cuneiform and cuboid tarsals
Nerve supply:
from sciatic nerve (tibial branch)
Action:
plantar flexes and inverts foot; supports inner medial longitudinal arch of foot

Peroneus longus

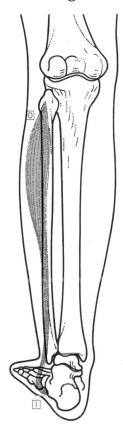

Position:
down outside of upper part of back of lower leg
Origin:
head and upper shaft of fibula
Insertion:
first metatarsal and first cuneiform tarsal on sole of foot
Nerve supply:
from sciatic nerve (superficial peroneal branch)
Action:
plantar flexes and everts foot; supports transverse and outer longitudinal arches of foot

Peroneus brevis

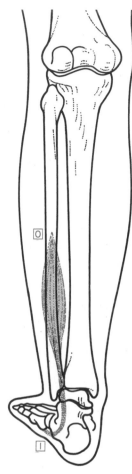

Position:
down outside of lower part of
back of lower leg
Origin:
lower part of shaft of fibula
Insertion:
fifth metatarsal
Nerve supply:
from sciatic nerve (superficial
peroneal branch)
Action:
plantar flexes and everts foot;
supports longitudinal arches
of the foot

Flexor digitorum longus

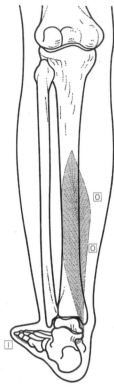

Position:
on inside of back of lower leg
Origin:
shaft of tibia
Insertion:
distal phalanges of four outer
toes
Nerve supply:
from sciatic nerve (tibial
branch)
Action:
plantar flexes and inverts
foot; flexes the toes; supports
inner longitudinal arch of
foot

Flexor hallucis longus

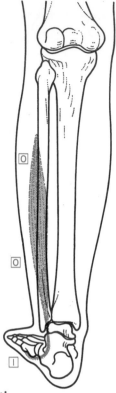

Position:
on outer side of back of lower
leg
Origin:
shaft of lower part of fibula
Insertion:
on underside of distal
phalanx of big toe
Nerve supply:
from sciatic nerve (tibial
branch)
Action:
plantar flexes and inverts
foot; flexes the big toe;
supports inner longitudinal
arch of foot

 List the muscles which support the arches of the foot. In each
case, name the arch(es) they support.

Muscles and tendons of the hand

TENDONS

The flexor and extensor muscles which bend and straighten the
fingers occur in the forearm and not in the hand. The long
tendons from these muscles pass to the ends of the fingers. The
tendons are surrounded by protective synovial sheaths and are
held in place by fibrous bands or fasciae, called the transverse
and dorsal carpal ligaments. The palmar aponeurosis is a flat
wide tendon into which the tendon of the Palmaris longus
muscle is inserted. The palmar aponeurosis is triangular in shape
and occupies the middle of the palm.

MUSCLES

The hand contains only very small muscles. The flexor of the
thumb and the adductor and abductor muscles moving the
thumb and fingers occur in the hand. The thenar eminence

Figure 5.7   *Front of hand (palmar surface)*

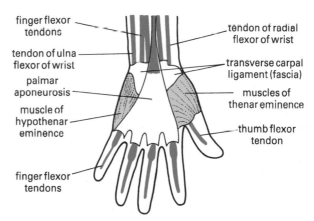

Figure 5.8   *Back of hand*

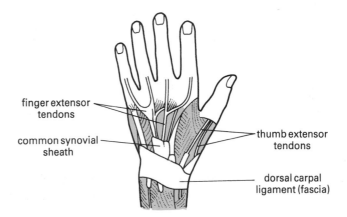

consists of the muscles moving the thumb while the hypothenar eminence on the medial side consists of the muscles moving the little finger. The adductor muscles of the eminences enable the hand to grip objects. Although these muscles are small, they have a very rich nerve supply allowing very fine control. This allows the variety of grips needed to handle both small and large objects. They are supplied by the median nerve.

Muscles and tendons of the foot

TENDONS

The tendons from the flexor and extensor muscles in the leg cross the ankle into the foot. Each toe has an extensor tendon on its upper surface (dorsum) and a flexor tendon on the under (plantar) surface.

LIGAMENTS

The tendons from the leg muscles are held in place at the ankle by transverse crural and cruciate crural ligaments.

The spring ligament connects the calcaneum to the navicular tarsal. It resists the flattening of the inner longitudinal arch of the foot. The long plantar ligament connects the calcaneum to the metatarsals and resists the flattening of the outer longitudinal arch. These ligaments take the strain during walking.

Figure 5.9   *Foot (dorsum)*

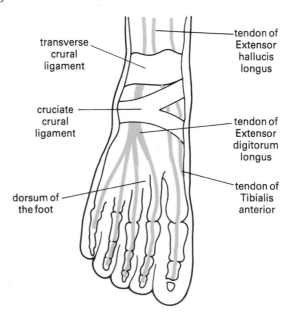

transverse crural ligament

cruciate crural ligament

dorsum of the foot

tendon of Extensor hallucis longus

tendon of Extensor digitorum longus

tendon of Tibialis anterior

MUSCLES

There is an extensor muscle to the four larger toes on the dorsum of the foot, which has its origin on the upper surface of the calcaneum. The plantar muscles make up the fleshy part of the sole of the foot and are the flexors, adductors and abductors of the toes. Clawed toe results from loss of control of the flexors and extensors of the foot. Deep peroneal and plantar nerves supply the foot muscles.

Figure 5.10   *Foot (plantar surface)*

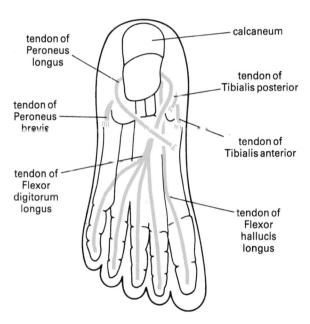

calcaneum

tendon of
Peroneus
longus

tendon of
Tibialis posterior

tendon of
Peroneus
brevis

tendon of
Tibialis anterior

tendon of
Flexor
digitorum
longus

tendon of
Flexor
hallucis
longus

EFFECTS OF EXERCISE ON MUSCLES

Circulation

Exercising muscles stimulates blood and lymph flow, as it generates heat which dilates blood capillaries and causes movements which push the fluid along veins and lymph vessels. This improved circulation removes toxic waste products and supplies nutrients more rapidly, allowing the muscle to function more effectively.

ATP

Exercising a muscle increases the number of mitochondria in the muscle fibres. Mitochondria are the cell organelles which produce ATP, the immediate source of energy for contracting muscle fibres.

Strength

Muscle which is not regularly exercised will atrophy (waste away). Exercise increases the strength of muscles and the flexibility of joints. It improves posture and can help to prevent low back pain. Excessive or unsuitable exercising causes muscle fatigue and minor injury to muscles, tendons and ligaments.

EFFECTS OF MASSAGE ON MUSCLES

Circulation

Massage produces frictional heat which warms the skin and dilates the blood capillaries. This speeds up the circulation of blood and supplies nutrients to the muscle more rapidly. During massage the stroking movements towards the heart assist the return of venous blood and lymph to the heart. Toxic waste products in the muscle tissue are therefore removed more rapidly, so massage reduces muscle fatigue.

Relaxation

Massage will increase muscle relaxation, releasing tension which may be straining ligaments or tendons. Massage does not cause muscular contractions so it does not strengthen muscle.

Contra-indications to massage

The presence of inflammation in a muscle or in the skin covering it, highly vascular skin conditions, or a hypersensitive skin prone to allergic reactions, all contra-indicate massage treatment. Painful joints, where there could be structural damage to a tendon or ligament, should not be massaged.

 Describe the good effects of exercise on muscles which massage is unable to produce.

CHAPTER 6

The Nervous System

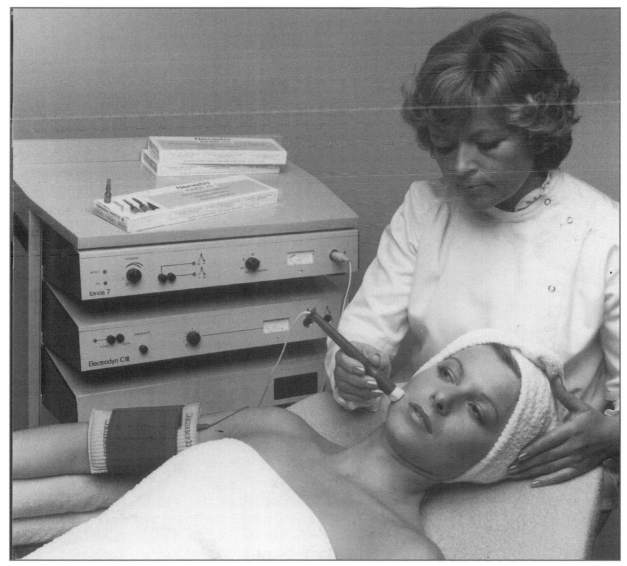

Galvanic iontophoresis

FUNCTIONS OF THE NERVOUS SYSTEM

The nervous system provides the most rapid means of communication between the various parts of the body. It stimulates muscular movements and co-ordinates all the body's activities. Co-ordination requires feedback, so that the level of response is related to the strength and direction of the stimulus.

The nervous system combines with the endocrine system to maintain homeostasis – keeping the body in a steady state. It senses changes outside and inside the body by means of its sense organs, interprets the changes in the central nervous system, then initiates actions to maintain homeostasis.

SUMMARY

The nervous system co-ordinates the body's activities and acts with the endocrine system to maintain homeostasis.

Nervous tissue

Nervous tissue is composed of two types of cells, neurons and neuroglia. The neurons are the structural and functional units conducting the nerve impulse. Neurons are unable to undergo cell division and reproduce themselves. When destroyed they cannot be replaced, although some damaged neurons can be repaired. The neuroglia has a supporting and protective function.

NEURON STRUCTURE

Each neuron consists of a cell body from which impulse-conducting processes extend. The cell body has a central nucleus and granular cytoplasm containing mitochondria and a Golgi body. The rough endoplasmic reticulum and ribosomes form characteristic Nissl granules in neurons. The cytoplasm also contains thin fibres called neurofibrils.

The slender processes extending from the neuron cell body are of two types, dendrons and axons. Dendrons have short branches called dendrites and conduct impulses inwards towards the cell body. One or many dendrons may be present in a single neuron. An axon is a longer process, branching at the end, which conducts impulses outwards away from the cell body. Each neuron has a single axon composed of axoplasm.

MYELIN SHEATH

The axon may be surrounded by a fatty non-conducting sheath of myelin, secreted by Schwann cells of the neuroglia. Such axons are said to be myelinated. The myelin sheath insulates the axon to prevent loss of the electrical impulse and increases the speed at which the impulse is conducted. At intervals there are gaps in the myelin sheath called nodes of Ranvier. On the outside of the myelin sheath is a membrane called the neurilemma.

 Explain the function of:
(a) the myelin sheath
(b) neuroglia
(c) dendrons

NERVE FIBRE

An axon and its sheaths is known as a nerve fibre. The axons from a large number of neurons are arranged in bundles and covered with connective tissue sheaths, forming nerves.

TYPES OF NEURON

There are three types of neurons: sensory, motor and interneurons.

• Sensory neurons carry impulses from sensory receptors to the brain and spinal cord. They usually have one process from the cell body which divides into an axon and a dendron, and are said to be unipolar.

• Motor neurons carry impulses from the brain and spinal cord to effectors (muscles and glands). They have several branched dendrons and a single axon, and are said to be multipolar.

• Interneurons (association or connector neurons) carry impulses from sensory neurons to motor neurons and occur only in the brain and spinal cord. They are multipolar, often with a short axon (stellate).

Figure 6.1   *Types of neurons*
(a)   *Motor neuron (multipolar)*
(b)   *Sensory neuron (unipolar)*
(c)   *Interneuron (stellate)*

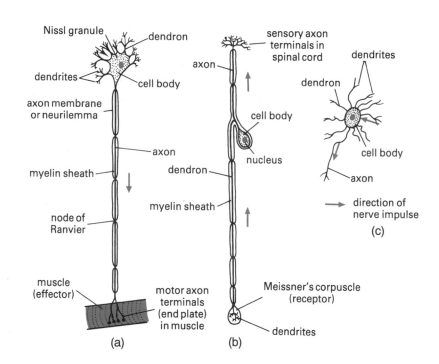

SUMMARY

Nervous tissue is composed of neurons which are cells conducting nerve impulses. Neurons are of several types and their axons may be surrounded by a myelin sheath.

 List eight structural components of a multipolar motor neuron.

The nerve impulse

A nerve impulse is electrical in nature, and is produced when a neuron is stimulated.

RESTING POTENTIAL

When a neuron is not conducting an impulse, the inside of the cell membrane is negatively charged, while the outside of the cell membrane is positively charged. Thus there is a potential difference between the two sides of the cell membrane, which is said to be polarised. The non-conducting condition of a neuron is known as resting potential.

ROLE OF IONS

The electrical charges are due to the proportions of negatively and positively charged ions inside and outside the neuron. The ions are derived from two salts, sodium chloride and potassium chloride, which split up, or ionise, in solution to form positive sodium (Na^+) and potassium (K^+) ions, and negative chloride (Cl^-) ions. There are also many negatively charged protein ions inside the neuron. The potassium ions are mostly inside the neuron, while the sodium ions are mostly outside.

Figure 6.2   *Resting potential in an axon*

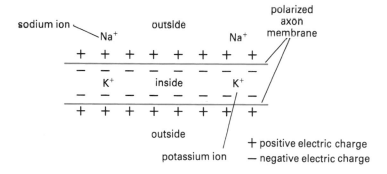

ACTION POTENTIAL

If a stimulus of sufficient strength is applied to a neuron, an impulse passes through it along the axon. As the impulse passes, the charges on the membrane at that point are momentarily reversed, so the membrane depolarises. The outside of the cell membrane becomes negatively charged and the inside becomes positively charged. This reversal is due to the movements of sodium and potassium ions through the cell membrane. The conducting condition of the neuron is known as action potential.

Figure 6.3 *Action potential in
an axon*

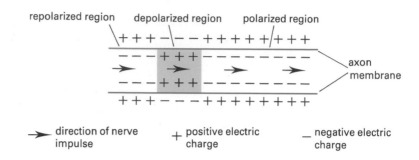

REFRACTORY PERIOD

After the impulse has passed, the membrane becomes polarised
again. The time taken for the membrane to repolarise is the
refractory period of the neuron and is about 3 milliseconds. The
neuron is unable to transmit another impulse until the end of
the refractory period.

PROPERTIES

The speed of transmission of a nerve impulse is greater in axons
with a larger diameter and where they are myelinated. The
response of a neuron to a stimulus follows the all-or-none law.
Below a particular strength of stimulus or threshold, no action
potential is generated. Above the threshold there is a full-sized
action potential. If a series of below-threshold stimuli are applied
to a neuron in quick succession, an impulse may be generated by
their cumulative effect. This property is known as summation.

SUMMARY

The nerve impulse is electrical in nature and is caused by movement
of ions through the axon membrane.

Synapses

The junction between two neurons is called a synapse. It occurs
where the end of the axon of one neuron lies close to a dendrite
of the other neuron, leaving a narrow gap, the synaptic cleft,
between the two. This gap has to be crossed for the impulse to
pass from one neuron to the other.

CHEMICAL TRANSMITTERS

Electrical impulses are unable to cross the gap and must be converted into chemical transmitters. The end of the axon bears a synaptic knob, containing mitochondria to provide energy and many vesicles containing the chemical transmitter substance, usually acetylcholine. The synaptic knob ends in a presynaptic membrane, bounding the synaptic cleft. On the opposite side of the cleft is the postsynaptic membrane of the dendrite of the next neuron.

Figure 6.4   *Conduction of nerve impulse across synapse*

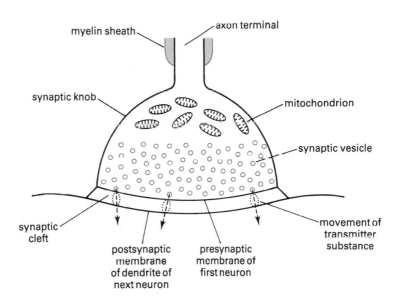

The arrival of an electrical impulse at the synaptic knob causes the release of transmitter substance from vesicles which become attached to the presynaptic membrane. The transmitter substance crosses the synaptic cleft and becomes attached to receptor sites on the postsynaptic membrane and depolarises it. Thus an action potential is generated and an electrical impulse passes through the neuron to the next synapse. Synapses cause nerve impulses to pass in one direction only through the neuron.

MOTOR END PLATE

A special kind of synapse occurs at a nerve-muscle junction known as a motor end plate (see figure 6.1a).

SUMMARY

A synapse is a junction between two neurons, across which a chemical impulse passes in one direction only.

 Q | What is the function of a synapse?

The reflex arc

REFLEX ACTIONS

The simplest type of nervous activity is a reflex action. This is an automatic rapid response to a particular stimulus, with no conscious involvement of the brain. Examples of reflex actions are the knee jerk when the patellar ligament is tapped, and the contraction of the pupil in response to a bright light shining on the eye. Coughing, sneezing, and the secretion of saliva are also reflex actions.

REFLEX PATHWAY

The conduction pathway of the impulse causing a reflex action is called a reflex arc, and one simple type involves just three neurons. A sensory receptor picks up a stimulus and triggers an

Figure 6.5   *Patellar reflex (knee jerk)*

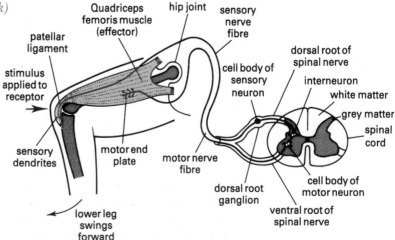

impulse in a sensory neuron. The impulse crosses the synapse to an interneuron in the spinal cord. A second synapse passes the impulse to a motor neuron whose motor end plate synapse passes on the impulse which makes the muscle contract. There are thus five parts to a simple reflex arc: a receptor, three conducting neurons, and an effector (the muscle). Where the interneuron is in the spinal cord, a spinal reflex occurs, e.g. the patellar reflex.

 Give examples of reflex actions associated with:
(a) the eye
(b) the digestive system
(c) the nose

VOLUNTARY ACTIONS

Voluntary actions are more complicated than the involuntary reflex actions, as the control centres of the brain modify the response. From the spinal cord the sensory impulse passes up to the brain, which may inhibit the immediate reflex response in the light of stored memory and intelligence. A motor response then passes down the spinal cord and appropriate muscles are stimulated to produce a conscious, reasoned reaction to the original stimulus.

SUMMARY

Reflexes are the body's main method of maintaining homeostasis, as they give a rapid countering response to changes in the internal and external environment.

THE SENSORY SYSTEM

The ability to sense stimuli is vital for an individual's survival. Sensation is a state of awareness of the external and internal environment of an individual. Perception is the conscious knowledge of a sensory stimulus.

Stimuli

Stimuli are picked up by receptors and converted into nerve impulses. Stimuli may be light rays, sound waves, temperature changes, touch, pressure or chemical substances. All sense receptors contain the dendrites of sensory neurons and respond to a stimulus of relatively low intensity. Receptors may be single cells, as in the skin, or part of a complex sense organ like the eye.

Perception

Many sensory nerve impulses pass to the brain to produce a conscious sensation. Some sensory impulses that end in the spinal cord can initiate muscle contractions, but do not produce conscious sensations. Conscious sensations undergo projection – although they are perceived by the brain, they appear to come from the point of stimulation. Thus, one appears to feel heat on the area of skin warmed by an infra-red lamp, but the feeling of warmth is actually in the brain.

The perception of a sensation may disappear if the stimulus is prolonged. On entering a bath of hot water the skin feels as if it is burning, but this sensation quickly decreases. This is known as adaptation and is due to synapse fatigue. The sensation of wearing clothes and jewellery is also quickly lost as a result of adaptation.

Types of receptor

Receptors may be classified according to their position in the body.

- Exteroceptors occur near the body surface and detect changes in the external environment.

- Visceroceptors occur in blood vessels, the food canal and other internal organs (viscera). Sensations from these receptors are felt as pain, pressure, hunger, thirst and nausea.

- Proprioceptors occur in muscles, joints, tendons, ligaments and the internal ear (organ of balance). They give information about the state of muscular contraction, the position of bones and tension of the joints, so defining body position and movements. This is known as the kinesthetic sense.

Where in the body would you expect to find the following?
(a) a motor end plate
(b) a myelin sheath
(c) transmitter substance
(d) a proprioceptor

General senses

General senses involve a simple receptor and occur throughout the body. Cutaneous (skin) sensations and the kinesthetic sense are general senses. Cutaneous sensations include light touch, deep pressure, cold, heat and pain (see chapter 3). Some parts of the skin contain many more receptors than others. The most sensitive areas with the greatest density of receptors are the eyelids, finger tips, lips and nipples. Cutaneous receptors are simple, consisting of the dendrites of sensory neurons that may or may not be enclosed in a capsule. In the hair root, the dendrites form a network but are not enclosed in a capsule. Meissner's and Pacinian corpuscles have connective tissue capsules enclosing the dendrites.

PAIN RECEPTORS

Pain receptors are the dendrites of certain sensory neurons which respond to excessive stimuli of any type as a sensation of pain. They do not undergo adaptation, unlike the receptors for touch and temperature sensations, as pain sensations must not be ignored in order to identify danger. The sensory impulses for pain all pass to the brain.

ANAESTHESIA

Anaesthesia is the loss of feeling. It may occur over a limited area of skin due to nervous disease, 'freezing' by solid carbon dioxide, or by local anaesthetics. When only loss of the sense of pain is meant, the correct term is analgesia, and pain-killing drugs are analgesics. The brain can produce natural analgesics known as endorphins which inhibit pain impulses.

HYPERAESTHESIA

Hyperaesthesia is over-sensitiveness to touch and contra-indicates beauty therapy treatments. It is a symptom of certain nervous diseases such as neuralgia. The pain occurs in the skin above a sensory nerve, for example in the skin above the trigeminal cranial nerve of the face following an attack of shingles.

Special senses

SENSE ORGANS

Special senses involve complex receptors called sense organs which are localised in the head. The eye supplies information about the shape, size and colour of objects, and their movements. It also informs the brain about the direction and intensity of the light reaching the eye. The chemical senses of smell and taste are perceived by the nose and taste buds of the tongue respectively. The ears contain sound receptors for hearing, as well as the receptors concerned with balance.

Explain what is meant by the terms:
(a) kinesthetic sense
(b) sensory adaptation
(c) hyperaesthesia

THE CENTRAL NERVOUS SYSTEM

The central nervous system comprises the spinal cord and brain, the meninges (membranes surrounding the brain and spinal cord) and the cerebro-spinal fluid.

Spinal cord

FUNCTIONS

The spinal cord has several functions. It allows spinal reflex actions, forming part of the conducting pathway. It conveys sensory impulses from one region of the spinal cord to another and from the skin and muscles of the trunk and limbs to the brain.

STRUCTURE

The spinal cord is a long-cylindrical organ with a tapering end. It runs from the brain to the second lumbar vertebra. It passes through the vertebral foramina of the vertebrae, which give protection to the delicate nervous tissue. The cord is divided into right and left halves. It has a central cavity, the spinal canal, continuous with the cavities of the brain and containing cerebro-spinal fluid.

Pairs of spinal nerves emerge from the spinal cord between adjacent vertebrae, each nerve being formed by the fusion of a dorsal and a ventral root (see figure 6.5).

The meninges

POSITION

The meninges are three membranes covering the outside of the spinal cord and brain. The outer membrane is thick and fibrous, the middle one is thinner, while the very thin inner membrane contains the blood vessels which nourish the nervous tissue.

Between the outer membrane and the bony wall of the vertebral canal is the epidural space. It contains adipose tissue, to pad the cord, and blood vessels. Local anaesthetics can be injected into this space during childbirth to relieve severe labour pains. Between the middle and inner membranes is a space containing cerebro-spinal fluid.

FUNCTIONS

The functions of the spinal meninges are to form a protective covering round the spinal cord and to retain the nutritive cerebro-spinal fluid.

Cerebro-spinal fluid

This fluid circulates through the ventricles (cavities) of the brain, the spinal canal and the space between the middle and inner membranes of the cranial and spinal meninges.

COMPOSITION

It is a clear, colourless, watery fluid, containing white blood cells and dissolved glucose, salts, proteins and urea. It diffuses out of the blood contained in networks of capillaries lining the ventricles of the brain.

FUNCTIONS

The functions of the cerebro-spinal fluid are to supply nutrients from the blood to the brain cells, to act as a shock absorber, and to keep the cranial volume constant.

The brain

The brain is the enlarged front end of the spinal cord, developing in three regions as fore, mid and hindbrain. It is protected by the cranial bones of the skull and covered by the cranial meninges, which are continuous with the spinal ones.

Figure 6.6   *Brain (vertical section)*

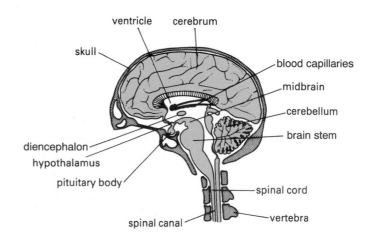

FUNCTIONS

The functions of the brain are those of a nervous control centre. It receives impulses from all the sense receptors and interprets them in its sensory association centres. It also sends motor impulses to the effector organs (muscles and glands). Its association and motor centres co-ordinates the body's movements, allowing it to function efficiently as a whole and to develop skills. The brain controls feeding, sleeping, temperature regulation, drinking and the salt/water balance of the body. It stores information in the memory, so that behaviour can be modified by past experience. It also has association centres concerned with emotional and intellectual processes.

STRUCTURE

The brain is divided into four main parts: the brain stem, the cerebellum, the diencephalon and the cerebrum. The brain contains a number of cavities called ventricles that communicate with one another, with the space between the middle and inner meninges and with the spinal canal. The cerebro-spinal fluid circulates through all these cavities. A superficial layer of nerve cells known as a cortex occurs in the cerebrum and cerebellum. The brain is well supplied with blood vessels in the inner meningeal membrane, as it needs a continuous supply of oxygen and glucose to maintain consciousness and life.

- The brain stem is the region just above the spinal cord. It controls involuntary reflex actions. The cardiac, respiratory and vasomotor centres regulate heart beat, breathing and diameter of blood vessels respectively. It also controls coughing, sneezing, swallowing, vomiting and hiccuping. It carries nerve fibres from the spinal cord to the anterior parts of the brain.

- The cerebellum is part of the hind brain and occurs posteriorly at the level of the brain stem. It is the motor co-ordinating centre of the brain. It maintains posture and allows the co-ordinated movements required in muscular skills. It receives motor impulses from the cerebrum and sensory impulses from the proprioceptors in the muscles and joints. Information about the position of the head in relation to the rest of the body reaches the cerebellum from the inner ear receptors. The cerebellum is then able to generate the muscle contractions needed to maintain balance.

- The diencephalon, which includes the hypothalamus, is part of the forebrain. It relays the sensory impulses reaching the brain to the cerebrum. The hypothalamus lies near the pituitary gland and controls many of the body's homeostatic mechanisms, such as body temperature, water content, thirst and appetite. It controls the autonomic nervous system which regulates the heart rate, the emptying of the bladder and the movement of food through the food canal. It links the functioning of the nervous and endocrine systems via the pituitary gland. It also maintains the pattern of wakefulness and sleep.

- The cerebrum forms the major part of the forebrain and is the largest of the brain regions. Over its surface is the highly folded cerebral cortex.

Explain the functions of the hypothalamus in controlling the body's
activities.

Figure 6.7   *Areas of the cerebral cortex (side view)*

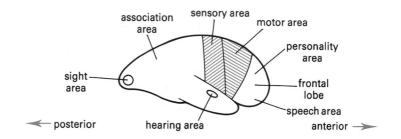

The cerebral cortex is divided up into areas of three main types.

(a)   Motor areas towards the anterior end control the main
pathways for muscular movement.

(b)   Sensory areas posterior to the motor areas interpret sensory
impulses.

(c)   Association areas at the posterior end of the cortex and in
the anterior frontal lobes are concerned with intellectual
processes of thought and memory, emotions and
personality traits.

In the cerebral cortex, activity of the neurons making up the
grey matter generates brain waves. These can be detected and
recorded to produce an electroencephalogram (EEG).
Abnormal brain activity, as in epilepsy, shows up on an EEG.

SUMMARY

The brain is the nervous control centre which co-ordinates all the
body's activities.

THE PERIPHERAL NERVOUS SYSTEM

Nerves are bundles of axons (nerve fibres) surrounded by a
connective tissue sheath, which carry impulses to and from the
central nervous system. The peripheral nervous system includes

mainly those nerves involved in voluntary actions. The 12 pairs of cranial nerves originate from the brain inside the skull which they leave via foramina. The 31 pairs of spinal nerves originate from the spinal cord and leave between the vertebrae.

Cranial nerves

Some of these nerves are mixed, containing both motor and sensory axons, while others are either sensory or motor. Most cranial nerves are confined to the head and neck, but the tenth pair have branches in the trunk. Details of the fifth and seventh cranial nerves are given in table 6.1 and figure 6.8.

Table 6.1   *Cranial nerves*

No.	Name	Branches	Type	Role
V	Trigeminal		mixed	
		Ophthalmic	sensory	Receives impulses from skin of front of scalp, forehead, upper eyelid, eyeball and upper part of the nose
		Maxillary	sensory	Receives impulses from the upper jaw, palate, lower part of the nose, lower eyelid and cheek
		Mandibular	mixed	Receives sensory impulses from the lower jaw, floor of the mouth and skin in front of the ear; takes motor impulses to the muscles of mastication (masseter temporalis and pterygoid)
VII		Facial	mixed	Receives sensory impulses of taste; supplies the muscles of facial expression
		Temporal	motor	Takes motor impulses to auricular, frontalis, orbicularis oculi and corrugator muscles
		Zygomatic	motor	Takes motor impulses to the orbicularis oculi muscles
		Buccal	motor	Takes motor impulses to the procerus, buccinator, orbicularis oris, zygomaticus and levator muscles of mouth
		Mandibular	motor	Takes motor impulses to the lower lip and chin supplying risorius, mentalis and triangularis muscles
		Cervical	motor	Takes motor impulses to the platysma muscle

Figure 6.8 *Distribution of fifth and seventh cranial nerves to the face (side view)*

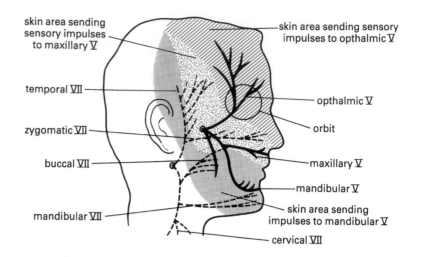

> **Q** List the names and branches of cranial nerves which supply the muscles moving the mouth and lips.

Spinal nerves

Each spinal nerve has two points of attachment, or roots, to the spinal cord. These are the dorsal root carrying sensory axons whose impulses are passing inwards, and the ventral root carrying motor axons whose impulses are passing outwards. A short distance from the spinal cord, the two roots combine to form a mixed spinal nerve, which is surrounded by a fibrous sheath. The dorsal root has a swelling, or ganglion, containing the cell bodies of the sensory neurons (see figure 6.5).

GROUPS

The 31 pairs of spinal nerves are named according to the region of the spinal cord from which they emerge. There are:

- eight pairs of cervical nerves;
- twelve pairs of thoracic nerves;
- five pairs of lumbar nerves;
- five pairs of sacral nerves;
- one pair of coccygeal nerves.

Each spinal nerve divides into several rami (branches) just beyond the point where its two roots join. The posterior rami supply the muscles and skin of the back.

PLEXUSES

Some of the anterior rami join up with those of adjacent nerves to form plexuses (networks). There are four main plexuses on each side of the body.

- The cervical plexuses of the neck supply the skin and muscles of the head, neck and upper region of the shoulders. The phrenic nerves to the diaphragm come from the cervical plexus.

- The brachial plexuses at the top of the shoulders supply the skin and muscles of the arms, shoulders and upper chest.

- The lumbar plexuses occur between the waist and hip bone and supply the front and sides of the abdomen wall and part of the leg. The femoral nerves, passing down the front of the thighs to the flexor muscles of the thigh and extensor muscles of the leg, are the largest nerves from the lumbar plexuses.

- The sacral plexuses at the base of the abdomen supply the buttocks and some leg muscles. The sciatic nerves from these plexuses are the largest nerves in the body and supply muscles of the legs and feet. The sciatic nerves pass from the buttocks down the back of the thighs and give branches to the lower legs and feet. (For the nerve supply to individual muscles, see chapter 5).

Most thoracic nerves pass directly to the structures they supply in the chest wall. Each spinal nerve has two thin branches, the rami communicans, which link it with the autonomic nervous system.

Q Give the position and functions of the following:
(a) the sciatic nerve
(b) the phrenic nerve

THE AUTONOMIC NERVOUS SYSTEM

The autonomic nervous system controls the involuntary activities of smooth and cardiac muscle, and of glands. It is largely concerned with motor reflexes and is regulated by centres in the brain stem, hypothalamus and cerebral cortex of the brain, to which it sends impulses.

Divisions

The autonomic nervous system has two divisions, or sets of nerves, known as sympathetic and parasympathetic, which usually have opposite effects. The opposite effects result from the different chemical transmitters secreted at the nerve/effector synapse. Parasympathetic nerve endings produce acetylcholine. Sympathetic nerve endings produce noradrenalin, which has similar effects to those of the hormone adrenalin.

In general, the effects of the sympathetic division are to increase the body's use of energy, for example during exercise or stress. The effects of the parasympathetic division are concerned with energy conservation. Together they maintain homeostasis, as one division counteracts the effects of the other – one acting as an 'accelerator' and the other as a 'brake' for example.

Functions

Some of the functions of the autonomic nervous system are shown in table 6.2.

Table 6.2   *Functions of the autonomic nervous system*

Organ (effector)	Parasympathetic division	Sympathetic division
Heart	Slows the rate	Accelerates the rate
Bronchioles	Constricts	Dilates
Arteries supplying the skeletal muscles	Dilates	Constricts
Sphincters of the food canal	Relaxes (opens)	Contracts (closes)
Bladder	Relaxes the wall	Contracts the wall
Pupil of the eye	Constricts	Dilates
Arrector pili muscles of the hairs		Contracts (gooseflesh)
Sweat glands		Increases secretion of sweat

 Q   Explain how the autonomic nervous system controls the rate of the heart beat.

--- SUMMARY ---

The autonomic nervous system acts with the endocrine system to maintain homeostasis by regulating the body's physiology.

SUBSTANCES THAT AFFECT THE NERVOUS SYSTEM

Drugs

SEDATIVES

Sedatives are drugs that reduce nervousness and excitement by their action on the central nervous system. One group are the tranquillisers, used to treat anxiety.

HYPNOTICS

Hypnotics are drugs which induce sleep. One group are the barbiturates, although these have been largely replaced by tranquillisers. Both barbiturates and tranquillisers are addictive if prescribed for long periods of time.

NARCOTICS

Narcotics are drugs producing a condition of stupor. Opium drugs such as morphine and heroin have this effect. These drugs, too, are addictive.

ANALGESICS

Analgesics act by inhibiting impulses of pain. Aspirin and paracetamol are commonly used to treat minor pains. Too frequent use of aspirin can damage the lining of the food canal, and too frequent use of paracetamol can cause liver damage.

STIMULANTS

Stimulants act by stimulating the sympathetic nervous system. Amphetamines, which are drugs related to the hormone adrenalin, are stimulants and also cause weight loss. As they are addictive, they should not be used as slimming aids. Caffeine from coffee is a brain stimulant, as it speeds up transmission across synapses.

Nerve poisons

These are substances which have adverse effects on the nervous system.

ALCOHOL

Alcohol (ethanol) is a depressant, having a narcotic and sedative action. It affects the intellectual faculties of the brain, reducing self-control. Larger amounts of alcohol dull sense perception and slow the transmission of nerve impulses. Co-ordination of muscular movements is affected, causing clumsiness and slurring of speech. High alcohol consumption has dangerous social consequences by inducing violent behaviour and seriously reducing driving ability. Excess consumption finally results in heavy sleep or stupor, prolonged until the alcohol absorbed has been oxidised.

METHANOL

Methanol (methyl alcohol) is present in methylated spirit and has effects on the body similar to those of ethanol. It is, however, even more toxic, having a pronounced adverse effect on the nervous system. In large quantities it causes neuritis, affecting the optic nerves particularly and resulting in blindness.

LEAD

Lead is a nerve poison. The general sources of the lead absorbed by the nervous system are tetraethyl lead from petrol exhaust gases and lead salts in soft drinking water that has been standing in lead pipes. Lead poisoning causes mental and behavioural impairment. It causes tremors and paralysis due to nerve damage, usually starting in the muscles on the back of the wrist, and causing 'wrist drop' as an early symptom.

CHAPTER 7

The Digestive System

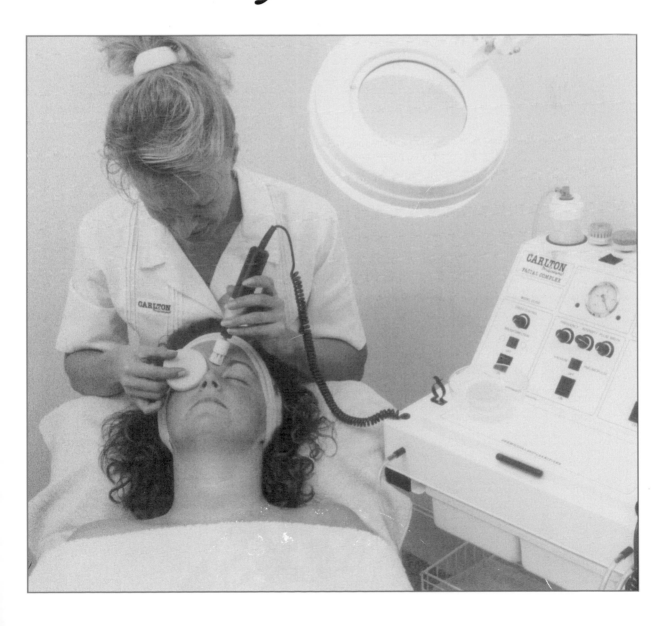

NUTRIENTS

The digestive system is involved in obtaining the chemicals required to sustain life. The chemicals required by the body for energy and warmth, growth and repair, and protection against disease, are called nutrients. There are six groups of nutrients which must be supplied in our food and drink. Carbohydrates and fats are the nutrients required for energy, proteins, water and mineral salts are used in tissue building, while vitamins are protective in function.

Carbohydrates

The main function of carbohydrates is to provide energy. They are also a source of body fat. Carbohydrates are compounds of the elements carbon, hydrogen and oxygen. Sugars, starches and celluloses are the three groups of carbohydrates which occur in food.

SUGARS

Sugars are white crystalline solids which dissolve in water, and usually taste sweet:

- Monosaccharides, such as glucose and fructose, are simple sugars. Glucose is the sugar present in blood, and other carbohydrates are converted into glucose during digestion

Figure 7.1 *Structure of*
carbohydrate molecules
(a) Monosaccharide: glucose
(b) Disaccharide: maltose
(c) Polysaccharide: starch

(a) formula $C_6H_{12}O_6$
the molecule has a 6-membered ring structure

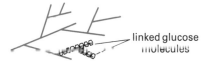

(b) formula $C_{12}H_{22}O_{11}$
the molecule has two 6-membered rings joined through an oxygen atom by the removal of water

(c) chains of linked glucose units form a bush-shaped molecule

linked glucose
molecules

and metabolism. Glucose also occurs in some fruits, such as grapes and figs. Fructose is the sweetest of the sugars and occurs in honey and fruits.

- Disaccharide sugars, such as sucrose, maltose and lactose, consist of two monosaccharides linked together by the removal of a water molecule. Sucrose is present in sugar cane, sugar beet, carrots and fruits. It is formed by linking a glucose with a fructose molecule. Maltose is malt sugar from barley grains and is not very sweet. It is formed by linking two glucose molecules. Lactose is the sugar present in milk.

STARCHES

Starches are polysaccharides – composed of large numbers of glucose units linked together by the removal of water molecules. The compact, bush-like starch molecules contain straight-chain amylose units and branched-chain amylopectin units. They are storage products. Starches occur in granules inside the cells of cereals, potatoes and root vegetables. The starch granules are enclosed by a membrane which is destroyed by cooking. Starch is insoluble in water, but cooked starch forms a colloidal suspension. Glycogen is the starch formed in the body from glucose. It is stored in liver cells as star-shaped granules, and also in muscles.

CELLULOSES

Celluloses are fibrous polysaccharides built up from glucose units. Together with pectin, they form the cell walls of plants and are present in cereal bran, root vegetables and hard fruits. Cellulose is not broken down by human digestive juices but forms roughage, or dietary fibre.

UNREFINED CARBOHYDRATES

Unrefined carbohydrates, supplied by potatoes, pasta, pulses, wholegrain foods, fresh fruit and vegetables, are converted relatively slowly into glucose during digestion. Glucose is therefore absorbed into the blood over a longer period. These foods also contain fibre, giving bulk so a person's appetite is quickly satisfied.

Refined carbohydrates, such as glucose and cane sugar, are quickly absorbed into the blood and provide instant energy, but leave the body feeling unsatisfied.

Lipids

Lipids are fatty materials which function as an energy source. They have a higher energy value than carbohydrates as they contain less oxygen in their molecules. Fats can be stored in the body, the subcutaneous fat insulating the body against heat loss as well as providing an energy reserve. Phospholipids and cholesterol have the important function of forming cell membranes.

Lipids contain carbon and hydrogen as well as oxygen, and are organic substances which are insoluble in water. The lipids include triglycerides (fats and oils), phospholipids, sterols (cholesterol) and steroid hormones and vitamins.

TRIGLYCERIDES

Triglycerides are built up from three fatty acid molecules combined with glycerol. Many different fats occur in food, varying in the particular fatty acids they contain.

- **Saturated fats** contain fatty acids lacking double bonds, because all the possible sites for hydrogen atoms in the fat molecule are filled. They are stable solid fats, containing palmitic acid (in cocoa butter), stearic acid (in lard) and butyric acid (in butter).

- **Monounsaturated fats** have one double bond providing an unfilled site for two hydrogen atoms in the molecule. They are liquid at room temperature and not as stable as saturated fats. They gradually oxidise in the air, becoming rancid. Monounsaturated fatty acids (e.g. oleic acid) occur in olive oil and in avocados.

- **Polyunsaturated fats** have two or more double bonds in their fatty acids and are oily liquids. They oxidise in the air, becoming rancid. Polyunsaturated fatty acids, e.g. linoleic and arachidonic acids, occur in sunflower, corn and soya oils, and in fish oils.

Triglycerides form the neutral fat deposits in the body. They are transported in the blood in the form of lipoprotein particles. These have a core of triglycerides and cholesterol, with an outer envelope of phospholipids and protein to disperse the fat. The waxes forming sebum and ear wax are formed from triglycerides.

Animal fats, containing mainly saturated fatty acids, occur in dairy produce, egg yolk, red meat and bacon. Oily fish contain polyunsaturates.

Vegetable oils contain mainly unsaturated fatty acids, for example soft margarine contains around 60%.

> *Q* Compare the chemical structure of a starch molecule with that of a triglyceride.

PHOSPHOLIPIDS

Phospholipids form the middle layer of cell membranes and the myelin sheath round nerve fibres. The phospholipid molecule is similar to that of a triglyceride, but one of the fatty acid molecules is replaced by phosphoric acid. They are present in fish oils.

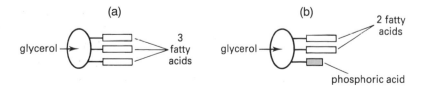

Figure 7.2   *Structure of lipid molecules*
(a)   Triglyceride (fat or oil)
(b)   Phospholipid

CHOLESTEROL

Cholesterol is a complex lipid formed from saturated fats. It is present in the blood and is a component of cell membranes. It is needed for the synthesis of several hormones (e.g. sex hormones) and the bile salts.

Proteins

FUNCTIONS

Proteins function as tissue building materials and are active components of biochemical reactions. They can be oxidised as an energy source if carbohydrate or fat is not available, but this results in tissue loss as protein is not stored in the body.

STRUCTURE

Fibrous proteins have long chain molecules. Examples of fibrous proteins are collagen (in connective tissue), myosin and actin (in muscle fibres), keratin (in skin, hair and nails) and fibrin (in blood clots). Other types of protein act as enzymes and antibodies, and as hormones (insulin and adrenalin). Protein forms part of the haemoglobin molecule which carries oxygen in the blood.

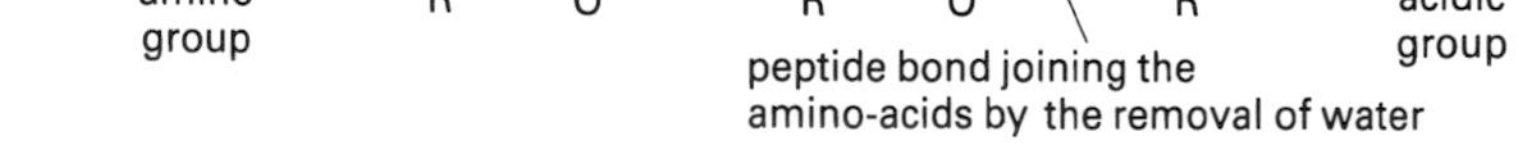

Figure 7.3   *Structure of protein molecules*
(a)   General formula for an amino acid
(b)   Polypeptide or protein

Proteins contain nitrogen in addition to carbon, hydrogen, and oxygen, and may also contain sulphur and/or phosphorus. They are built up from smaller molecules called amino acids which are linked by peptide bonds to form polypeptide chains. A large number of different proteins can be synthesised by varying the order and type of the amino acids in the polypeptide chain. Several polypeptide chains may be linked together, or the chains may be coiled into complex shapes. Heat causes proteins to 'denature' by altering the shape of the molecules.

AMINO ACIDS

There are around twenty different amino acids, divided into two types: essential amino acids which cannot be made by the body, and inessential ones made by converting other amino acids. The eight amino acids essential for adults are lysine, tryptophan, phenylalanine, methionine, valine, threonine, leucine and isoleucine. Among the inessential amino acids are glycine, tyrosine and alanine.

SOURCES

Animal proteins contain more of the essential amino acids than plant proteins, as the proteins of animals are more like those of man. Wheat protein is low in lysine, and maize protein is low in tryptophan. Plant proteins are described as being of low biological value because they do not contain the complete range of essential amino acids. Plant proteins occur in cereal products, legumes, pulses and nuts. Texturised vegetable protein (meat substitute) is also available. Animal proteins occur in meat, fish, cheese, milk and egg white.

Minerals

FUNCTIONS

The functions of minerals are to form components of body tissue (bone and blood); to take part in biochemical reactions involving enzymes; and to maintain the osmotic (salt/water) balance of the body fluids. Some eight major minerals are required in relatively large amounts, while only traces of several other minerals are necessary.

MAJOR MINERALS

The major minerals include calcium, iron, phosphorus, sulphur, sodium, potassium, chlorine and magnesium.

- **Calcium** is essential for the ossification of bones and teeth, for blood coagulation and for muscle contraction. It is also required for the normal functioning of cell membranes, transmitter release at nerve endings and glandular secretion. In an adult there is approximately 1 kg of calcium, of which 99% occurs in bone tissue from which it is constantly being withdrawn and replaced. The food sources of calcium include milk, cheese, bread, pilchards and green vegetables. It is also present in hard drinking water.

- **Iron** forms part of the blood pigment haemoglobin and the muscle pigment myoglobin. It is needed for the production of ATP in cells (see chapter 8). Iron is stored in the liver. Foods containing iron are liver, red meat, egg yolk, nuts, beans and dried fruits.

- **Phosphorus** occurs as the calcium salt (calcium phosphate) in bones and teeth. Phosphates are involved in the release of energy from glucose and form part of biologically active substances such as ATP and DNA. Phosphorus is present in most foods, and good sources are yeast extract, cheese, eggs, white fish, peanuts and wholemeal bread.

- **Sulphur** is a component of many structural proteins including the keratin of skin and hair. It occurs in egg yolk, fish, red meat and liver.

- **Sodium** and **chlorine** occur as sodium chloride (common salt) in all the body fluids. Salt is needed to maintain the body's osmotic balance. It is essential for the conduction of nerve impulses and prevention of muscle cramps. A high salt intake may be associated with high blood pressure, which may result in strokes. All processed foods contain salt, particularly bacon and kippers.

- **Magnesium** occurs in bones as magnesium phosphate and is involved in ossification. It is also needed for the activity of enzymes which release energy in the cell. It occurs in green vegetables and salads.

 Q Why is calcium an essential mineral in a balanced diet? List three foods which provide this nutrient.

TRACE MINERALS

Trace minerals required by the body are shown in table 7.1.

Vitamins

FUNCTION

The function of vitamins is to maintain good health. They are organic substances required in very small amounts which the body is (in most cases) unable to synthesise. Vitamins are involved in enzyme reactions forming part of the body's

Table 7.1   *Trace minerals required by the body*

Mineral	Food source	Role in the body
Cobalt	Liver	Forms part of the Vitamin B12 molecule
Copper	Eggs, cereals, fish and spinach	Required for the formation of haemoglobin; also part of an enzyme involved in melanin synthesis
Fluorine	Some drinking water	Makes tooth enamel more resistant to dental caries (decay)
Iodine	Fish	Forms part of the hormone thyroxin
Manganese	Tea, nuts, and cereals	Required for the formation of haemoglobin, and for enzymes concerned with growth, reproduction and lactation
Selenium	Meat, liver, milk, seafood and wholegrain cereals	Needed to protect cell membranes from damage by free radicals. Protects against breast cancer
Zinc	Protein foods	It is an activator of several enzymes and is necessary for growth; it is required for the synthesis of insulin; larger amounts are required by women taking the oral contraceptive pill

physiological processes. Many act as co-enzymes (enzyme activators).

SOLUBILITY

Vitamins are divided into two groups according to their solubility. The fat-soluble vitamins are A, D, E, and K, while the water-soluble ones include the B group and C. A large unnecessary intake of vitamin pills has little useful effect and results in their being excreted. Dietary supplements are useful in special cases.

FAT-SOLUBLE

Fat-soluble vitamins can only be absorbed from the food canal in the presence of fatty foods, in which they usually occur. Surpluses are stored in the liver and if taken in excess reach toxic levels, causing liver damage.

- **Vitamin A** (Retinol) is essential for dim-light vision, and the health of epithelia such as mucous membranes and skin epidermis. Vitamin A can be produced in the intestine from dietary carotene, an orange pigment in carrots and tomatoes. Other sources of the vitamin are fish liver oils, liver and kidney, eggs and dairy products. Beta-carotene taken as a dietary supplement can be toxic in excess.

- **Vitamin D** (Calciferol) is essential for maintaining the blood calcium level by increasing calcium absorption from food. It regulates the interchange of blood and bone calcium and thus affects the hardening of bones and teeth. Children and pregnant or lactating women require larger amounts of Vitamin D. Its dietary sources are fish liver oils, fatty fish, margarine and eggs. It is also formed in the skin by the action of ultra-violet rays in sunlight on a cholesterol derivative. It is toxic if an overdose is taken.

- **Vitamin E** (Tocopherol) inhibits the oxidation of polyunsaturated fatty acids that form part of cell membranes. It also protects the liver from damage by some toxic chemicals (e.g. carbon tetrachloride). It is present in egg yolk, milk, wheat germ, nuts and seeds.

- **Vitamin K** (Phylloquinone) is necessary for the production of prothrombin, which aids normal blood clotting. This vitamin occurs in leafy vegetables and cereals. It is also produced by bacteria in the intestine. Antibiotics which kill these bacteria prevent its production.

WATER-SOLUBLE

Water-soluble vitamins are absorbed along with water in the food canal. They include all the B complex and Vitamin C.

Vitamin B complex is a group of chemically varied substances which act as co-enzymes in the enzyme reactions of metabolism. All members of the group tend to occur in the same foods and cannot be stored by the body. Not all the B Vitamins are numbered.

- **Thiamin (B1)** is necessary for the steady release of energy from glucose. It is rapidly destroyed by heat. Sources are wholegrain cereals, yeast extract, eggs, liver, milk, vegetables and fruit.

- **Riboflavin (B2)** is essential for using the energy released from food. Its main source is milk, but riboflavin is destroyed if milk is exposed to the ultra-violet rays of sunlight. It is also in green vegetables, fish, meat and eggs.

- **Nicotinic acid** or **niacin (B5)** is also involved in the breakdown of glucose to release energy. It inhibits the production of cholesterol and assists in fat breakdown. Its source is wholegrain cereals, yeast extract, meat, liver, beans and nuts.

- **Pyridoxine (B6)** is an essential co-enzyme in protein metabolism, including the repair of body tissues. It also acts in fat metabolism. It is destroyed by heat. It is required in larger amounts by women taking the contraceptive pill. It occurs in wholegrain cereals, yeast extract, liver, meat, nuts, bananas, salmon, tomatoes and cabbage.

- **Cyanocobalamin (B12)** is a co-enzyme needed for the formation of red blood cells in the red bone marrow. It is also involved in amino acid metabolism. It is unusual in containing the mineral cobalt. Its source is liver, kidney, milk, eggs and cheese. Because it is not present in vegetable foods, a vegan diet will be deficient in this vitamin

- **Folic acid** is essential for the normal formation of red and white blood cells, and for the synthesis of DNA. It is required in larger amounts by women taking the contraceptive pill, and during pregnancy. It occurs in liver, raw leafy vegetables, oranges and bananas. It is also synthesised by bacteria in the food canal. Anticonvulsant drugs used to treat epilepsy destroy folic acid.

- **Pantothenic acid** is necessary for the release of energy from glucose and for the conversion of fats and amino acids to glucose. It is also needed for the synthesis of cholesterol and adrenal hormones. It occurs in kidney, liver, yeast extract, cereals and green vegetables.

- **Biotin** is necessary for the release of energy from glucose and for the synthesis of fatty acids. It occurs in liver, kidney, yeast extract and egg yolk. It is synthesised by bacteria in the food canal.

- **Vitamin C** (Ascorbic acid) is needed to maintain healthy connective tissue by its involvement in collagen formation. It prevents bleeding from small blood vessels, particularly those in the gums. It helps wounds to heal. It is rapidly destroyed by heat and by cooking food in water containing bicarbonate of soda. However, potatoes and green vegetables retain much of their Vitamin C if they are placed into boiling water, to which no bicarbonate of soda has been added, and cooked for the

Food	Nutrients								
	Sugar	Starch	Fat	Protein	Calcium	Iron	Vitamin A	Vitamin D	Vitamin A
Baked beans	▓	░	▓	▓					
Bread white		░	▓		▓	▓			
Bread Wholemeal	▓	░	▓	▓		▓			▓
Carrots (raw)	▓	░			▓		░		
Cheese			░	░	░		▓	▓	
Chicken			▓	░	▓				
Cornflakes	▓	░		▓	▓				
Cream			░		▓		▓		
Eggs			░	░	▓	▓	▓	░	▓
Fish (white)				░	▓				
Honey	░								
Liver			▓	░	▓	░	░	▓	
Meat (lean)			▓	░	▓	░			
Milk	▓				░		░	▓	
Oranges	░				▓				
Pilchards			░	░	▓			░	
Potatoes		░							
Yeast extracts					▓	▓			

Key

F = dietary fibre present   [ ] major source   [ ] minor source   [ ] absent

present

Vitamin K	Thiamin	Ribo-flavin	Niacin	Pyridox-ine	Cyanocob-alamin	Folic acid	Pantoth-enic acid	Biotin	Vitamin C	
										F
	minor	minor	major							
	major	minor	major	minor	minor	minor	minor			F
			minor						minor	F
		minor			minor			minor		
	minor		major							
	minor	minor	minor							F
	minor	minor	minor							
		major		minor	minor			major		
			minor	minor						
minor	major	major	minor	minor	major	minor	minor	major		
	major	minor	major	major	major					
	minor	major	minor		minor					
						minor			major	
	major								major	
	minor	minor	major	minor	minor		minor	minor		

minimum time. Fresh fruits, particularly citrus fruits and blackcurrants, are good sources of Vitamin C. Smokers need 40% more Vitamin C in their diet.

 Q | In which foods do the majority of the B group vitamins occur?

FREE RADICALS

Most essential minerals and vitamins are available in tablet form as dietary supplements to supply individual nutrient deficiencies. One such supplement has recently been developed to counter the effects of free radicals in the body.

Free radicals are atoms or molecules with unpaired electrons. They are very unstable and oxidise other molecules by taking electrons from them. They oxidise unsaturated fatty acids in this way, causing them to go rancid. As fats containing unsaturated fatty acids make up part of the structure of cell membranes (plasma, nuclear and mitochondrial membranes), free radicals damage these membranes and affect cell metabolism. It has been suggested that free radical damage to mitochondria is the key to the body changes which occur during ageing.

These free radicals may be produced during normal cell metabolism, ingested in food, or come from pollutants. They are destroyed in the body by peroxidase enzymes (which contain selenium) and by the antioxidant Vitamins A, C and E.

Water

Water forms about two-thirds of the body weight and is a major structural component. It is the solvent in which all the biochemical reactions of metabolism take place. Water acts as the suspending fluid for blood and lymph cells, and lubricates the tissues.

The evaporation of water in sweat cools the body, but excessive water loss can result from vomiting or diarrhoea, causing dehydration. At least one litre of water should be swallowed daily in a temperate climate. In addition to drinks, water is obtained from fruit and vegetables in the diet.

———————— **SUMMARY** ————————

Nutrients are the chemicals required by the body for energy and warmth, growth and repair, and protection against disease. They are supplied in the food that makes up an individual's diet. Carbohydrates and fats are the main nutrients providing energy. Proteins, minerals and water are needed for new tissue growth, while vitamins keep the body functioning healthily.

Sugars and starches are the carbohydrates providing energy, while cellulose provides fibre. Fats also provide energy and can be stored in adipose tissue. Proteins contain chains of amino acids and are used as tissue building units and as enzymes. Minerals either form part of the body structure or aid metabolism. The body's fluid balance is maintained by mineral salts and dietary water. Vitamins are biochemically important substances that the body is unable to synthesise for itself. The small quantity of each vitamin required must therefore be obtained from the diet.

DIET

Balanced diet

A balanced diet contains all six main nutrients in adequate amounts for energy, growth, reproduction and protection of the body. The precise amount of each nutrient needed will vary for each individual, but recommended amounts for various groups of people have been proposed. The current recommended daily allowances for women and girls are shown in table 7.3.

Factors to take into account when advising on a balanced diet relate to individual nutritional requirements. The energy requirement varies with the age, sex and occupation of the person.

ENERGY VALUE

The energy value of a nutrient is obtained by burning a known weight of it in a bomb calorimeter. The heat given out on burning the nutrient increases the temperature of a known weight of water. From this data, the amount of heat energy can be calculated. It is measured either in kilocalories (kcal) or in kilojoules (kJ). A kilocalorie is the amount of heat needed to raise the temperature of 1 kilogram of water by 1 °C. 1 kcal is

Table 7.3   *Recommended daily allowances in the diet for women and girls*

Nutrient	Weight (in grams)
Protein	50.0
Total fat ($\frac{1}{3}$ saturated fat) ($\frac{2}{3}$ polyunsaturates)	75.0
Carbohydrates	275.0
Fibre	25.0–30.0
Calcium	0.5
Iron	0.012
Salt	not exceeding 9.0

equivalent to 4.2 kJ, so 4.2 kJ raise the temperature of 1 kg of water by 1 °C. Glucose, protein, fat and alcohol all produce energy when taken into the body, but fats have the highest energy (calorific) value.

Table 7.4   *Energy values of nutrients*

Weight g	Nutrient	Energy value kcal	kJ
1	Glucose	3.75	16
1	Protein	4.00	17
1	Fat	9.00	37
1	Alcohol	7.00	29

The recommended daily energy intake from foods for women and girls is 2,000 kcals or 8,400 kJ.

DIETARY FIBRE

Dietary fibre is supplied by unrefined carbohydrates, vegetables and fruit. A high-fibre diet has advantages in promoting health.

- Because of fibre's capacity to absorb water and swell, faeces are bulkier and softer, making them easier to eliminate without straining. This prevents constipation and haemorrhoids (piles).

- The presence of fibre in food makes it less viscous so that it moves more rapidly through the alimentary canal. This makes appendicitis, hiatus hernia, gall bladder disease and diverticular colon disease less likely.

- Carcinogens (cancer causing materials) present in faeces have less time to attack the gut lining, reducing the likelihood of bowel cancer.

- Fibre supplies a large part of the food for the symbiotic bacteria in the small intestine. Some of the products produced by these bacteria are beneficial, such as B group vitamins.

- Diabetes is helped by a high-fibre diet as it reduces the surge in blood glucose following a meal.

 List the advantages of a high-fibre diet.

DEFICIENCY DISEASES

Malnutrition is the result of having a diet which is inadequate or not balanced. If all the nutrients are present in inadequate amounts, then undernutrition, leading to eventual starvation, results. If one particular nutrient is absent or in short supply, a deficiency disease may occur (see table 7.5). Equally, if too much of any one nutrient is present in the diet, malnutrition occurs.

 Which nutrient is associated with the following diseases?
(a) goitre
(b) osteoporosis
(c) scurvy
(d) polyneuritis
(e) dental caries

SPECIAL DIETARY NEEDS

Certain groups of people may have special dietary needs which contra-indicate the normal balanced diet.

- Teenage girls (under 18) generally show a decrease in physical activity so they use less energy. This will lead to overweight,

Table 7.5   *Deficiency diseases*

Deficient nutrient	Name of disease	Symptoms of the disease
Calcium	Rickets Osteomalacia Osteoporosis	Soft bones which become deformed in children Soft bones, with bowing of the legs Decrease in bone mass causing bones to break easily
Iron	Anaemia	The haemoglobin content of the blood is too low; it results in tiredness, breathlessness, depression
Fluorine	Dental caries	Tooth decay due to weakened tooth enamel
Iodine	Cretinism Goitre	Dwarfism and mental retardation in children Enlargement of the thyroid gland in the neck
Vitamin A	Night blindness Epithelial atrophy	Inability to see in dim light Scaly skin
Thiamin	Beri-beri Polyneuritis	Muscle paralysis affecting limbs and digestive system Reflexes related to the senses of kinesthesia and touch are impaired
Riboflavin	Cheilitis Cataract	Lips cracking, and sores in the corners of the mouth Impaired sight due to clouding of the lens of the eye
Niacin	Pellagra	Skin becomes dark and scaly; chronic diarrhoea
Pyridoxine	Dermatitis	Inflamed skin round eyes, nose and mouth
Cyanocobalamin	Pernicious anaemia Nerve cell degeneration	Red bone marrow is unable to form new red blood cells The axons of the nerve cells in the spinal cord degenerate
Folic acid	Macrocytic anaemia	Abnormally large red blood cells are produced
Vitamin C	Scurvy	Tender swollen gums which bleed; teeth become loose and fall out
Vitamin D	Rickets Osteomalacia	(see calcium)

particularly where high-energy snacks are frequently eaten, unless unrefined carbohydrates replace refined ones to provide 9,000 kJ of energy per day. Because of the need to build up bone mass, the recommended normal calcium intake should be doubled, so more low-fat milk, cheese and yogurt should be eaten. At least 0.5 kg of fruit and vegetables should be included in the daily diet to provide fibre, minerals and vitamins.

- Women with a very active lifestyle need more energy foods in their diet to supply 10,500 kJ. There will be a higher protein turnover from increased muscular activity, requiring extra protein in the diet. A higher proportion of dietary fat should be polyunsaturates. These form prostaglandins, which counter the effects of stress and may reduce premenstrual tension.

- Pregnant women need a diet containing more energy foods, protein, vitamins and minerals to provide for the growth and development of the foetus. The pregnant woman also needs to store fat subcutaneously for the future needs of the foetus, and for breast milk secretion. In the last ten weeks of pregnancy, foetal and placental growth and the extra fat laid down add 12.5 kg to the usual weight.

  The diet must provide 10,000 kJ of energy daily, preferably from unrefined carbohydrates and unsaturated fats. Extra Vitamin D and 1.2 g of calcium daily are needed for foetal bone formation. Increased iron and Vitamin C are needed, as the vitamin aids the absorption of iron required for the synthesis of haemoglobin. Supplements of folic acid and zinc prevent the birth defects of spina bifida and cleft palate from developing in the foetus. Women who have been taking the contraceptive pill in previous years may also need a Vitamin B6 (Pyridoxine) supplement.

- Women who are breast-feeding have daily energy requirements that are even higher than during pregnancy – 11,500 kJ are needed. The diet must provide extra protein and unsaturated fat, and have a high calcium, iron, and Vitamin A, D and C content. It is essential that at least two litres of water are swallowed daily in drinks, as over one litre will be needed for the breast milk. Highly spiced or strong tasting foods should be avoided as they can flavour breast milk.

- Post-menopausal women (over 60) suffer from increasing degenerative changes which affect their dietary requirements. The metabolic rate falls by 20% and, as the level of physical activity is reduced, obesity may occur. There is a gradual decline in body function and resistance to stress, and both the digestion and absorption of nutrients is progressively disrupted. Deficiencies of iron, zinc, folic acid and Vitamins B12, C and D commonly occur. Dietary supplements may therefore be needed. Shortage of iron and zinc may result in hair thinning. A reduced intake of energy foods to provide

8,000 kJ is sufficient, and this should be obtained mainly from unsaturated fats and unrefined carbohydrate which also supplies fibre. Older women also require less protein in the diet.

- Vegan and vegetarian diets do not provide the whole range of amino acids needed for protein synthesis unless vegetables are combined with grains, pulses and nuts. As milk, cheese and eggs form part of most vegetarian diets, these animal products will also supply essential amino acids. Vegans, who eat no animal products, need a supplement of the Vitamins B2, B12 and D.

- Many medically prescribed diets differ from the normal balanced diet. Diabetics have a diet of rigorously controlled carbohydrate intake. A high fibre content obtained from unrefined carbohydrates reduces surges in the blood glucose level.

Obesity

Obesity and overweight are the result of taking in more energy-providing nutrients than can be used up by the body's activities. The excess nutrients will then be converted into fat and deposited under the skin and round internal organs. Energy expenditure depends on a person's activity level and their metabolic rate (the rate at which their body uses energy just to keep alive). The metabolic rate varies, depending on age, body size, sex, environmental temperature and the hormone balance of the person.

PREVALENCE

Around 13% of men and 15% of women are obese, while 38% of men and 26% of women are overweight in the UK. To decide whether an individual's weight in relation to their height lies in the healthy, overweight or obese sectors, either a graph of weight against height can be used, or a body mass index can be calculated.

HEIGHT/WEIGHT RELATIONSHIP

Obesity occurs if a person is 20% over the maximum desirable weight. Using the graph in figure 7.4, a woman of height 1.625 m (5' 5") would be obese if she weighed over 68 kg (150 lb),

Figure 7.4   *Height/weight graph for women*

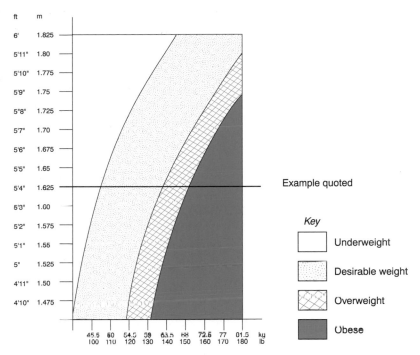

ft   m

6'   1.825

5'11"   1.80

5'10"   1.775

5'9"   1.75

5"8"   1.725

5'7"   1.70

5'6"   1.675

5'5"   1.65

5'4"   1.625   ———— Example quoted

5'3"   1.00

5'2"   1.575

5'1"   1.55

5"   1.525

4'11"   1.50

4'10"   1.475

45.5 60 54.5 59 63.5 68 72.5 77 81.5 kg
100 110 120 130 140 150 160 170 180 lb

Key

☐ Underweight

▧ Desirable weight

▨ Overweight

■ Obese

overweight if between 62 kg (138 lb) and 68 kg, and a healthy weight if she was between 47.5 kg (105 lb) and 62 kg.

BODY MASS INDEX

Body mass index (BMI) is calculated by dividing the weight of a person in kg by their height in m squared.

$$BMI = \frac{x\ kg}{y\ m^2}$$

A BMI of 20–25 is desirable, 25–30 is overweight, and above 30 is obese.

HEALTH HAZARDS

Even moderate obesity is a health hazard. It is a major factor predisposing a person to coronary heart disease, strokes, high blood pressure, varicose veins, diabetes, gallstones, hernias, arthritis and gout. Life expectancy is therefore considerably reduced by obesity.

SLIMMING DIET

Obesity can be treated by adopting a slimming diet and taking more exercise, provided the obesity has a dietary cause.

- Carbohydrates can be greatly reduced in the diet with no observable ill-effects. The blood glucose level will remain normal due to the action of the hormones insulin, adrenalin and glucagon (see chapter 13). A small amount of glucose is required for the complete oxidation of fats used as the alternative energy source. Unrefined carbohydrates should provide the necessary 4,200 to 6,300 kJ of energy, and sufficient fibre for healthy functioning of the digestive system.

- Fats must not be completely excluded from the diet, though saturated fats should be drastically reduced. Polyunsaturated fatty acids are essential for life, as arachidonic acid is converted into prostaglandins. These are lipids which regulate a variety of body processes including blood pressure and peristalsis. Fats also provide the fat-soluble Vitamins A, D, E and K.

- Proteins provided by lean meat and fish should be supplied daily in small quantities. Proteins are not stored by the body and have a short lifespan, so tissue deterioration sets in rapidly without them.

- All major and trace minerals, and both fat- and water-soluble vitamins must be present in a slimming diet to avoid deficiency diseases. A multivitamin and mineral dietary supplement is often advantageous. The amount of common salt (sodium chloride), however, should be reduced to prevent high blood pressure.

- Alcohol supplies additional energy so a sliming diet should preferably be alcohol free.

A slimming diet is seldom a lasting solution to obesity. New eating habits need to be adopted for the rest of the person's life in order to remain permanently at a healthy weight.

SUMMARY

Obesity and overweight are the result of taking in more energy-providing nutrients than can be used up by the body's activities. Obesity is one of the most important preventable causes of ill-health and premature death. It can be treated by adopting a slimming diet consisting of fibre-rich unrefined carbohydrates and low fat, alcohol and salt content. Essential minerals and vitamins must be included, by dietary supplements if necessary.

Give three health hazards of being overweight. What dietary advice would you give to a thirty-year-old obese client who wished to attain a healthy weight?

Eating disorders

ANOREXIA

Anorexia nervosa is a condition involving severe appetite loss and aversion to food. It results in serious weight loss and occurs mainly in young women who believe themselves to be overweight and carry dieting to excess. It is frequently accompanied by amenorrhoea (absence of menstruation). Anorexics always feel cold and have poor blood circulation. Soft downy hair grows all over the body.

Over-use of laxatives prevents water in the food from being absorbed by the colon. This produces a reduction in body weight due to water loss. The person becomes dehydrated which affects the fluid balance and may result in kidney failure or heart attack.

Emotional conflicts are often involved and secretive eating habits are adopted to hide the disease. The person has a distorted body image, believing that they are fat when they are in fact emaciated. Anorexics have very low self-esteem and the eating disorder dominates their life. The condition can develop into a serious nervous disorder, with a mortality rate of around 10%. Medical treatment may be required over several years.

BULIMIA

Bulimia nervosa is a condition where the patient eats enormous meals, then induces vomiting or takes laxatives. Acid vomit damages tooth enamel, and retching may rupture the oesophagus.

THE DIGESTIVE PROCESS

Digestion

Some of the nutrients contained in food are not in a suitable form for absorption by the body, as they do not dissolve in water. Such nutrients must be digested to convert them into simpler soluble substances. Most carbohydrates, fats and proteins need digesting. Minerals and some vitamins are already water-soluble and do not need digesting.

The digestion and absorption of food occurs in the alimentary canal (food canal). Food is pushed along this long tubular structure by the squeezing movements of its walls which are known as peristalsis. Ingestion is the act of taking food into the alimentary canal through the mouth. Elimination (defaecation) is the expulsion from the alimentary canal of the undigested food remains. It occurs through the anus.

During the process of digestion, food is broken down mechanically by the teeth and peristaltic churning movements.

Enzymes

Food is also chemically broken down by a series of digestive juices. Most of these juices contain enzymes, biological catalysts which speed up chemical reactions in the body without being destroyed themselves. Enzymes are proteins synthesised by living glandular cells. They are most active at body temperature (37 °C) and at a specific pH value.

 Define the following terms:
(a) vitamin
(b) enzyme
(c) peristalsis

THE DIGESTIVE ORGANS

The digestive organs consist of the alimentary canal and the accessory organs, which include the teeth, tongue, salivary glands, liver, gallbladder and pancreas.

The alimentary canal

WALL

The wall of the alimentary canal has the same basic structure along its length, having four layers or tunics. On the outside is the serosa tunic, a serous membrane which is part of the peritoneum which attaches the alimentary canal to the wall of the abdominal cavity. Below the serosa is the thick muscularis tunic consisting of smooth muscle as a longitudinal layer outside and a circular layer inside. An autonomic nerve plexus controlling peristalsis occurs between the two muscle layers. Below the muscle layer is the submucosa, a layer of connective tissue which contains many blood vessels. On the inside, lining the lumen or food cavity, is the mucosa consisting of a thin layer of smooth muscle, the muscularis mucosa, attached to a mucous membrane. The mucous membrane is stratified in regions needing protection against friction from the food, or simple in regions where absorption of nutrients occurs.

Figure 7.5   *Structure of wall of alimentary canal (small intestine region)*

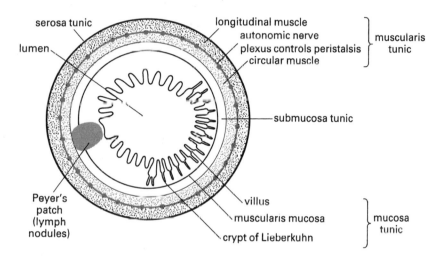

The alimentary canal is divided into several regions of varying length and width, described below.

BUCCAL CAVITY

The buccal cavity is the space inside the mouth, bounded by the cheeks, hard and soft palates and the tongue. It is lined by stratified squamous epithelium. Hanging below the soft palate is the uvula, on each side of which are the palatine tonsils. The lingual tonsils are at the base of the tongue. The tonsils are part of the lymphatic system (see chapter 12).

> **Q** Describe the structure of the ileum wall.

PHARYNX

The pharynx (throat) links the buccal cavity to the oesophagus (gullet) and is lined with stratified squamous epithelium. Although it is both an air and a food passage, when food is being swallowed breathing is temporarily stopped as the larynx (air passage) is closed by the epiglottis. Swallowing begins as a voluntary action, aided by the tongue, but further movement of the food is involuntary by peristalsis.

OESOPHAGUS

The oesophagus is a long narrow tube passing through the thorax, which it leaves through a hole in the diaphragm called the hiatus. Hiatus hernia is the protrusion of the lower end of the oesophagus and the upper part of the stomach into the thoracic cavity through an enlargement of the hiatus. It occurs mainly in women over 50 years of age, as a result of previous pregnancy, obesity or continual lifting of heavy weights. The oesophagus is lined by a stratified squamous epithelium and secretes mucus as a lubricant to aid peristalsis. Just below the diaphragm it opens into the stomach.

STOMACH

The stomach occurs in the upper left region of the abdominal cavity. It is a curved enlargement of the alimentary canal, divided into four regions: the cardia, fundus, body and pylorus.

- The upper region, or cardia, is separated from the oesophagus by the cardiac sphincter, a ring-shaped muscle which, on contracting, narrows the opening between the oesophagus and the stomach. It relaxes during swallowing so that food can pass into the stomach. It contracts to retain food in the stomach, but relaxes when the reflex action of vomiting occurs.

- Above and to the left of the cardia is the fundus of the stomach.

- Below is the large central region or body of the stomach, where the mucosa lies in large folds (rugae) which smooth out as the stomach fills.

- The stomach then narrows at the pylorus region, where it opens into the small intestine. The pyloric sphincter is a ring of muscle controlling this opening. It contracts to retain food in the stomach for around three to four hours, by which time the food has been converted into a creamy suspension called chyme.

The stomach mucosa contains gastric glands with three types of cells:

(a) peptic cells at the base of the glands, which secrete pepsinogen;

(b) oxyntic cells which secrete hydrochloric acid that activates pepsinogen to form the enzyme pepsin;

(c) goblet cells at the top of the glands which secrete a thick mucus to protect the stomach wall from damage by the acid and enzyme in the gastric juice. Very vigorous peristaltic movements in the stomach churn the food and mix it with the gastric juice.

Figure 7.6   *Digestive organs (transverse colon removed)*

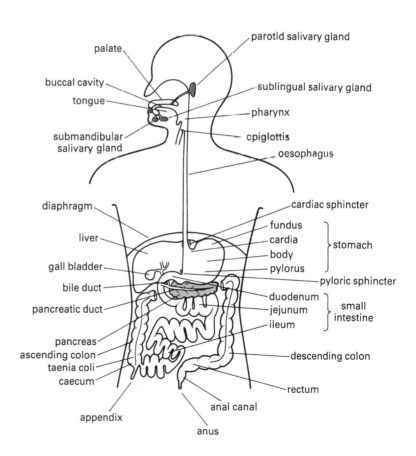

SMALL INTESTINE

The small intestine is divided into three parts: the duodenum, the jejunum, and the ileum. The duodenum begins at the pyloric sphincter and is 25 cm long. It merges with the narrower jejunum, which is 2.5 m long and leads into the ileum, whose length is 3.6 m. The coils of the small intestine are bound together and to the abdominal wall by a membrane, the mesentery, which is part of the peritoneum.

- The walls of the small intestine contain glands which secrete a digestive juice from deep pits in the mucosa called crypts of Lieberkuhn. In the duodenum only, the submucosa contains Brunner's glands which secrete an alkaline mucus to neutralise stomach acids and protect the wall of the duodenum from ulceration.

- The mucosa of the small intestine has small finger-like projections called villi, which increase the internal surface area enormously to aid the absorption of digested nutrients. The villi are covered by a simple columnar epithelium so that nutrients can pass through easily. The epithelial cells have tiny microvilli projecting from their free surface, which further increase the absorptive area. Goblet cells occur amongst the epithelial cells to secrete mucus. Each villus contains a central lymphatic duct, surrounded by a network of blood capillaries.

- Lymph nodules in groups called Peyer's patches occur in the mucosa and submucosa of the ileum. They act as a defence against harmful bacteria in the alimentary canal.

Figure 7.7   *Villus in small intestine*

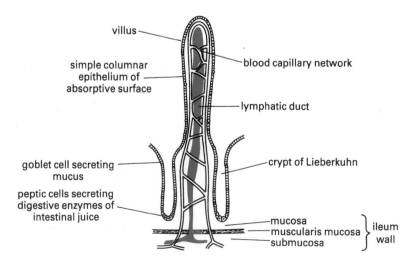

| Q | Explain the functions of:
(a) the pyloric sphincter
(b) the mesentery
(c) villi |

LARGE INTESTINE

The large intestine is 1.5 m long and twice as wide as the small intestine. It extends from the ileum to its opening at the anus. It is divided into four regions: the caecum, the colon, the rectum, and the anal canal.

- The opening into the caecum from the ileum is guarded by a fold of membrane called the ileocaecal valve. The caecum is 6 cm long and ends in a narrow, closed tube 8 cm long, called the vermiform appendix. At the other end the caecum leads into the colon. The caecum and appendix have no known function in human digestion.

- The colon has ascending, transverse and descending portions, ending in the pelvic colon which leads into the rectum. It is 1.3 m long. The longitudinal muscle of its wall consists of three strips only, the taenia coli, which are shorter than the colon in length and pucker its wall. There are no villi in the mucosa, which is bounded by a simple columnar epithelium containing goblet cells to secrete mucus.

- The rectum is the continuation of the colon and lies anterior to the sacrum in the pelvic cavity. It is 20 cm long and its last few centimetres form the anal canal.

- The anal canal has longitudinal folds in its highly vascular lining. Inflammation of the anal veins results in haemorrhoids (piles). At the external end of the anal canal is the anal sphincter, which contracts to close the anus. The sphincter consists of an internal ring of smooth muscle and an external ring of skeletal (voluntary) muscle. The anus normally remains closed except during the elimination of the undigested food remains (faeces).

The accessory organs

TEETH

The teeth of the permanent dentition occupy sockets in the maxillae and mandible. Teeth are composed of bone-like dentine, and consist of a crown above the gum and a root embedded in the socket. The crown has a thin covering of very hard enamel, while the root is covered by a layer of cement. The tooth socket is lined by a fibrous periodontal membrane attached to the cement, which anchors the tooth in the jaw and acts as a shock absorber. In the centre of the dentine is a pulp cavity. Pulp is a connective tissue containing nerves and blood vessels which enter the tooth through the root.

The 32 teeth vary in shape and function, and can be represented by a dental formula viz: $i\frac{2}{2}$ $c\frac{1}{1}$ $p\frac{2}{2}$ $m\frac{3}{3}$, giving the numbers of teeth of each type on one side of the jaws.

- Incisors (i) are chisel-shaped teeth used to cut food.

- Canines (c) are pointed and tear food.

- Premolars (p) and molars (m) have flattened surfaces with small projections called cusps, and grind or crush food.

TONGUE

The tongue forms the floor of the buccal cavity. A fold of mucous membrane called the lingual frenulum is attached to the underside of the tongue to anchor it in the buccal cavity. The surface of the tongue is roughened by small projections called papillae, and it carries taste buds which respond to chemical stimuli (sour, salt, bitter and sweet).

SALIVARY GLANDS

Three pairs of salivary glands open into the buccal cavity.

- The parotid pair lie below and in front of the ears, on top of the masseter muscle. Their ducts open opposite the upper second molar teeth.

- The submandibular pair occur posteriorly below the tongue. Their ducts open behind the middle lower incisors.

- The sublingual pair occur anteriorly below the tongue and have several ducts opening into the floor of the buccal cavity.

The parotids are compound tubuloacinar glands, while the other two pairs are of the compound acinar type. The glands produce a digestive juice called saliva, but the secretions of the individual glands vary. The parotids secrete a thin, watery liquid containing the enzyme salivary amylase (pytalin). The submandibulars also secrete this enzyme, but as they produce mucus the secretion is thicker. The sublingual secretion contains mainly mucus.

Saliva contains 99.5% water and provides the solvent for food. It is slightly acidic due to the action of mouth bacteria on food debris, with a pH between 6.5 and 6.9. The mucus in saliva lubricates the food so that it is easily swallowed. The secretion of saliva is a reflex action in response to taste stimuli from the tongue. The smell and sight of food also stimulate saliva secretion.

 Q | Describe the composition and action of the secretion produced by the salivary glands.

LIVER

The liver occurs on the right side of the abdominal cavity under the diaphragm, to which it is attached by the falciform ligament. It is a large, red, glandular organ, covered by a fibrous capsule and composed of several lobes. It has a small left lobe and a larger right lobe which is subdivided into caudate and quadrate lobes.

- The liver consists of a large number of lobules, which are hexagonal blocks of hepatic cells. The vertical plates of hepatic cells radiate from a central hepatic vein branch in each lobule. The hepatic veins return blood to the heart from the liver.

- The blood supply to each lobule comes from two vessels. The hepatic artery brings oxygen-containing blood from the heart, while the hepatic portal vein brings digested food from the small intestine. Branches of these vessels occur in spaces between the liver lobules.

- Between the plates of hepatic cells in the lobules are narrow channels called canaliculi. The hepatic cells secrete the digestive juice bile into the canaliculi, which carry it to the bile ducts between the lobules.

- Bile is a greenish alkaline fluid containing bile salts (sodium bicarbonate, glycocholate, and taurate) and the bile pigments bilirubin and biliverdin produced from worn out red blood cells.

- Alternating with the canaliculi are similar spaces called sinusoids, in which blood passes from the hepatic artery and hepatic portal vein branches to the central hepatic vein branches.

Figure 7.8   *Blood supply of liver lobule*
(a)   Side view
(b)   Cross-section

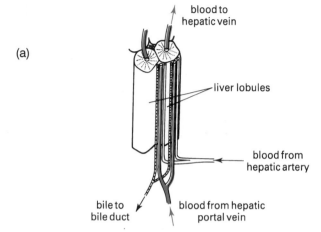

(a)

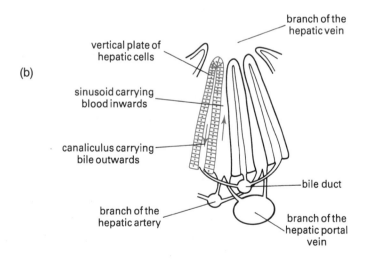

(b)

GALL BLADDER

The gall bladder is a sac on the underside of the liver. Its inner wall is thrown into folds which allow it to expand as it fills with bile from the liver. Contraction of its muscular wall forces the stored bile into the main bile duct which opens into the duodenum.

PANCREAS

The pancreas is a compound tubuloacinar gland lying below the stomach. It contains small clusters of glandular epithelial cells of two types.

• One type, the islets of Langerhans, are endocrine glands secreting the hormones insulin and glucagon into the blood stream.

• The other type, the acini, are exocrine glands secreting pancreatic digestive juice which passes down the pancreatic duct to the duodenum.

Just before reaching the duodenum the pancreatic duct joins the bile duct, both ducts opening together just below the pyloric sphincter.

CHEMICAL DIGESTION

The food broken down by the teeth is rolled round the buccal cavity by the tongue and mixed with saliva.

Peristalsis

Each swallowed food mass (bolus) then travels the length of the alimentary canal by peristaltic movements.

Digestive juices

The food is acted upon by a series of digestive juices which chemically break it down into simpler soluble nutrients.

Regulation

The smell and sight of food, and its presence in the alimentary canal, stimulate the autonomic nervous system and the secretion of certain hormones, which regulate the ordered secretion of the digestive juices.

End products

The end products of this chemical digestion are simple sugars from carbohydrates, amino acids from proteins, and fatty acids and glycerol from fats. The actions of the digestive juices are shown in table 7.6.

Table 7.6   *Chemical digestion in the alimentary canal*

Region where digestion occurs	Digestive glands	Digestive juice	Enzymes present	Food acted on	Nutrients produced
Buccal cavity (continuing in oesophagus)	Salivary (three pairs)	Saliva (slightly acid)	Salivary amylase	Cooked starch	Maltose sugar
Stomach	Gastric (in stomach wall)	Gastric (acid)	Pepsin (activated by acid)	Protein	Peptides
Duodenum	Pancreas	Pancreatic (alkaline)	Trypsin (activated by enterokinase)	Protein and peptides	Dipeptides and amino acids
			Pancreatic amylase	Starch	Maltose sugar
			Lipase	Fats	Fatty acids and glycerol
	Brunner's (in duodenal wall)	Intestinal (alkaline)	Protease	Protein and peptides	Amino acids
	Liver	Bile (alkaline)	None	Bile salts act on fats	Emulsified fat
Jejunum and Ileum	Crypts of Lieberkuhn (in intestine wall)	Intestinal (slightly alkaline)	Erepsin Lipase	Peptides Fats	Amino acids Fatty acids and glycerol
			Maltase Amylase Lactase (Enterokinase)	Maltose Starch Lactose (Trypsinogen)	Glucose Maltose Simple sugars (Trypsin)

 Q Describe the composition and functions of bile.

ABSORPTION

The soluble nutrients from food are able to diffuse through the mucosa of the alimentary canal wall and enter the body's transport systems, the blood or lymph vessels.

In the stomach

The stomach absorbs alcohol, which enters the blood capillaries in the stomach wall. Absorption of alcohol occurs very rapidly once it has been consumed, particularly when the stomach is empty.

In the small intestine

The small intestine absorbs most of the nutrients through the villi, which contain smooth muscle and are able to move about gently, to bring them into close contact with the digested food. Glucose and amino acids are absorbed by a combination of diffusion and active transport. They pass into the capillary networks of the villi which drain into the hepatic portal vein. Fatty acids and glycerol pass into the columnar epithelial cells of the villi by pinocytosis. Here they are converted back into fat droplets and enter the lymph vessels as a white emulsion. The fat is carried by the lymphatic system to the blood in the main veins. Fat-soluble vitamins are also absorbed in this way. Inorganic salts and water-soluble vitamins are absorbed into the blood capillary networks of the villi.

In the colon

The colon absorbs much of the water from the undigested food remains. If this material contains large amounts of dietary fibre, less water is removed from it and it remains much softer. The water-holding properties of fibre allow the soft undigested food remains to pass quickly through the intestine and be easily eliminated.

SYMBIONTS

Fibre (cellulose) can be broken down by bacteria in the large intestine, and some of the by-products are the gases carbon dioxide and methane, leading to some flatulence. Other by-products are some of the vitamins, e.g. folic acid and biotin. Such bacteria are described as symbiotic because both they, and their human carrier, obtain benefit from the association. The bacteria obtain food and a protected environment, while the person obtains extra nutrients. By the time the food remains reach the rectum they have become faeces.

METABOLISM

Metabolism involves all the chemical activities of the body and the use or production of energy.

Assimilation

Once nutrients have been absorbed from the alimentary canal and enter the blood, they are taken to the living cells of all the body's tissues and become involved in cell metabolism. This is known as nutrient assimilation.

Carbohydrate metabolism

Glucose is the end product of carbohydrate digestion. It is used by living cells as the preferred source of energy. The level of glucose in the blood is kept constant by the activity of the hepatic cells of the liver, regulated by the pancreatic hormones and adrenalin. Excess glucose is either converted into glycogen and stored in the hepatic cells, or converted into fatty acids and carried by the blood to the body's fat deposits for storage.

If the diet contains insufficient carbohydrate for the body's needs, stored glycogen and fat are converted back to glucose by the liver to maintain the blood glucose level. Thus the liver has a homeostatic function: keeping the blood glucose level constant.

 Q Distinguish between (a) absorption and (b) assimilation, in relation to carbohydrate nutrients.

Fat metabolism

The end products of fat digestion are fatty acids and glycerol, used as an energy source in addition to glucose. In a normal balanced diet, 35% of the body's energy comes from fat. The liver cells can convert glycerol to glucose, which is then used as described above. Fatty acids cannot be converted into glucose, but are broken down by a series of chemical changes called beta-oxidation. Incomplete breakdown of fatty acids (ketosis) produces an increased level of blood ketones (e.g. acetone) which are harmful. Ketones may escape from the blood into the lungs and appear in the breath. This commonly happens in diabetics. Excess fat in the diet is stored in the body's fat deposits.

Protein metabolism

The end products of protein digestion are amino acids. In the body cells they are built up into new protein molecules required for building new tissues and for enzyme synthesis. If there is no other energy nutrient available, protein can be broken down by the liver and used to produce energy.

DEAMINATION

The first stage in protein breakdown is called deamination, during which the nitrogen-containing amino group is removed, and converted into urea to be excreted in the urine. The rest of the amino acid molecule is used to provide energy. Surplus amino acids from the dietary proteins cannot be stored by the body, so they too are deaminated and used for energy. Proteins extracted from worn out cells are broken down into their constituent amino acids in the liver and used similarly. There is a continuous turnover of proteins in the body cells.

Functions of the liver in metabolism

As a result of its functions in carbohydrate, fat and protein metabolism, the liver produces a lot of heat from chemical reactions. This heat is transferred to the blood which distributes it to cooler parts of the body.

The liver also synthesises cholesterol. Excess cholesterol from dietary fats is excreted in the bile, where a high concentration may produce gallstones during storage. The liver secretes a chemical which stimulates the red bone marrow to produce new red blood cells. This chemical can only be secreted if Vitamin B12 is available. The liver also breaks down worn out red blood cells forming the bile pigments in the process. The veins in the liver act as a blood reservoir, so the liver stores blood. The liver synthesises the plasma proteins of the blood.

Sex hormones are broken down in the liver once they are no longer required. The liver stores minerals such as iron, copper and potassium, and Vitamins A, D, E, K and B12. It can deal with some poisons, converting them into less toxic substances or storing them to prevent harm to more sensitive tissues.

 List six major functions of the liver.

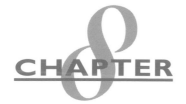

CHAPTER 8

The Respiratory System

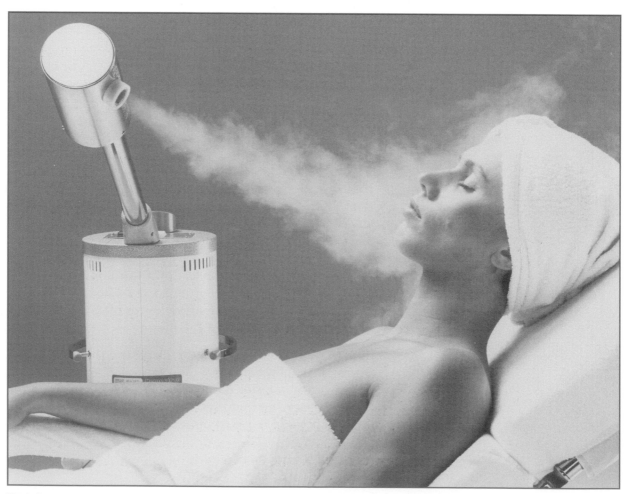

Facial steamer

RESPIRATION

Respiration is the process by which the body obtains a supply of energy by breaking down nutrients. This process occurs in every living cell of the body tissues and is part of cell metabolism.

Aerobic and anaerobic

The chemical reactions involved in cell respiration may be aerobic, if oxygen is required, or anaerobic if they occur in the absence of oxygen. Anaerobic respiration occurs in the cells of actively contracting muscle, while resting muscle cells respire aerobically. The cells of other tissues respire aerobically all the time. The complete chemical breakdown of glucose molecules to supply energy occurs in the presence of oxygen. Anaerobic respiration results in the partial or incomplete breakdown of glucose molecules and releases less energy. Respiratory enzymes act as catalysts during the chemical breakdown of energy foods in all the living body cells.

During aerobic cell respiration, carbon dioxide is liberated and oxygen is used up. The tissues therefore require a continuous supply of oxygen from the blood. As carbon dioxide is acidic and toxic to living cells, the blood must continuously remove it from the tissues, together with other toxic waste products. The oxygen supply is obtained from the air, and the carbon dioxide is expelled into the air. Table 8.1 shows the way the composition of the air is changed by human respiration.

Table 8.1   *Composition of air*

Gases in the air	Composition in volumes %	
	Air breathed in (inspired)	**Air breathed out (expired)**
Oxygen	21	17
Carbon dioxide	0.03	4
Water vapour	variable	increased
Nitrogen	78	78
Rare gases	0.9	0.9

The process by which air enters and leaves the body is known as breathing or ventilation. External respiration is the exchange of gases between the lungs and the blood. Internal respiration is the exchange of gases between the blood and the living cells of the body tissues.

SUMMARY

The release of energy from nutrients occurring in living cells is called respiration. Where the process requires oxygen, as in most tissues, aerobic respiration occurs. If energy is released in the absence of oxygen, as in contracting muscle, anaerobic respiration occurs.

 Distinguish between aerobic and anaerobic respiration. In each case, give one example of a tissue in which the process occurs.

RESPIRATORY ORGANS

The air must be brought into contact with a vascular respiratory surface, where the exchange of oxygen and carbon dioxide gases can occur during external respiration. Substantial amounts of water will evaporate from such a surface. To prevent dehydration by reducing evaporation, the respiratory surface occurs inside the lungs. A system of tubes connects the lungs to the outside air. The nose, nasopharynx, pharynx, larynx, bronchi, and the bronchioles and alveoli of the lungs, form the respiratory organs.

Figure 8.1   *Section through head to show respiratory organs (side view)*

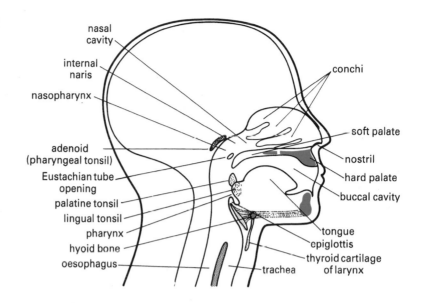

Nose

STRUCTURE

The nose consists of two nasal cavities, opening to the outside at the nostrils (external nares). Internally the nasal cavities connect with the nasopharynx by two internal nares. A vertical partition, the nasal septum, separates the nasal cavities which are roofed by the nasal bones and nasal cartilage. The floor of the nasal cavities is formed by the palate.

The ethmoid conchi and turbinate bones subdivide each nasal cavity into three groove-like air passages lined with a mucous membrane containing ciliated and goblet cells. These scroll-shaped bones provide a large surface area for the membrane. The mucus secreted traps dust and bacteria entering with the air, and the outward beating of the cilia keeps dirt out of the lungs.

FUNCTIONS

The functions of the nose are to moisten, warm and filter the air breathed in. It acts as the organ of smell and as a resonating chamber for the voice.

 Describe the structure and functions of the nose.

Nasopharynx

The nasopharynx is the upper part of the cavity behind the nose, and is lined with mucous membrane. The two Eustachian tubes from the middle ears open into it so that air pressure inside the ear can be adjusted to prevent damage to the ear drum.

ADENOIDS

The posterior wall of the nasopharynx carries the pharyngeal tonsil composed of lymphoid tissue. When enlarged it is known as the adenoids, and can block the internal nares and cause mouth-breathing, with the loss of the protective function of nose-breathing.

Pharynx

STRUCTURE

The pharynx (throat) is a continuation of the nasopharynx, extending to the larynx (voice box) in the neck. It is lined with a protective stratified squamous epithelium. The palatine and lingual tonsils occur on its lateral walls.

FUNCTIONS

The functions of the pharynx are to act as both an air and a food passage, and as a resonating chamber for the voice.

Larynx

STRUCTURE

The larynx is a short passage connecting the pharynx to the trachea (windpipe). It opens from the pharynx at a slit-like glottis. Its walls are supported by nine pieces of cartilage, one of which is the thyroid cartilage or Adam's apple. These cartilages hold the air passage permanently open.

EPIGLOTTIS

The epiglottis is a leaf-shaped piece of cartilage lying on top of the larynx. It closes the glottis when food is swallowed, which prevents food going down the wrong way and blocking the air passage.

VOCAL CORDS

Two pairs of folds in the larynx wall form the vocal cords on each side of the glottis. When the muscles attached to these cords contract, the space between them is narrowed. When air passes the vocal cords, they vibrate and cause sound waves in the air in the pharynx, nose and buccal cavity.

Trachea

The trachea extends into the thorax from the larynx, and is a narrow tube 11 cm long. Its wall is composed of three layers. On the inside is a pseudostratified ciliated epithelium which secretes mucus. The middle layer is composed of elastic connective tissue. The outer layer contains approximately 20 C-shaped bands of hyaline cartilage to keep the trachea permanently open. The open ends of the cartilages are posterior, so that where the trachea touches the oesophagus, food boluses in the oesophagus can bulge slightly into the trachea as they are swallowed.

 Describe the structure of the tracheal wall. How is the structure of the wall related to the function of the trachea?

Bronchi

The two bronchi are formed by forking of the lower end of the trachea. They carry the air into the lungs. The right bronchus is only half as long as the left bronchus and is nearly vertical. The walls of the bronchi are lined by a ciliated columnar epithelium and, like the trachea, contain C-shaped cartilages to hold them open.

Lungs

POSITION

The lungs lie on each side of the thoracic cavity, extending from the clavicles to the diaphragm. They are roughly conical in shape and both are lobed. The right lung has three lobes and the left lung has two. Each lung is enclosed in a pleural membrane and another pleural membrane lines the thoracic cavity.

Between the pleura there is a cavity containing a lubricating fluid, allowing the lungs to slide freely over the thoracic wall during breathing. The medial surface of each lung contains a vertical slit called the hilus. The pulmonary blood vessels, nerves and bronchi enter or leave the lung at the hilus. The left lung has a cardial notch, a medial depression into which the heart fits.

Figure 8.2   *Respiratory organs of the thorax (anterior view)*

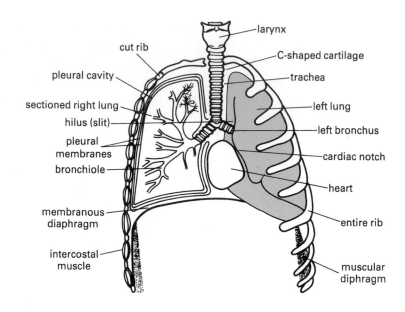

BRONCHIOLES

Within the lungs each bronchus subdivides forming a tree-like system of bronchioles, which become progressively narrower. The walls of the wider bronchioles are supported by small plates of cartilage, while those of the narrower terminal bronchioles contain smooth muscle but no cartilage supports. The columnar ciliated epithelium lining the walls of the wider bronchioles changes to a squamous epithelium in the terminal bronchioles, where no goblet cells secreting mucus are present.

ALVEOLI

Alveoli are cup-shaped cavities within the lungs. They are lined by a thin film of water, essential for dissolving oxygen from the alveolar air. The alveoli are grouped round an air space, the alveolar duct, which leads from a terminal bronchiole.

Figure 8.3   *Functional unit of the lung*

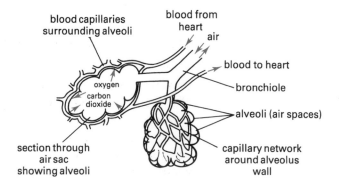

The alveolar wall consists of two types of epithelial cells. It is a simple squamous epithelium with interspersed septal cells, which are cuboid and secrete a detergent-like chemical to lower the surface tension of the water film and allow the alveoli to expand so that air can enter. Phagocytes (dust cells) also occur in the alveolar wall to remove foreign particles which have entered the lungs.

On the outer side of the alveolar wall is a network of blood capillaries, linking branches of the pulmonary arteries with branches of the pulmonary veins. The lungs contain around 300 million alveoli and provide an enormous respiratory surface for the exchange of gases.

SUMMARY

The respiratory organs are a system of tubes and spaces which bring atmospheric air into contact with a respiratory surface where the gases oxygen and carbon dioxide can be exchanged between the air and the blood.

 Q What is the function of each of the following?
(a) pleural membranes
(b) septal cells
(c) phagocytes

BREATHING OR VENTILATION

Breathing or ventilation is the passage of air into and out of the lungs, known as inspiration and expiration respectively.

Pressure and volume changes

The pressure inside the thoracic cavity is increased to cause expiration and decreased to cause inspiration. The pressure changes are brought about by volume changes of the thoracic cavity. Reducing the volume of the thorax increases the pressure on the lungs, leading to expiration. Increasing the volume of the thorax reduces the pressure on the lungs by causing a partial vacuum which draws air into the lungs during inspiration.

RESPIRATORY MUSCLES

These volume changes are caused by the external intercostal muscles between the ribs, and the diaphragm muscle. The muscles contract to cause inspiration and relax to cause expiration. Contraction of the external intercostal muscles lifts the ribs and pushes the sternum forward. This increases the dimensions of the thorax from back to front and increases its circumference. Contraction of the radiating diaphragm muscles flattens the diaphragm by decreasing its surface area, and increases the dimensions of the thorax from top to bottom.

Figure 8.4   *Changes in volume of the thorax*
(a)   Due to intercostal muscles
(b)   Due to diaphragm muscles

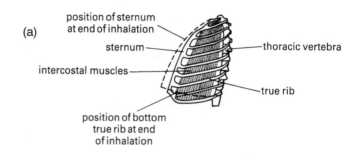

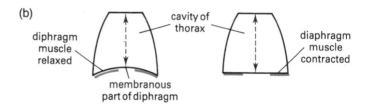

Both sets of muscles relax to decrease the volume of the thorax. The ribs then slope downwards and the sternum moves inwards, reducing the circumference of the thorax. The stomach and liver push the relaxed diaphragm upwards so that it bulges up into the thoracic cavity. The respiratory muscles contract and relax alternately, so inspiration and expiration alternate.

RESPIRATORY VOLUMES

A respiratory centre in the brain stem controls these reflex breathing movements. A person at rest takes in and gives out only 0.5 litre of air with each breath. This is known as the tidal volume. The tidal volume multiplied by the rate of respiration per minute is called the minute volume. The number of breaths per minute varies between 12 and 20, so the minute volume varies between 6 litres (0.5 × 12) and 10 litres (0.5 × 20). The total lung capacity is about 5 litres of air while the tidal volume is only 0.5 litre, so only one-tenth of the air is exchanged during each quiet breath.

By taking a deep breath, an extra 3 litres of air will enter the lungs and be expelled when breathing out. The 3.5 litres of air entering and leaving the lungs during deep breathing is the vital capacity. It is the maximum volume of air that can be exchanged during breathing. The remaining 1.5 litres of air which is not expelled is the residual volume. The lungs therefore never collapse completely during ventilation. The functional residual capacity is the air remaining in the lungs throughout normal quiet breathing. These volumes are measured by an instrument called a recording spirometer which produces a tracing similar to that in figure 8.5.

Figure 8.5   *Recording spirometer tracing*

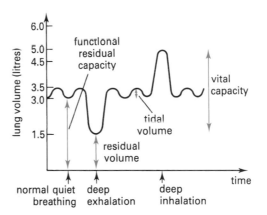

SUMMARY

Breathing (ventilation) is the passage of air into and out of the lungs. Respiratory muscles contract to reduce pressure on the lungs increasing their volume so that air is drawn in. When the muscles relax the lungs are compressed and air is forced out. The brain stem controls these reflex breathing movements. The volume of air exchanged is greater during a deep breath than in a normal quiet breath, but some air always remains in the lungs to prevent their collapse.

Distinguish between residual volume, minute volume and tidal volume, in relation to breathing.

EXTERNAL RESPIRATION

This is the exchange of the gases oxygen and carbon dioxide between the blood in the capillaries covering the alveoli walls and the air in the alveolar cavities.

Pulmonary circulation

The deoxygenated blood entering the lungs in the pulmonary arteries becomes oxygenated as it flows through the capillaries, then returns to the heart in the pulmonary veins. This movement of the blood, from the heart to the lungs and back again, is known as the pulmonary circulation.

Gaseous diffusion

The enormous surface area of the alveoli and the narrowness of the blood capillaries gives the maximum surface exposure for

Figure 8.6   *External respiration*

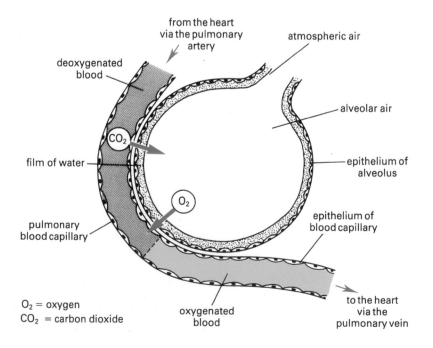

O_2 = oxygen
CO_2 = carbon dioxide

gaseous exchange. The thinness of the alveolar and blood capillary walls allow the dissolved gases to diffuse across very readily. Diffusion of the oxygen and carbon dioxide depends on the difference in the amount of each gas present in the alveolar air and in the blood. As there is more oxygen in the alveolar air and less in the blood, oxygen will diffuse into the blood. The higher concentration of carbon dioxide in the deoxygenated blood in the pulmonary capillaries causes it to diffuse into the alveolar air spaces.

SUMMARY

External respiration occurs in the alveoli of the lungs. Oxygen diffuses from the air in the alveoli into the blood in the capillaries surrounding the alveoli walls, while carbon dioxide diffuses in the opposite direction.

INTERNAL RESPIRATION

This is the exchange of oxygen and carbon dioxide between the blood and the living cells of the body tissues. During this process the oxygenated blood in the tissue capillaries becomes deoxygenated.

Figure 8.7   *Internal respiration*

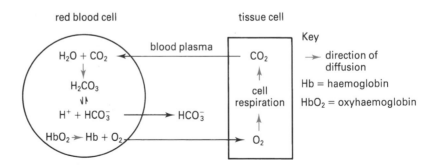

Gaseous diffusion

The different concentrations of oxygen and carbon dioxide in the blood and body cells results in gaseous exchange by diffusion. Oxygen diffuses from the blood into the body cells, and carbon dioxide formed in the body cells diffuses into the blood.

 Q | Distinguish between external and internal respiration.

Role of haemoglobin

Inside the red blood cells, oxygen is carried by haemoglobin as bright red oxyhaemoglobin. Where living tissue cells are using up oxygen rapidly so the oxygen concentration in the cells remains low, oxyhaemoglobin readily releases its oxygen. The oxygen dissolves in the blood plasma and diffuses into the tissue cells. The deoxygenated haemoglobin is purple in colour.

Role of enzyme

Carbon dioxide diffuses in solution from the living tissue cells into the blood in the tissue capillaries. The red blood cells contain an enzyme which speeds up the reaction between carbon dioxide and water to form carbonic acid.

$$CO_2 + H_2O \xrightarrow{\text{enzyme}} H_2CO_3$$

The carbonic acid splits up into ions, forming positive hydrogen ions (H^+) and negative hydrogen carbonate ions (HCO_3^-).

$$H_2CO_3 \rightleftharpoons H^+ + HCO_3^-$$

The hydrogen carbonate ions can readily pass through the wall of red blood cells so they diffuse out into the blood plasma because of the concentration gradient between the red cells (high) and the plasma (low).

SUMMARY

Internal respiration occurs in the body tissues. Oxygen from the blood in the tissue capillaries diffuses into the living cells of the tissue, and carbon dioxide from the cells diffuses into the blood.

METABOLIC RATE

The rate at which the body produces energy by breaking down nutrients is the metabolic rate. This is affected by various factors. It increases during exercise, nervous stress and high body temperature. It decreases during relaxation and sleep.

Basal metabolic rate (BMR)

The body requires a certain amount of energy daily just to keep alive – to maintain its basal metabolism. Basal metabolic rate (BMR) is a measure of how fast the body cells break down energy nutrients to release enough energy just to stay alive. The rate of oxygen consumption and carbon dioxide production are convenient ways of measuring BMR, which accounts for around 60% of the daily energy expenditure.

Respiratory quotient

The volume of carbon dioxide produced, divided by the volume of oxygen used up in a definite time, is called the respiratory quotient (RQ).

$$RQ = \frac{\text{volume of } CO_2 \text{ produced}}{\text{volume of } O_2 \text{ used}}$$

During aerobic respiration, if the energy nutrient is solely glucose, equal volumes of oxygen and carbon dioxide are exchanged and the RQ = 6/6 = 1.

$$C_6H_{12}O_6 + 6\ O_2 \rightarrow 6\ CO_2 + 6\ H_2O$$
$$\text{(glucose)} \qquad \underbrace{\qquad\qquad}$$
$$\text{(equal volumes)}$$

When triglyceride (fat) alone is the energy source, as more oxygen is used up than carbon dioxide produced, the fraction is less than one and the RQ = 0.7. When protein alone is the energy source, the RQ = 0.99. Using a mixture of these three energy sources gives an RQ of between 0.8 and 0.9. A balanced diet gives an RQ of 0.85, showing that both carbohydrates and fats are used as energy sources.

Aerobic pathway

In most body cells, aerobic respiration occurs. Glucose is first broken down to pyruvic acid by a series of anaerobic reactions called glycolysis. The further breakdown of pyruvic acid into carbon dioxide and water cannot occur unless oxygen is present, and is the aerobic phase of the process.

ATP

The energy released from the glucose molecules is stored in ATP molecules. In all the living body cells, ADP molecules and phosphate ions are present. The energy released from the breakdown of glucose is used to join a phosphate ion to an ADP molecule by a high energy bond. This forms an ATP molecule, which stores the energy temporarily. When the cell requires energy for its metabolism, ATP molecules release it by breaking their high energy bonds, and reforming ADP molecules and phosphate ions.

(i)   ADP + phosphate + energy (from glucose) → ATP

(ii)   ATP → ADP + phosphate + energy (for cell's use)

 Q | What is the molecule which temporarily stores energy for use in the cell? From what components is this molecule formed?

RELAXED MUSCLE

When a muscle is not contracting, the breakdown of glucose occurs only slowly as very little energy is required by the muscle. The blood supplying the muscle is able to bring sufficient oxygen for the complete breakdown of glucose to carbon dioxide and water to occur by aerobic respiration.

Anaerobic pathway

CONTRACTING MUSCLE

During anaerobic respiration, which occurs in vigorously contracting muscle cells, glucose is incompletely broken down, as the blood is unable to supply oxygen fast enough for aerobic respiration to occur. The glucose is first converted to pyruvic acid, which is then partially broken down into lactic acid. About 80% of the lactic acid is carried to the liver by the blood. In the liver it is converted back into glucose which can be used again as an energy source. Some of the lactic acid accumulates in the muscle tissue causing muscle fatigue.

OXYGEN DEBT

This toxic lactic acid must eventually be removed by breaking it down into carbon dioxide and water by reactions requiring additional oxygen, known as the oxygen debt. After vigorous exercise, deep breathing occurs to obtain this extra oxygen to pay back the oxygen debt.

SUMMARY

The metabolic rate can be obtained by measuring the rate of oxygen consumption or carbon dioxide production as the body cells break down energy nutrients. Energy is released during a series of biochemical reactions known as a metabolic pathway, which may be aerobic or anaerobic. The energy released is stored in ATP molecules and later released in living cells which require energy for their metabolism.

 Describe the process of respiration in a vigorously contracting muscle cell.

DISORDERS OF THE RESPIRATORY SYSTEM

All the following disorders contra-indicate facial massage and electrical muscle stimulation

- **Rhinitis** is inflammation of the mucous membrane lining the nasal cavities and covering the conchi. The membrane swells and blocks the free flow of air through the nose. There is increased secretion of a watery mucus.

- **Hay fever** is an allergic reaction to foreign proteins, usually those in pollen. The respiratory membranes become inflamed and a watery fluid exudes from the eyes and nose. The allergy has a genetic cause. It runs in families and is related to asthma and eczema.

- **Bronchial asthma** is an allergic reaction to foreign proteins, either eaten or breathed in, such as wheat products or house dust. It is characterised by attacks of wheezing and difficulty in breathing. It is caused by spasms of the smooth muscle in the walls of the bronchioles, which partly closes their air passageway. The bronchi often become clogged with mucus. Breathing out is especially difficult during these spasms.

- A **common cold** is a rhino-viral infection of the mucous membrane lining the nasal cavities. This predisposes the membrane to further attack by bacteria, which cause the secretion of thick mucus in place of the clear nasal discharge of the viral infection. Sore throat, sneezing, slight fever and headache commonly occur. It is most readily transmitted by touching with contaminated fingers, rather than by droplet infection from sneezing and coughing. Frequent hand washing, and avoiding touching the face, particularly the eyes and nose, are the best preventive measures against transmitting the virus to others.

- **Influenza** is a viral infection of the respiratory system causing a feverish illness. It is readily transmitted by droplet infection, particularly during the first few days of the illness. The symptoms are a raised temperature, shivering, sore throat, cough and eye pain. Viral pneumonia can be a serious complication. Antibiotics are ineffective in destroying the virus. Flu injections will protect vulnerable people during epidemics.

 Name two respiratory disorders which are allergic reactions and two which are viral infections.

SMOKING AND HEALTH

Irritants

If tobacco smoke is inhaled, solid particles and tar droplets enter the trachea and bronchi. The irritant chemicals from the smoke kill the cilia of the epithelial cells lining the upper respiratory passages, and cause the goblet cells to secrete excessive mucus. As the cilia become ineffective, mucus impregnated with solid particles and tar droplets remains in the bronchial tubes instead of being carried upwards towards the pharynx. Attempts to clear this mucus result in 'smoker's cough'.

The irritant chemicals trapped in the lungs slowly destroy the alveoli, greatly reducing the surface for gaseous exchange. Emphysema results. The loss of elasticity in the lungs causes them to be permanently inflated as the alveoli are replaced by fibrous connective tissue. The lungs then tend to succumb to other respiratory infections, such as bronchitis or pneumonia. Prolonged contact with the irritant chemicals may finally cause lung cancer. Giving up smoking at any time reduces the chance of dying from lung cancer.

Carbon monoxide

The raised level of carbon monoxide in tobacco smoke reaches the blood and is irreversibly combined with haemoglobin to form carboxyhaemoglobin. This means that the blood has less haemoglobin for carrying oxygen, which reduces the supply to the extremities. This can make limb amputations necessary. The permeability of the blood vessels is increased, leading to a higher rate of fatty deposition in the arteries (atherosclerosis), with an increased risk of coronary heart disease. Carbon monoxide may be one of the factors involved in hypertension (high blood pressure).

In pregnancy

Women who smoke during pregnancy produce babies up to 0.23 kg lighter than average, and are more likely to miscarry or have a still-born child.

Addiction

Nicotine is the drug present in tobacco smoke which causes addiction, as it is a 'mood altering' drug. The nicotine passes from inhaled smoke through the alveoli walls in the lungs into the blood, which carries it to the brain. Here it acts as a stimulant, increasing the activity of the brain and increasing the heart rate by up to fifteen beats per minute.

Passive smoking

The smoke exhaled by tobacco smokers contains many dangerous chemicals such as carbon monoxide, cyanide, arsenic and benzine. The smoke coming directly from a cigarette between puffs contains an even higher proportion of these toxic substances. These pollutants are breathed in by others sharing the room or home, and are particularly harmful to young children. They are believed to be causal factors in bronchitis, pneumonia, cot death and glue ear in young children. In adults they cause an increased risk of heart disease, stroke, cancer of the mouth, oesophagus and lung, emphysema, bronchitis and stomach ulcers.

SUMMARY

Smoking has harmful effects on the respiratory passages, lungs, blood, arteries, heart and limbs. It also harms the foetus during pregnancy.

  Describe the harmful effects of tobacco smoke on:
(a) bronchi
(b) blood
(c) a foetus

The Urinary System

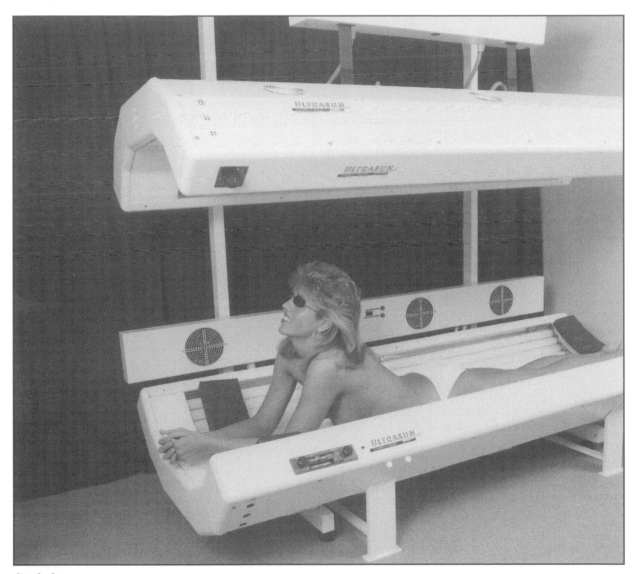

Sunbed

FUNCTION OF THE URINARY SYSTEM

The primary function of the urinary system is the regulation of the composition and volume of the blood, which involves both excretion and osmoregulation. Both these processes contribute to homeostasis by preventing marked changes in blood composition.

SUMMARY

The urinary system maintains a stable internal environment for the body tissues by regulating the composition of the blood.

Excretion

WASTE PRODUCTS

The metabolism of nutrients results in the production of waste products in the living cells of the body tissues. If these waste products accumulated in the tissues and organs they would become toxic, preventing the body from functioning efficiently. Ill-health, and finally death, would occur. The blood collects up these waste products and removes them from the tissues. The toxic substances which must be removed during excretion are carbon dioxide, urea and uric acid.

SOURCES

Carbon dioxide is a waste product of glucose metabolism and is excreted by the lungs. Urea is formed from the nitrogen waste of protein deamination, while uric acid is a waste product of DNA breakdown. These two waste products are mainly excreted by the urinary system, but small amounts are also excreted by the skin in the sweat. Gout is a hereditary condition where there is an abnormally high level of uric acid in the blood which the kidneys are unable to remove. Crystals of uric acid are deposited in the joints, particularly the big toe joints, causing considerable pain.

SUMMARY

The removal of the toxic waste products of metabolism is known as excretion.

 List three toxic waste products and explain how each one originates during cell metabolism.

Osmoregulation

SALT/WATER BALANCE

Excess of some essential materials, such as water and mineral salts, must be removed if the body is to maintain a correct balance between its water and salt content. The urinary system is involved in this process, but the osmotic (salt/water) balance is also affected by water loss through the skin (in sweat), lungs (in expired air) and alimentary canal (in faeces).

SUMMARY

The process of maintaining the correct balance between the body's water and salt content is known as osmoregulation.

 Define the following:
(a) deamination
(b) excretion
(c) osmoregulation

ORGANS OF THE URINARY SYSTEM

The organs of the urinary system are the two kidneys connected by the two ureters to the urinary bladder. A single urethra connects the bladder with the exterior urinary opening. In addition, there are the renal arteries and veins which carry blood to and from the kidneys.

Figure 9.1 *Organs of the urinary system*

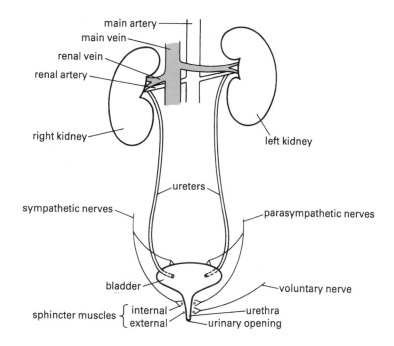

Kidneys

POSITION

The two kidneys are attached to the posterior body wall on either side of the vertebral column between the twelfth thoracic and third lumbar vertebrae, i.e. just above the waist. They lie outside the peritoneum, the membrane lining the abdominal cavity. The right kidney is placed slightly lower than the left kidney, to provide space for the liver which lies on the right side of the abdominal cavity and superior to the kidney. The kidneys are protected by the eleventh and twelfth pairs of ribs and are anchored to the body wall by an outer thin layer of fibrous connective tissue.

> **Q** | Describe the position of the two kidneys in the body.

Externally, the kidneys are two bean-shaped dark red organs, which are approximately 11 cm long, 6 cm wide and 2.5 cm thick. Their medial surface is concave and contains a notch called the hilum. A ureter leaves each kidney at the hilum and the renal blood vessels, lymph vessels and nerves connect with the kidney there. Each kidney is surrounded by a transparent fibrous membrane, the renal capsule. Adipose tissue is deposited on the outside of this membrane, so the kidneys are embedded in a fatty layer for cushioning and heat insulation.

Figure 9.2 *Internal structure of the kidney*

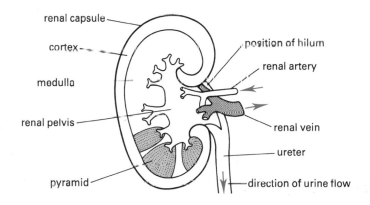

Internally, the kidney is divided into two regions, the cortex and the medulla. The outer cortex is dark red in colour, while the inner medulla is reddish-brown. Within the medulla are a number of triangular pyramids, with their apices directed towards the hilum. A large cavity called the renal pelvis occurs in the region of the hilum. The ureter is a continuation of the renal pelvis.

Each kidney is composed of around one million functional units called nephrons. Each nephron is associated with networks of blood capillaries and branches from the renal arteries (arterioles) and renal veins.

NEPHRON STRUCTURE
Nephrons are very small thin-walled tubes with a cup-shaped

Bowman's capsule at one end, which encloses a knot of blood capillaries called a glomerulus. Blood enters the glomerulus from a branch of the renal artery called an afferent arteriole and leaves by an efferent arteriole. Below the capsule the nephron tubule has three distinct regions. A coiled proximal convoluted tubule is followed by a U-shaped loop of Henle and a coiled distal convoluted tubule. Each nephron opens into a common collecting duct.

The capsules and convoluted tubules of the nephrons lie in the cortex of the kidney. The loops of Henle and the collecting ducts lie in the medulla. The common collecting ducts open into the renal pelvis at the apex of a pyramid.

Figure 9.3   *Nephron and its blood supply*

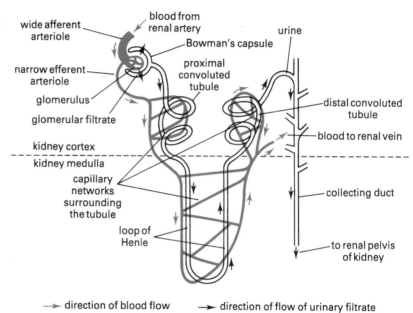

CAPSULE

The wall of the Bowman's capsule is composed of a single layer of podocyte cells which have foot-like projections wrapped around the capillaries of the glomerulus and resting on their basement membrane.

TUBULE

The wall of the proximal convoluted tubule is lined by a simple cubical epithelium, the cells having microvilli on their free surface. The wall of the descending limb of the loop of Henle is lined by a simple squamous epithelium, while the wall of the ascending limb has a simple cubical epithelium. The cubical epithelium lining the distal convoluted tubule is without microvilli. A simple cubical epithelium also forms the wall of the collecting ducts.

BLOOD VESSELS

Capillary networks surround each region of the nephron tubule. These capillaries originate from the efferent arteriole leaving the glomerulus, and drain into a branch of the renal vein.

 Where in the urinary system would you find the following?
(a) microvilli
(b) podocytes
(c) simple squamous epithelium

Ureters

Each ureter is a narrow tubular extension of the renal pelvis. Like the kidneys, the ureters lie outside the peritoneum. They enter the posterior surface of the bladder at separate openings. Their function is to carry the waste product or urine from the kidney to the bladder.

Bladder

STRUCTURE

The bladder is a hollow muscular organ situated in the pelvic cavity. Its muscular wall is highly extensible and is lined on the inside by transitional epithelium which is able to stretch. The bladder opens at its base into a tube, the urethra. This opening is surrounded by internal and external sphincter muscles.

CONTROL

The internal sphincter is controlled by the autonomic nervous system. As the bladder fills with urine its wall stretches and eventually stimulates a parasympathetic reflex which relaxes the internal sphincter muscle and contracts the bladder. The external sphincter is controlled by the conscious part of the brain, so its relaxation is a voluntary action not an involuntary reflex. The external sphincter normally relaxes following the relaxation of the internal sphincter. Urination (micturition) then occurs. Thus emptying the bladder is brought about by a combination of involuntary and voluntary nerve impulses.

 Q | Explain the mechanism by which urination is controlled.

Urethra

STRUCTURE

The urethra is a narrow tube leading from the floor of the bladder, and opening at the body surface. It opens close to the vaginal opening and anus in the female, and at the tip of the penis in the male. It carries urine to the exterior in both sexes, and in the male it carries the reproductive fluid (semen) also.

CYSTITIS

Cystitis is an inflammation of the wall of the bladder. It causes frequent and painful urination, producing a burning pain in the urethra. It is caused by a bacterial infection, usually E coli bacteria from the intestine. These bacteria are present on the skin around the anus and, in women, can easily enter the urethra and reach the bladder. Careful hygiene in the anal region is important in preventing this infection.

As the organism grows less well when urine is dilute, the liquid intake should be increased, particularly in hot climates where sweating concentrates urine. Extra fluid is necessary both when treating an acute attack and as a preventive measure against further attacks.

FORMATION OF URINE

Urine

Urine has an average pH of 6, so it is slightly acid. It contains 95% water by weight, 2% urea, 0.05% uric acid, 0.05% ammonia,

0.35% sodium ions and small amounts of other salts. Its yellow colour is due to a pigment formed from the breakdown of haemoglobin.

 List the soluble components of urine in order of increasing percentage by weight.

The factors influencing the volume of urine produced are the salt/water (osmotic) balance, the blood pressure, high external temperature or feverish illnesses, diet and emotional state.

- The salt/water balance in the blood is controlled by the hormones aldosterone and ADH. It affects the volume of urine produced as explained below.

- When blood pressure falls the homeostatic control mechanism causes more water to be reabsorbed into the blood, increasing its volume and raising the blood pressure. The volume of urine will therefore be reduced.

- When the body temperature increases more water is lost from the body by sweating. The volume of urine is therefore reduced to compensate for the extra water loss.

- A diet with a high salt content results in more water being reabsorbed in the kidney, as the blood has a higher osmotic pressure. This reduces the volume of urine produced. Where large amounts of liquid are swallowed, the volume of urine will obviously be increased. Some chemicals known as diuretics (present in tea, coffee and alcoholic drinks) increase urine volume by partially inhibiting the reabsorption of water from the nephron tubule.

- Emotional states, such as nervousness, result in increased production of urine.

 Explain how (a) decreased blood pressure and (b) increased body temperature influence the volume of urine produced.

The two processes occurring in the kidney which are responsible for the formation of urine are ultra-filtration and reabsorption.

Ultra-filtration

CAPSULE

Ultra-filtration occurs in the Bowman's capsules of the nephrons. It occurs because the efferent arteriole taking blood from the glomerulus is narrower than the afferent arteriole bringing blood to it. As blood is held back in the glomerular capillaries, the blood pressure there becomes much higher than normal. The increased pressure forces the fluid part of the blood (plasma) through the capillary wall pores and into the space within the capsule wall. Blood cells and plasma proteins remain in the glomerulus, as they are too large to pass through the walls of the capillaries and Bowman's capsule.

GLOMERULAR FILTRATE

The fluid filtered into the space within the capsule wall is called the glomerular filtrate. This contains a number of substances which are useful to the body, as well as the toxic waste materials which were being carried by the blood.

SUMMARY

Ultra-filtration in the nephron capsule separates a glomerular filtrate from the blood.

Reabsorption

Reabsorption of the useful constituents of the glomerular filtrate occurs through the wall of the nephron tubule. The reabsorbed substances pass into the blood contained in the capillary networks surrounding the nephron tubule.

OSMOTIC PROCESS

In the proximal convoluted tubule, glucose, water and some sodium ions are reabsorbed. In the loop of Henle, more sodium ions are reabsorbed, greatly increasing the osmotic pressure of the blood in the capillaries surrounding the tubule. The higher osmotic pressure increases the blood's ability to absorb water from the glomerular filtrate passing through the distal convoluted tubule and collecting ducts. Water passes back into the blood by osmosis. The remaining liquid leaving the tubule is now urine.

DIABETES

Altogether, all the glucose and 99% of the water in the glomerular filtrate is reabsorbed by the blood. In diabetics not all the glucose is reabsorbed, so some occurs in the urine.

 What is the role of each of the following in the formation of urine?
(a) glomerulus
(b) loop of Henle
(c) efferent arteriole
(d) distal convoluted tubule

OSMOREGULATION

Osmoregulation, the control of the relative amounts of sodium salts and water in the blood, is thus carried out by the nephron tubule.

HORMONAL CONTROL

This osmoregulatory activity of the nephron is controlled by hormones and is homeostatic in nature. Aldosterone, a hormone secreted by the adrenal glands, stimulates increased sodium reabsorption from the tubule into the blood. ADH (anti-diuretic hormone) secreted by the posterior lobe of the pituitary gland, stimulates increased reabsorption of water from the tubule into the blood and therefore reduces the volume of urine and the frequency of urination.

—————— SUMMARY ——————

The nephron tubule reabsorbs useful substances from the glomerular filtrate, which then becomes urine as it leaves the kidney from the renal pelvis.

 Name the two hormones which bring about the homeostatic control of the salt/water balance in the blood. Explain the role of each hormone in this regulatory process.

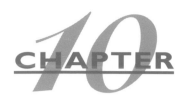

CHAPTER 10

Body Fluids

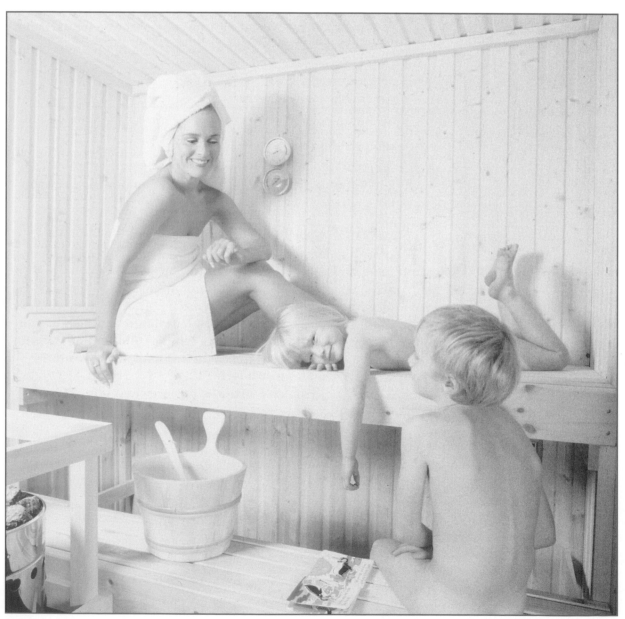

Sauna

DISTRIBUTION

The body fluids form between half and three-quarters of the body weight. About two-thirds of the body fluid is intracellular, occurring inside the body cells. The remaining one-third lies outside the cells in vessels, ducts and body spaces, and is extracellular. It includes the blood and lymph, cerebrospinal fluid, urine, glomerular filtrate (in the kidney tubules), synovial fluid (in the joints), tears, saliva and other digestive juices, the fluid in the pleural cavity surrounding the lungs, and tissue fluid bathing the cells.

The body fluids are separated from one another to form distinct fluid compartments of variable size. A fluid compartment may be as small as the inside of a single cell, where it is bounded by the cell membrane. The spaces inside the heart and blood vessels form a very large compartment.

HOMEOSTASIS

Homeostatic mechanisms keep the volume of fluid in each compartment constant, in spite of the fact that water can readily move from one compartment to another.

Fluid balance

When the body is in fluid balance, it contains the correct volume of water in each of its fluid compartments to allow normal functioning of the body.

OSMOSIS

The fluid balance in the various compartments is maintained by osmosis – the transfer of water through the semi-permeable membranes separating each fluid compartment. As the body must contain a constant volume of water to maintain fluid balance, water intake must be equal to water loss.

Water is obtained from food and drink, and also from cell metabolism as water is formed during many of the chemical reactions which occur. Water is lost from the kidneys in urine, from the skin in sweat, from the lungs in the water-saturated expired air, and from the rectum in the faeces.

OSMOREGULATION

In the hypothalamus of the brain there is an osmoregulation centre which is sensitive to the osmotic pressure of the blood. The osmotic pressure of the blood increases if the volume of water in the blood plasma falls. This increase in osmotic pressure of the blood leads to a sensation of thirst, so the person will take more water into the body by drinking. Water loss is reduced by the production of less urine due to the action of ADH (antidiuretic hormone) on the kidneys. If large quantities of liquid are drunk, the osmotic pressure of the blood will decrease and water loss by the production of large volumes of urine will restore the fluid balance.

DEHYDRATION

Some diseases result in considerable water loss leading to marked dehydration of the body tissues. Vomiting and diarrhoea cause abnormally large water loss from the alimentary canal. Feverish illnesses, which cause considerable sweating, result in great water loss from the skin. Severe dehydration is corrected by drinking water containing sugar and a little salt. Water containing sugar is more readily absorbed by the alimentary canal than pure water. The salt is required to replace the sodium ions lost in sweat, faeces and vomit.

 What is meant by 'fluid balance'? What is the physical process which maintains this balance? Name a condition which is the result of fluid imbalance.

Salt balance

ELECTROLYTES

The osmotic pressure of the body fluids is also determined by some of the solutes present in them. Some of these solutes are electrolytes, chemicals which split up or ionise in water, to form electrically charged ions. Salts, acids, bases and some proteins are electrolytes. Many essential minerals are present as salts, such as calcium phosphate and sodium and potassium chlorides, and occur as ions in the body fluids. These salts help to maintain the osmotic pressure of the blood and other body fluids.

SODIUM IONS

Sodium ions are particularly important in this respect. The amount of sodium excreted in the urine is controlled by the hormone aldosterone. If the sodium concentration of the blood falls, less sodium is removed by the kidney tubules due to the action of aldosterone.

Acid/base balance

pH

Some electrolytes help to regulate the acid/base balance, or pH, of the body fluids. A stable pH is required for normal cell metabolism. The enzymes which speed up the chemical reactions of metabolism will only function effectively at a particular pH. The majority of enzymes are most active at a slightly alkaline pH between 7.35 and 7.45, known as the optimum pH. Some of the digestive enzymes, which do not act inside cells, function best at a lower or higher pH.

BUFFERS

To keep the pH approximately constant, substances called buffers occur in the body fluids. Hydrogen carbonate (bicarbonate) and phosphate ions are two important buffers in the blood. Because the presence of large amounts of carbon dioxide from cell respiration makes the blood increasingly acidic, the blood pH is lowered to below 7. The carbonic acid produced when carbon dioxide reacts with water in the blood plasma is taken up by the buffers, so the pH rises again.

RESPIRATORY CENTRE

An increased rate of breathing will remove carbon dioxide from the blood more rapidly and help to increase its pH. The respiratory centre in the brain stem is stimulated by a drop in blood pH. It triggers the increased rate of breathing which restores the acid/base balance.

  Define the following:
(a) an electrolyte
(b) a buffer
(c) pH

BLOOD

Structure

Blood is a red viscous body fluid, composed of a liquid plasma in which several types of cells are suspended. Plasma is a pale yellow liquid, 91% of which is water. The remaining 9% consists of dissolved solids, of which 7% are plasma proteins and the remaining 2% are salts, glucose, amino acids, waste products, hormones and antibodies.

PLASMA PROTEINS

The plasma proteins are of three main types: clotting agents, albumins and globulins.

- The clotting agent fibrinogen is converted into insoluble threads of fibrin when blood clots and is produced in the liver. Prothrombin is another plasma protein which acts as a clotting agent.

- Albumins form over half of the plasma proteins and are largely responsible for the viscosity of the blood. Together with electrolytes, albumins help to regulate blood volume by determining the osmotic pressure of the blood, which maintains the fluid balance. By their effect on blood volume, they have an important function in maintaining blood pressure. Albumins are formed by the liver.

- The third type of plasma proteins are the globulins. All antibodies are globulins. Antibodies can locate and destroy the foreign proteins present in disease-producing organisms (pathogens). Gamma globulins, for example, destroy the measles and hepatitis viruses. Other globulins are used to transport other materials in the blood. Iron is carried in the blood to the bone marrow, combined with a globulin called transferrin. Globulins are formed either in the liver or by white blood cells.

ERYTHROCYTES

Erythrocytes or red cells are the most numerous cells in the blood. Five million or so occur in every mm^3 of blood. They give the blood its colour and increase its viscosity. Each cell is a biconcave disc, 8 μm in diameter, and is without a nucleus. The outer cell membrane encloses a solution of the oxygen-carrying pigment haemoglobin, a purple iron-containing compound which becomes bright red oxyhaemoglobin when it absorbs oxygen. The biconcave shape of the erythrocyte provides a large surface area for absorbing oxygen.

Erythrocytes are formed in red bone marrow and survive for about three months. They then break down and are destroyed in the liver, where their haemoglobin is converted into bile pigments and the iron retained and recycled.

Figure 10.1   *Three types of cell found in human blood (not to scale). From left to right: erythrocyte (8 μm diameter), leucocyte (10 μm diameter) and thrombocyte (2 μm diameter)*

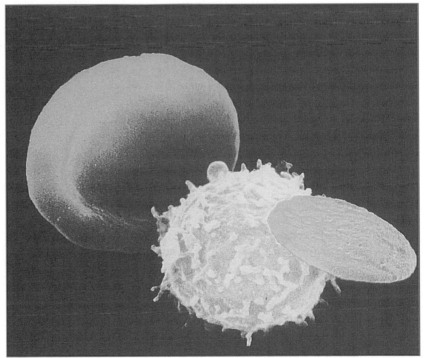

LEUCOCYTES

Leucocytes are white blood cells and are fewer in number than red blood cells. Their diameter is around 10 µm so they are slightly larger than red blood cells. They have an irregular spherical shape and contain a nucleus. Some types carry out amoeboid movement and engulf bacteria by phagocytosis. They then secrete lysozymes (enzymes) into vacuoles which are formed, to destroy the engulfed bacteria. Other types of leucocytes secrete antibodies which react with foreign proteins (antigens). These antigens may be chemicals released by bacteria (toxins), or they may be attached to the outside of the cell membrane of bacteria, viruses or foreign red blood cells, etc.

There are two main groups of leucocytes called polymorphonuclear and mononuclear types, which have differently shaped nuclei.

(a)   Polymorphonuclear leucocytes (polymorphs) have a lobed nucleus and granular cytoplasm. They form around three quarters of all leucocytes. They can migrate through the walls of small blood vessels to reach sites of infection. They carry out phagocytosis, engulfing and destroying bacteria until their lysozyme granules are used up. When loaded with killed bacteria, they die, forming pus. Their life span is approximately three weeks, but in the event of a bacterial infection it is much shorter. New polymorphs form in the red bone marrow.

Figure 10.2   *Leucocytes*
(a) Polymorph
(b) Lymphocyte
(c) Monocyte

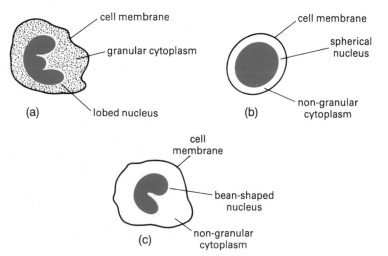

(b) Mononuclear leucocytes have a spherical nucleus and their cytoplasm is without granules. One type, the lymphocytes, form antibodies to destroy antigens. Another type, the monocytes, are phagocytic, producing lysozymes continuously. In the tissues, monocytes develop into macrophages and destroy invading bacteria. Mononuclear leucocytes are produced in lymphoid tissues, e.g. the lymph nodes and spleen.

THROMBOCYTES

Thrombocytes are small disc-shaped cell fragments shed from large cells in the red bone marrow. They are surrounded by membrane but have no nucleus, and are about 2 μm in diameter. They prevent fluid loss by aiding the clotting of blood. They will also adhere to form plugs at small wounds such as pinpricks. They have a short lifespan of one or two weeks.

State four characteristics of:
(a) erythrocytes
(b) leucocytes

Functions

Between 4 and 5 litres of blood occur in the female body, and an additional litre is present in males.

TRANSPORT

Blood has the major function of moving substances round the body, providing a transport system:

- Oxygen is carried in the erythrocytes, loosely attached to the haemoglobin pigment they contain to form oxyhaemoglobin. In tissues where the oxygen content is low, oxygen is released and diffuses out of the erythrocytes into the blood plasma, and then into the tissues. A low concentration of haemoglobin in the blood causes anaemia. In the lungs, where the concentration of oxygen in the alveolar air is much higher than in the blood, oxygen gas, dissolved in the water film lining the alveoli, diffuses into the blood. Oxygen is then absorbed by the haemoglobin in the erythrocytes.

- Carbon dioxide is carried partly by the erythrocytes and partly in the plasma, either as dissolved gas or as hydrogen carbonate ions. Carbon dioxide is formed in the tissues as a result of cellular respiration and diffuses into the blood. In the lungs, the carbon dioxide diffuses out of the blood into the alveolar air spaces, where its concentration is lower. Some nitrogen gas also diffuses in solution from the alveolar air spaces into the blood plasma, especially when the body is subjected to high pressures as in sub-aqua sports.

- Absorbed nutrients are transported in the blood from the small intestine to the liver and then to the body cells. Normally the blood contains a regulated amount of glucose to ensure that all tissues, particularly the brain tissue, have enough glucose to survive. The normal level of blood glucose (before meals) is between 810 and 990 mg/litre of blood. An abnormally high level of blood glucose is known as hyperglycaemia and causes cell damage. The constant level of blood glucose is homeostatically controlled by the hormones insulin, adrenalin and glucagon. Other nutrients required for cell metabolism and tissue building are transported to the tissues by the blood.

- Nitrogen waste from protein metabolism is carried by the blood from the tissue cells to the liver. Here the nitrogen waste is converted into the less toxic urea and carried to the kidneys to be excreted.

- Hormones produced by endocrine glands are transported by the blood to their target organs, in which they induce a response.

- Heat is also distributed round the body in the blood. As the blood passes through actively working organs, such as contracting muscles or the liver, it is warmed. The blood travels on to the colder parts of the body which absorb some of the heat. Surplus heat is lost from the blood via the skin blood vessels

PROTECTION

Another major function of the blood is to protect the body against pathogens. The leucocytes carry out this function by means of phagocytosis and antibody production.

- Antibodies destroy pathogens by attaching themselves to the cell membrane of the pathogen and causing it to burst (lysis) or by making the pathogens clump together (agglutinate). This protective method is known as the immune reaction.

- Immunity is the ability to resist disease, and innate immunity is present at birth. Adaptive immunity against specific pathogens can be acquired. An attack on the body by the pathogen results in the formation of the specific antibody by the lymphocytes. This antibody destroys the pathogen and its toxins, and may then remain in the blood for a considerable time. Any further attack by the same pathogen will be dealt with by the existing antibodies, so the person has acquired immunity to that particular disease. New antibodies against the pathogen can also be produced very rapidly.

  Active artificial immunity can be conferred by injecting a small amount of material from a pathogen. This material is called a vaccine. The lymphocytes are stimulated to form the relevant antibody by the vaccine. Immunity to influenza is obtained by this method.

- An allergy is an exaggerated immune response to a type of antigen called an allergen, to which most people show no reaction. The antibodies to allergens such as pollen, house dust, fur and food components are made in the lymph nodes and circulate in the blood. The antibodies become attached to cells in the skin and mucous membranes of the buccal cavity and respiratory ducts, making these tissues hypersensitive. On contact with an allergen, the hypersensitive cells release histamine causing an inflammatory allergic reaction.

SUMMARY

The blood has two major functions, acting as a transport system and protecting the body against disease. It carries oxygen, nutrients, hormones and heat to all living cells, and removes carbon dioxide and nitrogen waste from the tissues. The white blood cells destroy invading pathogens by phagocytosis or by producing chemicals called antibodies.

 What is meant by the following terms?
(a) immunity
(b) antibody
(c) allergen

Clotting

Clotting, or coagulation, of the blood prevents fluid loss from damaged blood vessels and blocks the entry of pathogens.

MECHANISM

When the blood thrombocytes are exposed to air at the site of a wound, a complex sequence of chemical reactions begins. It results in the conversion of the soluble plasma protein fibrinogen into a network of insoluble fibres of fibrin. Erythrocytes become entangled in the fibrin network to form a blood clot. The clotting of blood occurs faster at higher temperatures, which speed up the rate of chemical changes.

Clotting requires three blood components (thrombocytes and the two plasma proteins fibrinogen and prothrombin) and two nutrients (Vitamin K and calcium). Figure 10.3 shows the main stages in blood clotting.

Figure 10.3   *Main stages in blood clotting*

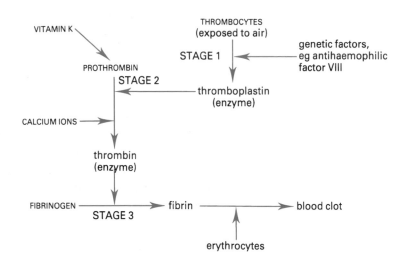

HAEMOPHILIA

There are genetic factors involved in clotting. One of these is antihaemophilic factor VIII produced in the liver, which affects the thrombocytes. In the absence of this factor, the blood does not clot and the disease of haemophilia occurs.

THROMBOSIS

After a clot forms, the remains of the blood plasma without its clotting proteins is called serum. Normally clotting does not occur inside undamaged blood vessels, as antithrombic substances are present in the blood. These substances are enzymes which can dissolve fibrin if it forms unnecessarily. However, if the inside of a blood vessel becomes rough by the occurrence of atherosclerosis, clotting can occur inside an intact vessel. Such a clot is known as a thrombosis, and it may block a narrow blood vessel and prevent blood reaching an organ. Where this happens in the coronary artery to the heart, a coronary thrombosis is said to occur and a heart attack may result.

 Distinguish between thrombocytes and prothrombin. In which process are they both involved?

Blood groups

In human blood the red cells carry antigens on their cell membranes. These antigens vary from person to person and their occurrence is due to inherited genes. An individual's blood can be classified as belonging to a particular blood group, depending on the antigens present. About 20 such blood groups occur, of which the ABO and Rhesus groups are the best known.

ABO SYSTEM

In the ABO system the red cells in an individual's blood carry one, both or neither of two antigens A and B. Where A is present but B is absent, the blood belongs to group A. Where B is present but A is absent, the blood belongs to group B. Where both antigens occur the blood is of the AB type, and where neither antigen occurs the blood belongs to group O.

In blood plasma, antibodies to the two antigens occur, but an individual never carries the antibody to any antigen present on their own red cells. Group A blood plasma therefore carries anti-B but not anti-A antibodies. Group O blood plasma carries both anti-A and anti-B antibodies.

A and O are the commonest blood groups in the UK. AB is a very rare blood group. If, during a blood transfusion, group A or group AB blood (with red cells carrying the A antigen) are given to a patient with group B or group O blood (who has anti-A antibodies in his/her plasma), the transfused red cells will be damaged and agglutinate, as the two types of blood are incompatible.

Table 10.1   *Blood groups of the ABO system*

Blood group	Antigens present on red cells	Antibodies present in plasma
A	A	anti-B
B	B	anti-A
AB	A and B	
O		anti-A and anti-B

RHESUS SYSTEM

In the Rhesus system, about 85% of white people and 99% of black people have an antigen called the Rhesus factor (or D-antigen) on their red blood cells and are said to be Rhesus positive. The rest of the population do not carry the antigen and are Rhesus negative. If the tissues of a Rhesus negative person come in contact with the Rhesus antigen, they will form an antibody against it which will be carried in their blood. If Rhesus positive blood is given to a Rhesus negative patient during a blood transfusion, the patient will form the antibody to destroy the Rhesus positive red cells, with often fatal results.

During pregnancy, when a Rhesus negative woman bears a Rhesus positive foetus, problems may occur. In the last month of pregnancy, or at birth, small amounts of foetal blood may get into the mother's circulation and cause her to form the antibody to the Rhesus antigen on the foetal red cells. At this late stage the current foetus may not be greatly harmed, but subsequent Rhesus positive babies will develop haemolytic disease (blue babies) due to the destruction of their red cells. This can be prevented by injecting the mother with an anti-Rhesus factor globulin (anti-D antiserum) immediately after the birth of each Rhesus positive baby. This globulin coats any escaped Rhesus positive foetal red cells, blocking the Rhesus positive antigen and preventing the mother from forming the antibody which will damage the foetus' blood.

 A person requiring a blood transfusion has blood of the type Group AB Rhesus negative. Explain why blood from a Group O Rhesus positive donor could not be used for the transfusion.

LYMPH

Structure

Lymph is a clear, colourless, watery fluid resembling blood plasma. It contains all the components of blood plasma (salts, nutrients, waste products, hormones and antibodies) in similar concentrations except for the plasma proteins, which occur in lower concentrations in lymph (4% instead of 7%). The large size of the molecules of some plasma proteins prevent them from filtering through the cells forming the capillary walls, so they remain in the blood plasma. Lymph contains fibrinogen and can therefore clot to form a whitish coagulation.

Floating in the lymph are leucocytes of the lymphocyte type.

Functions

After a meal, the lymph leaving the small intestine contains droplets of fat absorbed through the villi. The fat droplets produce a white emulsion instead of a colourless solution, so the lymph appears milky. One of the functions of lymph is to transport absorbed fat to the liver. Another function is to prevent water-logging of the tissues.

 What is lymph? How does its composition differ from that of blood?

TISSUE FLUID

Structure

Tissue fluid, like lymph, contains all the components of blood plasma except the plasma proteins of large molecular size. It is a clear, colourless, watery fluid containing nutrients (glucose, fatty acids, amino acids and mineral ions), dissolved oxygen and hormones which it supplies to the living cells of the tissues for their metabolism. It also contains dissolved carbon dioxide and nitrogen waste which it removes from the tissue cells where these waste products of metabolism are produced.

Function

The tissue fluid permeates the spaces between the cells in all the body tissues and is in contact with their cell membranes. It functions as the link between the blood and the living cells of the body tissues.

THE RELATIONSHIP BETWEEN BLOOD, LYMPH AND TISSUE FLUID

Hydrostatic pressure

The pumping action of the heart forces the blood against the walls of the arteries, creating a hydrostatic pressure (water pressure) known as the blood pressure. As the blood enters the much narrower blood capillaries, the hydrostatic pressure rises, forcing water through the thin capillary walls from the blood plasma. This reduces the blood volume so the hydrostatic pressure of the blood in the capillaries falls. At the same time, smaller molecules dissolved in the water (glucose and hormones) are carried through the blood capillary walls to the surrounding tissues. The blood cells and plasma proteins with very large molecules are unable to pass through the capillary walls and remain in the blood.

The fluid leaving the blood capillaries is the tissue fluid. This comes into close contact with the living cells of the tissues, allowing exchange of materials to occur between them.

Osmotic pressure

The blood remaining inside the capillaries has an increased osmotic pressure due to the loss of water and retention of plasma proteins. It therefore absorbs back some of the tissue fluid until the osmotic pressure bringing water into the blood capillaries is equalled by the hydrostatic pressure of the blood which forces plasma out of the capillaries.

Lymph flow

Any tissue fluid which is not reabsorbed into the blood capillaries enters the lymphatic capillaries through their selectively permeable walls and becomes the lymph. On average, 100 ml of lymph is formed per hour. The lymphatic vessels eventually drain into a main vein at the base of the neck and the lymph is returned to the blood.

 Describe the process of tissue fluid formation.

Figure 10.4   *Relationship between blood, lymph and tissue fluid*

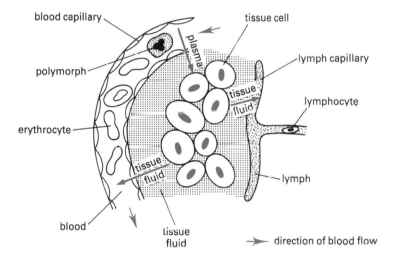

Oedema

Since the lymph transport back to the blood is not very efficient, standing for long periods causes swollen feet and ankles. The plasma proteins of large molecular size do gradually leak out of the blood vessels into the tissue fluid of the feet, thus reducing the osmotic pressure of the blood. Tissue fluid return is then slowed, causing it to accumulate in the tissues of the feet. Lymph return to the blood can be aided by gravity on 'putting one's feet up'. Oedema is the excessive accumulation of fluid in the tissues, leading to puffy local swellings. The delivery of nutrients to the tissue cells from the blood via the tissue fluid occurs much more slowly in oedematous tissue, as the nutrients have to diffuse greater distances to reach the cells.

Oedema is an example of fluid-imbalance, and has a number of possible causes. Standing for long periods is one cause. There may be an obstruction in the lymphatic drainage pathway, such as an infected swollen lymph node. An increased permeability of the blood capillary walls may occur due to histamine release from damaged cells. The escape of tissue fluid from the blood capillaries will then be too rapid for its removal by the lymphatic system, where the rate of flow is slow. Cell damage may be due to a sprain or an insect sting, when considerable oedema can occur in the region of the injury.

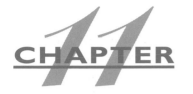

CHAPTER 11

The Cardio-vascular System

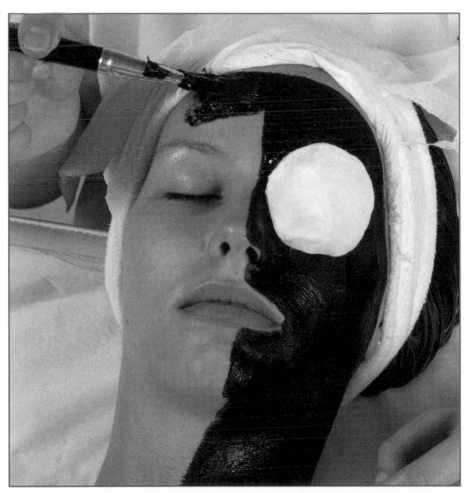

Face mask

TRANSPORT

A rapid transport system is needed to supply body cells with oxygen and nutrients and to remove toxic waste materials. A continuous closed system of blood vessels carry the transport medium, the blood, which flows in one direction round the body. The circulation of blood through the blood vessels is maintained by the heart, a muscular pump.

THE HEART

Position

The heart occurs in the thorax, between the lungs. It is set obliquely, two-thirds of the heart lying to the left of the mid-thoracic line, fitting into the cardiac notch of the left lung. The heart is enclosed in a membranous pericardium, so that it lies in a pericardial cavity which contains a watery fluid to prevent friction as the heart moves.

Structure

The heart is a hollow conical organ 12 cm long and composed of cardiac muscle (see chapter 5). It is divided into right and left halves by a vertical septum. Each half consists of an upper atrium (auricle) and a lower ventricle. Over the outside of the heart there is a network of blood vessels which are branches of the right and left coronary arteries and veins. They supply the heart muscle. The blood in the main veins enters the two atria of the heart and leaves in the main arteries from the two ventricles. The ventricles have much thicker walls than the atria to generate the pressure forcing the blood through the arteries.

Figure 11.1   *Structure of the heart*

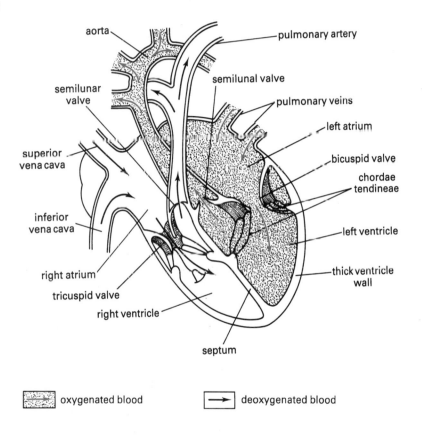

VALVES

Internally there are a number of valves in the heart to ensure that blood always flows in one direction. There are valves between the atria and ventricles on each side. These valves are flaps of tough tissue attached to the muscle of the ventricle walls by chordae tendinae, which prevent the valves being forced up into the atria by the pressure of blood in the ventricles. The valve on the left side of the heart has two flaps and is known as the

bicuspid (mitral) valve. That on the right side has three flaps and
is the tricuspid valve. There are valves between the ventricles and
main arteries called semilunar valves. They consist of groups of
three pockets projecting internally round the inside of the artery
wall. If they fill with blood trying to return to the heart, they
bulge into the lumen and close the artery.

 Q Describe the function of each of the following structures.
(a) pericardium
(b) coronary artery
(c) chordae tendineae

Circulation of blood through the heart

PULMONARY CIRCULATION

There is a double circulation of blood through the heart. In the
pulmonary circulation between the heart and lungs, blood
travels from the right ventricle to the lungs in the pulmonary
artery. It returns to the left atrium of the heart in the pulmonary
vein.

SYSTEMIC CIRCULATION

In the systemic circulation between the heart and all other body
systems except the lungs, blood travels from the left ventricle
through the aorta and returns from the body tissues to the right
atrium of the heart in the venae cavae (caval veins).

OXYGENATED AND DEOXYGENATED BLOOD

The left side of the heart contains oxygenated blood, which has
been brought to the heart from the lungs in the pulmonary
circulation. The right side of the heart contains deoxygenated
blood, which has been brought to the heart from the body
tissues in the systemic circulation.

SYSTOLE AND DIASTOLE

As the heart beats, contraction or systole of the atria increases
the pressure of blood inside the atria and forces open the
bicuspid and tricuspid valves. The blood is sucked into the
relaxed ventricles as the atrial systole forces blood through the
valves. The atria relax once the blood has entered the ventricles,
undergoing atrial diastole.

Contraction or systole of the ventricles then occurs, increasing the blood pressure inside the ventricles. The pressure rises to 120 mm of mercury in the left ventricle, but is lower in the right ventricle. The pumping action of the left ventricle is so strong that it can be felt as the pulse in arteries a considerable distance from the heart. The normal pulse rate varies between 60 and 80 beats per minute, with 72 beats as the average pulse rate. The pressure of the blood during ventricular systole forces open the semilunar valves so that blood can enter the arteries. The ventricles relax once the blood has entered the arteries, and ventricular diastole occurs until the next contraction. During diastole the pressure of blood in the ventricles falls to zero.

SUMMARY

The heart is a muscular organ which acts as a pump, driving blood through the blood vessels. This pumping action of the heart is felt as the pulse in the arteries. In the heart, deoxygenated blood is confined to the right side and oxygenated blood to the left, and two streams of blood circulate through the heart simultaneously. The pulmonary stream goes from the heart to the lungs and back, while the systemic stream goes from the heart to the rest of the body organs and back.

Blood enters the two atria of the heart from veins and leaves the two ventricles of the heart in arteries. Valves ensure that blood always flows in one direction through the heart, from atria to ventricles to arteries.

  Distinguish between systole and diastole in relation to the heart.

Blood pressure

Blood pressure is always maintained in the arteries, however, and does not fall to zero, due to contraction of their muscular walls. The blood pressure in the aorta at ventricular diastole is 80 mm of mercury, although that in the pulmonary artery is much lower. Less pressure is required in the pulmonary artery as the pulmonary circulation pathway is much shorter than that of the systemic circulation. In the systemic circulation, normal blood pressure is 120 mm of mercury at systole and 80 mm of mercury at diastole, usually expressed as 120/80. Blood pressures above these values indicate hypertension, and above 140/95 may result in a stroke or heart attack. Blood pressure is measured in the upper arm by an instrument called a sphygmomanometer.

Control of the heart beat

CARDIAC CYCLE

The cardiac muscle of the heart contracts and relaxes with an inherent rhythm known as the cardiac cycle. It beats without any direct stimulus from the nerves and can continue to beat when removed from the body, if it is in a suitable supporting fluid. A single cardiac cycle lasts 0.75 seconds. During a cardiac cycle, electrical changes occur in the heart which can be measured and displayed as an electrocardiogram (ECG).

Figure 11.2   *The cardiac cycle*

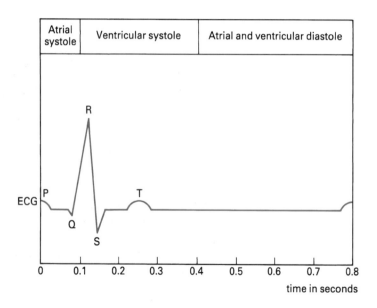

Peaks of electrical activity occur when heart muscle is contracting during systole. The QRS wave occurs at ventricular systole and the P wave at atrial systole. Electrical activity is low when the heart muscle is relaxed during diastole. There is a short pause at the end of each cycle before the next cycle begins.

NODES

There are two regions in the heart where the electrical activity causing contraction starts. These regions are two small patches of tissue called nodes. The sinu-auricular node (SAN), called the

pacemaker, is in the wall of the right atrium. The auriculo-
ventricular node (AVN) occurs near the tricuspid valve. From
the nodes, electrical activity spreads through the rest of the heart
muscle causing contractions. The pacemaker causes the heart to
beat automatically at a regular rate.

Figure 11.3 *Heart showing nodes and autonomic control*

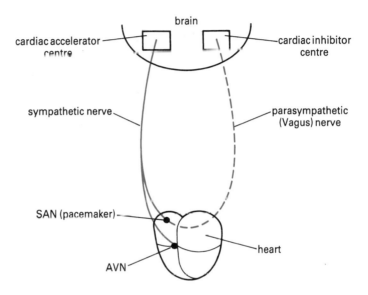

AUTONOMIC CONTROL

Nerve impulses from the autonomic nervous system can alter this
regular rate. They can act as a 'brake' or inhibitor, slowing down
the heart, or as an accelerator, speeding up the heart rate. These
nerve impulses come from cardiac inhibitor and accelerator
centres in the brain stem.

A parasympathetic (vagus) nerve passes from the inhibitor
centre to the pacemaker (SAN) and its impulses slow down the
heart rate. A sympathetic nerve passes from the accelerator
centre to both the nodes and its impulses speed up the heart
rate. These autonomic nerves provide a homeostatic mechanism
for controlling heart rate. They allow the heart rate to be
adjusted to the most suitable level for the body's activity at any
one time.

HORMONAL CONTROL

The hormone adrenalin can also speed up the heart rate. This
hormone is secreted as a response to a temporarily stressful

situation resulting in fear or anger and requiring a 'flight or fight' response (see chapter 13), but it does not provide homeostatic control.

 What is the function of the following, in relation to heart beat?
(a) the vagus nerve
(b) an electrocardiogram
(c) the sinu-auricular node

BLOOD VESSELS

The blood vessels are tubular organs in which the blood is transported round the body. There are three types of blood vessels, arteries, veins and capillaries.

Arteries

FUNCTION

Arteries are vessels that carry blood away from the heart to the body tissues. The main arteries close to the heart are wider, while the branches of the main arteries which lie close to the body tissues are narrower and are known as arterioles.

WALL STRUCTURE

Arteries have a narrow lumen (central space for the blood) and a thick muscular wall, which is very elastic and is composed of three layers.

- The inner layer of the arterial wall is called the tunica intima. On the inside, in contact with the blood, is the smooth endothelium, composed of simple squamous epithelium. The rest of the intima consists of connective tissue and an internal elastic membrane, which gives the intima a convoluted outline.

- The middle layer or tunica media is the thickest layer of the artery wall. It contains smooth muscle fibres which allow the artery to contract in diameter, collagen fibres which strengthen the artery wall, and elastin fibres giving elasticity. Nerves from the sympathetic division of the autonomic nervous system supply this muscle layer.

- The outer layer or tunica adventitia is thinner than the middle layer and is composed of connective tissue. There are many elastin fibres and some collagen and smooth muscle fibres in this connective tissue, which also contains small blood vessels.

Arterioles have thinner walls, but they always have an endothelium and a layer of smooth muscle in them.

Figure 11.4 *Cross-section of an artery*

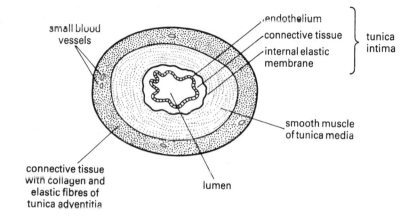

small blood vessels

endothelium
connective tissue
internal elastic membrane
} tunica intima

smooth muscle of tunica media

connective tissue with collagen and elastic fibres of tunica adventitia

lumen

BLOOD

The blood in the lumen of the artery moves in a series of spurts or pulses due to the heart beat. The contractile muscular walls also aid the circulation of blood between the pulses. The blood in an artery, therefore, is always under pressure. The arteries to the lungs (pulmonary arteries) carry deoxygenated blood, while the rest of the arteries carry oxygenated blood.

Q Describe the nature and function of an artery in blood transport.

Veins

FUNCTION

Veins are vessels which carry blood away from the body tissues and back to the heart, except in the case of portal veins. The hepatic portal vein carries blood away from the small intestine to the liver, before the blood returns to the heart in the hepatic vein (see chapter 7). The small veins leaving the tissues are called venules. They merge to form the larger veins.

WALL STRUCTURE

Veins have a larger diameter and a wider lumen than arteries, and their walls are much thinner and less muscular. Their walls have the same three layers as the walls of the arteries.

- The inner tunica intima is bounded by an endothelium which is unconvoluted. There is less elastic tissue present.

- The middle tunica media is a thinner, less muscular layer, containing collagen and elastin fibres.

- The outer tunica adventitia is a thick connective tissue layer with many collagen but few elastin fibres. It contains small blood vessels.

Figure 11.5   *Structure of a vein*
(a)   Cross-section
(b)   Vertical section showing a valve

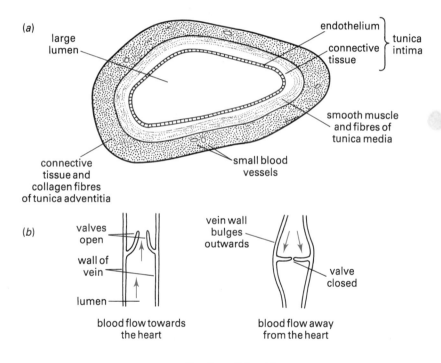

VALVES

The lumen of the veins is subdivided by groups of two or three semilunar valves which prevent backflow of blood. If backflow starts to occur, the pocket-shaped valves fill with blood, and bulge into the lumen obstructing it.

BLOOD

The blood in veins flows smoothly; there is no pulse and the blood pressure is low. The low pressure in the veins is not sufficient to counteract the force of gravity dragging the blood downwards in the veins of the legs when it needs to be travelling upwards. The upward movement of blood through the veins of the legs is due to the massaging effect of contractions of the skeletal muscles around them. Exercise thus aids venous return from the legs. The low blood pressure in the veins means that their walls do not need to be a strong as those of arteries.

VARICOSE VEINS

In people whose venous valves have become weak, often as a result of standing for long periods, the thin walls of the veins become pushed outwards and lose their elasticity through over-stretching. A vein damaged in this way is said to be varicose. Superficial veins in the leg often become varicosed, and so do those of the anal canal when the condition is known as haemorrhoids (piles). Exercise is an important factor in preventing varicose veins.

> *Q*   List four points of difference between the wall of the aorta and the wall of a large vein.

Capillaries

STRUCTURE

Capillaries are very narrow blood vessels which form networks in the tissues, linking arterioles to venules. The thin capillary walls

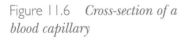

Figure 11.6   *Cross-section of a blood capillary*

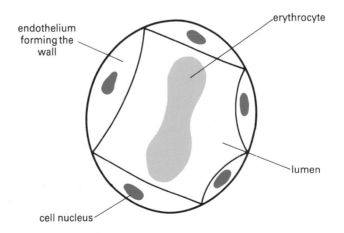

consist of an endothelium only, and the small lumen allows erythrocytes to pass only in single file. The capillary network is very well developed in very active tissues and organs, which are said to be highly vascular (e.g. liver, kidney, skin).

FUNCTION

The capillary network is very close to the living tissue cells, and exchange of substances between the blood and body cells takes place readily via the tissue fluid. Capillary blood pressure is less than that in the arterioles, but greater than that in the venules.

Vasomotor control

This is the nervous control of the diameter of blood vessels, especially the arterioles. In the walls of the carotid arteries, taking blood to the brain, are small sense organs called baroreceptors which are sensitive to increased blood pressure. Nerve impulses pass from these baroreceptors to a vasomotor centre in the brain stem. The vasomotor centre sends impulses to the smooth muscle in the tunica media of the arteriole wall via sympathetic nerves of the autonomic nervous system. These impulses are sent continuously and cause some contraction of the smooth muscle, giving a moderate amount of vasoconstriction (narrowing) of the arterioles at all times, which produces normal blood pressure. If the baroreceptors are stimulated by an increase in blood pressure in the carotid arteries, they send inhibitory impulses to the vasomotor centre. The centre then decreases the number of sympathetic impulses to the smooth muscle of the arteriole walls to below normal. More of the smooth muscle then relaxes, which allows the diameter of the vessel to increase and reduces blood pressure due to the vasodilation.

When the blood pressure in the carotid arteries is low the baroreceptors are not stimulated, so inhibitory impulses are not sent to the vasomotor centre. The centre then increases the number of sympathetic impulses to the smooth muscle of the arteriole walls causing vasoconstriction, which increases blood pressure to its normal value.

HOMEOSTASIS

This method of controlling blood pressure is a homeostatic mechanism, as it helps to restore the blood pressure to its

Figure 11.7   *Vasomotor control*

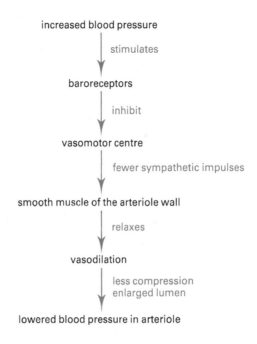

increased blood pressure

stimulates

baroreceptors

inhibit

vasomotor centre

fewer sympathetic impulses

smooth muscle of the arteriole wall

relaxes

vasodilation

less compression
enlarged lumen

lowered blood pressure in arteriole

normal level if it increases or decreases. Another method for controlling blood pressure involves the heart. Any increase in heart rate or force of contraction of the cardiac muscle will increase blood pressure. Any decrease in heart rate and force of contraction of the muscle will decrease blood pressure.

 What is meant by vasomotor control? Name the sense organs involved in this process and the position of the vasomotor centre.

THE ARTERIAL SYSTEM

Pulmonary circulation

The pulmonary artery, leaving the right ventricle of the heart, emerges from the top of the heart and immediately divides into right and left pulmonary arteries, taking deoxygenated blood to each lung.

Figure 11.8 *Pulmonary, systemic and portal circulations*

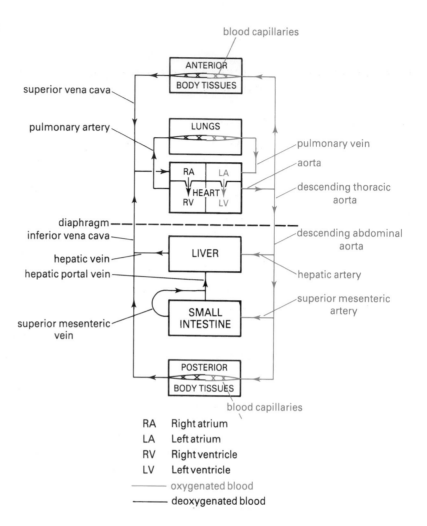

RA   Right atrium
LA   Left atrium
RV   Right ventricle
LV   Left ventricle
——— oxygenated blood
——— deoxygenated blood

Systemic circulation

The main artery, or aorta, carries oxygenated blood to the body tissues. On leaving the left ventricle, the aorta emerges from the top of the heart. The right and left coronary arteries to the heart muscle arise from the aorta, just above the point where it leaves the left ventricle. It continues anteriorly as the ascending aorta. It curves to the left forming the aortic arch, then passes posteriorly through the thorax and abdomen as a descending aorta. Each of these regions of the aorta gives off branches to the various body organs as shown in table 11.1.

Table 11.1   *Aorta and its branches*

Region of the aorta	Names of arteries branching from aorta	Region and organs supplied
Ascending	Right and left coronary	Heart muscle
Arch	Brachiocephalic, dividing into right common carotid and right subclavian	Right side of head and neck and top of arm
	Left common carotid	Left side of head and neck
	Left subclavian	Top of left arm
Descending thoracic	Series of L and R intercostals	Intercostal and chest muscles
	L and R superior phrenics	Upper surface of diaphragm
	L and R bronchials	Bronchi of the lungs
	L and R oesophageals	Oesophagus
Descending abdominal	L and R inferior phrenics	Lower surface of diaphragm
	Coeliac dividing into	
	hepatic	Liver
	splenic	Spleen and pancreas
	gastric	Stomach and oesophagus
	Superior mesenteric	Small intestine, caecum and upper parts of colon
	L and R suprarenals	Adrenal glands
	L and R renals	Kidneys
	L and R spermatic or ovarian	Testes or ovaries
	Inferior mesenteric	Lower part of colon and rectum
	L and R common iliacs dividing into	
	external iliacs	Legs
	internal iliacs	Buttocks, urinary bladder and reproductive ducts

Arteries of the head (Figure 11.10)

The common carotid artery on each side of the neck divides at the level of the larynx into two branches. An internal carotid artery passes through the temporal bone of the skull behind the ear and takes blood to the brain. An external carotid artery remains outside the skull and divides into facial, temporal and occipital arteries. These three arteries supply the skin and muscles of the face, side and back of the head respectively.

Figure 11.9 *Aorta and its branches*

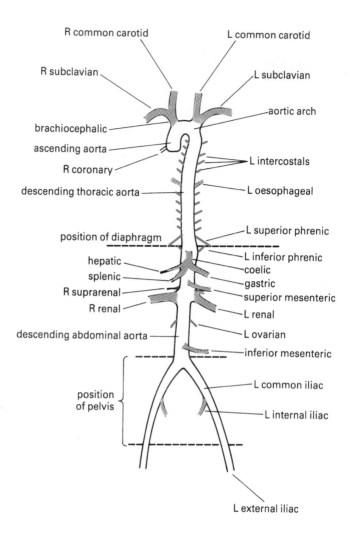

Arteries of the arm and hand (Figure 11.11)

The brachial artery of the upper arm is a continuation of the subclavian artery. Just below the elbow it divides into the radial and ulnar arteries, which pass down the lateral and medial sides of the forearm respectively and cross the wrist. The pulse can be felt in the radial artery in the wrist, proximally to the thumb. The radial and ulnar arteries are connected across the palm of the hand by a deep and a superficial palmar arch. Three palmar metacarpal arteries, and a digital artery to the thumb, arise from the deep palmar arch. Three digital arteries to the fingers arise from the superficial palmar arch.

Figure 11.10   *Main arteries of the head (side view)*

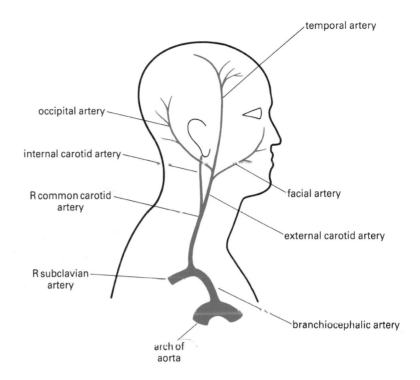

temporal artery

occipital artery

internal carotid artery

R common carotid artery

facial artery

external carotid artery

R subclavian artery

branchiocephalic artery

arch of aorta

Figure 11.11   *Arteries of the arm and hand (anterior view)*

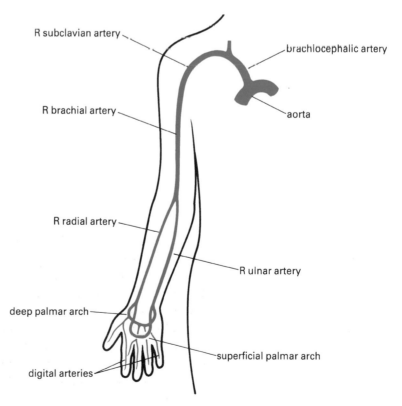

R subclavian artery

brachiocephalic artery

R brachial artery

aorta

R radial artery

R ulnar artery

deep palmar arch

superficial palmar arch

digital arteries

Arteries of the leg and foot (Figure 11.12)

Two external iliac arteries pass into the two thighs from the descending abdominal aorta and continue down the front of the thighs as the femoral arteries. Just below the knee, each femoral artery branches to form the anterior and posterior tibial arteries. A peroneal artery branches off each posterior tibial artery in the upper region of the calf. At the ankle, the anterior tibial artery becomes the dorsalis pedis artery on the dorsum of the foot. The posterior tibial artery divides at the ankle into medial and lateral plantar arteries on the plantar surface of the foot. These plantar arteries link up with the dorsalis pedis artery and give off digital arteries supplying the toes.

Q Where in the body do the following arteries occur?
(a) temporal
(b) peroneal
(c) subclavian
(d) plantar

Figure 11.12   *Arteries of the leg and foot (anterior view)*

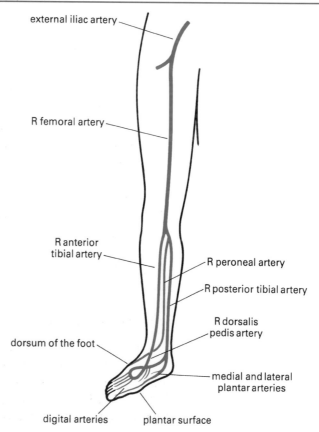

external iliac artery

R femoral artery

R anterior tibial artery

R peroneal artery

R posterior tibial artery

R dorsalis pedis artery

dorsum of the foot

medial and lateral plantar arteries

digital arteries   plantar surface

THE VENOUS SYSTEM

Pulmonary circulation

The pulmonary veins, which contain oxygenated blood from the alveolar capillaries of the lungs, return blood to the left atrium of the heart.

Systemic circulation

The systemic veins return deoxygenated blood to the right atrium of the heart through one of three large vessels. The veins of the arms, head, neck and thorax open into the superior vena cava (caval vein), the veins of the legs, pelvis and abdomen open into the inferior vena cava, and the coronary veins from the heart muscle open into the coronary sinus.

The deep veins supplying internal organs usually run parallel to the arteries and have the same names, for example the renal vein and renal artery supply the kidneys. Superficial veins occur just below the skin and are often visible, the purple colour of the deoxygenated haemoglobin showing through the thin walls.

Veins of the head

Blood is collected up from the scalp capillaries by the facial, temporal, occipital and posterior auricular veins, which run alongside similarly named arteries. These veins join to form an external jugular vein on each side behind and below the ear. The external jugular veins continue laterally down the neck and enter the subclavian veins. An internal jugular vein, bringing blood from the brain, descends on either side of the neck and enters the subclavian vein. The subclavian veins continue towards the heart as the brachiocephalic veins, after joining with the jugular veins. The brachiocephalic veins enter the superior vena cava.

Veins of the arm and hand

Blood in the digital veins from the fingers drains into the dorsal arch, leading to a dorsal venous network on the back of the hand. This venous network drains into superficial cephalic (lateral) and basilic (medial) veins in the forearm. There is another venous network on the palmar surface of the hand,

Figure 11.13   *Veins of the head*
(side view)

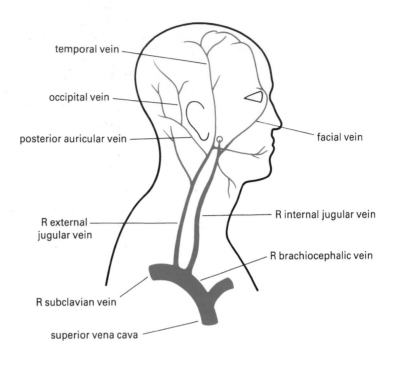

temporal vein

occipital vein

posterior auricular vein

facial vein

R internal jugular vein

R external
jugular vein

R brachiocephalic vein

R subclavian vein

superior vena cava

Figure 11.14   *Veins of the arm*
and hand (anterior view)

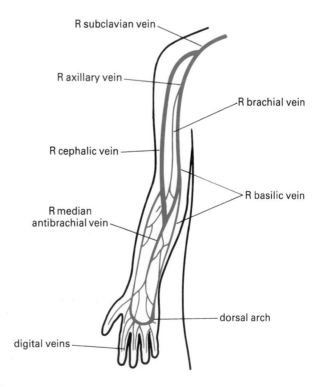

R subclavian vein

R axillary vein

R brachial vein

R cephalic vein

R basilic vein

R median
antibrachial vein

dorsal arch

digital veins

extending over the thenar and hypothenar eminences. This palmar network links up with the dorsal network into a median antibrachial vein, which passes up the anterior side of the forearm and joins the basilic vein at the elbow. The basilic vein is joined by a brachial vein in the upper arm to form the axillary vein. The axillary and cephalic veins join to form the subclavian vein at the top of each arm.

Veins of the leg and foot

The digital veins from the toes drain into a plantar arch on the sole of the foot and into a dorsal venous arch on the dorsum, from which dorsal pedis veins pass medially and laterally to the ankle. The main superficial veins of the leg are the saphenous

Figure 11.15   *Veins of the leg and foot (anterior view)*

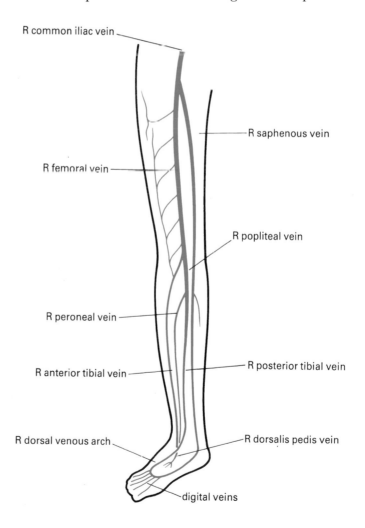

R common iliac vein

R saphenous vein

R femoral vein

R popliteal vein

R peroneal vein

R anterior tibial vein

R posterior tibial vein

R dorsal venous arch

R dorsalis pedis vein

digital veins

veins, which pass from the ankle medially up each leg to join with the external iliac veins. The saphenous veins frequently become varicosed.

The deep veins of the leg are the posterior tibial vein, passing up the back of the leg and joined by the peroneal vein, and the anterior tibial vein, passing up the front of the leg. These two deep tibial veins join below the knee to form the popliteal vein. Above the knee the popliteal vein continues up the back of the thigh as the femoral vein, which enters the external iliac vein. The blood from the leg is then returned to the heart in the inferior vena cava.

 Give the names of the following:
(a) the vessel taking blood to the left side of the head and neck
(b) the vessel bringing blood away from the kidneys
(c) the superficial medial vessel returning blood from the right foot and leg

Portal circulation

The hepatic portal vein contains blood which has absorbed nutrients from the intestine. It transports this to the liver, which controls the amount of each nutrient remaining in the blood. The hepatic portal vein is formed by the fusion of the superior mesenteric vein from the small intestine, the inferior mesenteric vein from the large intestine, and the splenic vein from the spleen, stomach and pancreas. The hepatic portal is the only vein in the body which does not return blood directly to the heart.

CONTRA-INDICATIONS

Disorders of the cardiovascular system which contra-indicate beauty therapy treatments such as massage and faradism are abnormal pulse rates, high blood pressure (hypertension), highly vascular skin conditions, varicose veins, angina pectoris (insufficient oxygen supply to the heart muscle) or the presence of an artificial pacemaker in the heart.

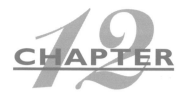

CHAPTER 12

The Lymphatic System

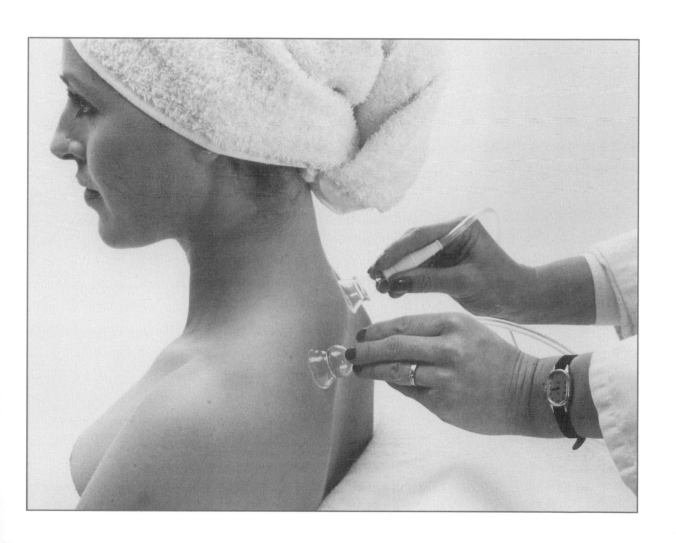

COMPONENTS

The lymphatic system comprises the lymph (see chapter 10) and the vessels in which it is transported, including lymph capillaries, lymphatics and the lymph ducts. Chains of small lymph glands or nodes occur along the lymphatics. The spleen, tonsils and thymus gland are three organs that form part of the lymphatic system. The lymphoid tissue of these structures is a specialised type of connective tissue.

FUNCTIONS

The functions of the lymphatic system are to drain tissue fluid from the organs and prevent oedema, and to return to the blood protein molecules which are unable to pass back through the blood capillary walls because of their large size. The lymphatic system also transports fats from the ileum, where they are absorbed by the villi, to the liver. Lymphocytes, which are part of the body's immune system, are produced by the lymphatic system.

 List five functions of the lymphatic system.

LYMPH CAPILLARIES

Position

Lymph capillaries occur in the spaces between the cells of all vascular body tissues, but are absent from the nervous tissue of the brain and spinal cord. They are narrow closed vessels which may form extensive networks.

Structure

Lymph capillaries are slightly larger in diameter than blood capillaries and are surrounded by collagen fibres on the outside. The lymph capillary wall is composed of simple squamous epithelium, forming an endothelium which is more permeable than that of a blood capillary wall. Some larger molecules, such as proteins, are able to pass into the lymph capillaries, although they cannot normally pass through the blood capillary walls.

Function

The lymph capillaries drain into an extensive system of larger lymph vessels, the lymphatics. The lymph capillaries remove tissue fluid and prevent oedema.

LYMPHATICS

Structure

Lymphatics resemble veins in structure. Their walls, though thinner, are composed of the same three layers that occur in veins. Lymphatics also contain internal valves to prevent backflow.

Lymph flow

The flow of lymph through the lymphatics is aided by skeletal muscle contractions, which have a massaging effect, and by respiratory movements. Exercise is therefore of great importance in maintaining lymph circulation. The rate of flow of lymph is very much slower than the rate of flow of blood in the blood capillaries.

Position

Lymphatics in the skin usually occur alongside veins. Lymphatics of the internal organs usually occur alongside arteries and form networks round them. Lymph nodes occur along the length of the lymphatics.

Describe the means by which lymph flow is maintained in the lymphatics.

LYMPH NODES

Position

Lymph nodes occur in groups, often concentrated in particular regions of the body, such as the neck and axillae. The groups of nodes are arranged in two sets, deep and superficial.

Structure

Lymph nodes are small oval structures varying between 1 mm and 25 mm in length. On one side of each node there is a slight depression called the hilum. Each node is surrounded by an external capsule of collagen fibres. Projecting inwards from the capsule are septa or trabeculae. The lymphoid tissue inside the node is divided into two regions, an outer cortex and an inner medulla.

Figure 12.1   *Structure of a lymph node*

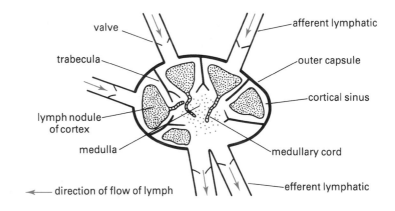

LYMPHOCYTES

The outer cortex contains blocks of lymphocytes called lymph nodules, which are separated from one another by the trabeculae. In the medulla the lymphocytes are arranged on collagen strands forming cords. The lymphocytes on the medullary cords produce antibodies. Some lymphocytes become detached and are carried out of the node by the lymph into the blood circulation. They will then destroy bacteria and their toxins in the tissues.

AFFERENT LYMPHATICS

Lymph nodes occur at the junctions of several lymphatics, and afferent lymphatics enter one lymph node at several points on its surface. The valves of the afferent lymphatics allow lymph to enter the series of irregular channels inside the cortex called the cortical sinuses. From here, the lymph diffuses into the medullary sinuses in the centre of the node between the cords.

MACROPHAGES

The sinuses are lined with phagocytic cells called macrophages which filter the lymph by ingesting bacteria, damaged cell material and unwanted proteins. If the lymph carries large numbers of bacteria due to an infection, some of the lymph nodes may enlarge and become painful. Infected lymph nodes may become blocked so that lymph is unable to drain away, causing local oedema.

EFFERENT LYMPHATICS

A smaller number of efferent lymphatics leave the lymph node from the region of the hilum. These vessels are a little wider than the afferent lymphatics, and their valves allow lymph to pass out of the node. The efferent vessels leaving a lymph node then enter another node in the chain, becoming afferent vessels.

 Q | Describe (a) the external appearance and (b) the internal structure of a lymph node.

Main groups of lymph nodes

Major groups of lymph nodes occur in the head and neck, in the axillae (armpits), in the groin, in the thorax and breasts, and in the abdomen. Tables 12.1 and 12.2 show the groups of lymph nodes in the head and neck and in the shoulders and axillae.

In the groin, superficial and deep inguinal lymph nodes occur, draining the pelvic region and the legs. The lymph nodes of the breast are described in chapter 14.

Figure 12.2   *Lymph nodes of the head and neck*

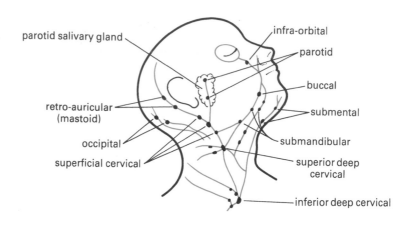

Table 12.1   *Groups of lymph nodes of the head and neck*

Name of node group	Position and areas drained
Infraorbital	Face: drains eyelids and conjunctiva of the eye
Buccal	Face: drains eyelids, nose and skin of the face
Mandibular	Face: drains chin, lips, nose, cheeks and tongue
Submental	Face: drains chin, lower lip and floor of mouth
Retroauricular (mastoid)	Side of head: drains skin of ear and temporal region of the scalp
Superficial cervical	Neck below ear: drains lower part of ear and parotid area
Occipital	Back of head: drains back of scalp and upper part of neck
Parotid	Face over parotid gland: drains nose, eyelids and ear
Superior deep cervical	Neck: drains posterior region of head and neck, tongue, larynx and oesophagus
Inferior deep cervical	Neck: drains posterior region of scalp and neck, superficial region of chest, and arm

Figure 12.3 *Lymph nodes of the shoulders and axillae*

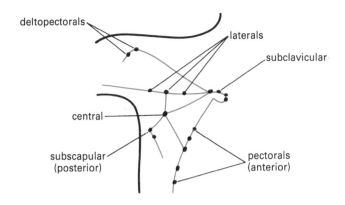

Table 12.2 *Groups of lymph nodes of the shoulders and axillae*

Name of node group	Position and areas drained
Deltopectorals	Shoulder below clavicle: drain the upper arm
Laterals	Axilla: drain the upper arm
Pectorals	Axilla: drain the skin and muscles of the thoracic wall and breast
Subscapular	Axilla: drain skin and muscles of the posterior region of the neck and thoracic wall
Central	Axilla: drains lateral, pectoral and subscapular nodes
Subclavicular	Axilla: drain deltopectoral nodes

 Name the body regions which are drained by the following lymph nodes:
(a) buccal
(b) superior deep cervical
(c) deltopectoral
(d) deep inguinal

LYMPH DUCTS

From each chain of lymph nodes the efferent lymphatics combine to form lymph trunks which empty into two main lymph ducts, the thoracic duct and the right lymphatic duct.

Thoracic duct

The thoracic duct is the main collecting duct of the lymphatic system. It receives lymph from the left side of the head, neck and thorax, and from the left arm and the whole of the abdomen and both legs. The lymph from the ileum containing absorbed fat also drains into the thoracic duct. The duct begins in the abdomen as a small dilatation, the cisterna chyli, in front of the second lumbar vertebra. It is approximately 40 cm in length and passes up through the thorax to open into the left subclavian vein.

Right lymphatic duct

The right lymphatic duct receives lymph from the right side of the head, neck and thorax, and from the right arm. It is very short, only 1.5 cm in length, and opens into the right subclavian vein.

Through these two lymph ducts the lymph is returned to the blood circulation via the subclavian veins.

> **Q** Explain how lymph in the lymphatics is finally returned to the blood circulation.

Figure 12.4   *Lymph ducts*

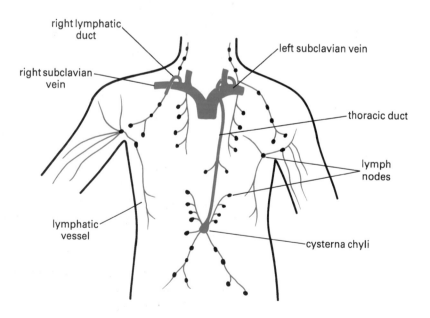

THE SPLEEN

Structure

The spleen is an oval organ, 12 cm in length. It lies on the left side of the upper abdomen between the fundus of the stomach and the diaphragm. It is a dark red highly vascular organ, surrounded by a fibroelastic capsule containing some smooth muscle. On the outside of the capsule is a serous membrane of the peritoneum, which allows the spleen to slide over other organs without damage.

Internally its structure is similar to that of the lymph nodes. It has trabeculae projecting inwards from the capsule, and a hilum through which the splenic artery and vein and the efferent lymphatics pass. The trabeculae form a framework consisting of bands of collagen and elastin fibres. The spaces between the trabeculae are filled with cells.

WHITE AND RED PULP

These cells belong to two different kinds of tissue called white and red pulp. The white pulp is lymphoid tissue arranged round arterioles. The clusters of lymphocytes in this tissue are called splenic nodules. The red pulp is closely associated with the branches of the splenic vein, and consists of small spaces filled with blood and cords of phagocytic cells which contain red pigment and red blood cells.

Functions

The functions of the spleen are to destroy bacteria and worn out red blood cells and platelets by phagocytosis (in the red pulp), and to form lymphocytes (in the white pulp). The spleen has such a large blood supply that it 'stores' blood, and will divert some of it if extra blood is required in the circulation due to haemorrhage. A sympathetic nerve causes the smooth muscle cells in the capsule to contract and squeeze out blood into the splenic vein.

 Where in the body would you find the following?
(a) the cisterna chyli
(b) white pulp
(c) the right lymphatic duct

THE TONSILS

The tonsils are patches of lymphoid tissue embedded in mucous membrane which occur at the back of the nose and throat. The pharyngeal tonsil occurs in the posterior wall of the nasopharynx and is known as the adenoids when it becomes enlarged. The palatine tonsils occur on each side of the uvula in the pharynx, and the lingual tonsils occur at the base of the tongue. The tonsils guard the opening into the respiratory passages, their lymphocytes acting as a defence against bacterial attack.

THE THYMUS GLAND

The thymus gland is a mass of lymphoid tissue in the thoracic cavity which occurs over the trachea and underneath the sternum. It is relatively large in children, but in adults the lymphoid tissue is replaced by fat and connective tissue. The thymus gland produces special lymphocytes which are involved in the body's immune system as they attack and destroy antigens.

PEYER'S PATCHES

Peyer's patches are groups of lymph nodules in the ileum wall. They provide a defence against bacteria which have entered the alimentary canal with the food.

 What are the functions of the following?
(a) the pharyngeal tonsil
(b) the spleen
(c) Peyer's patches

The Endocrine System

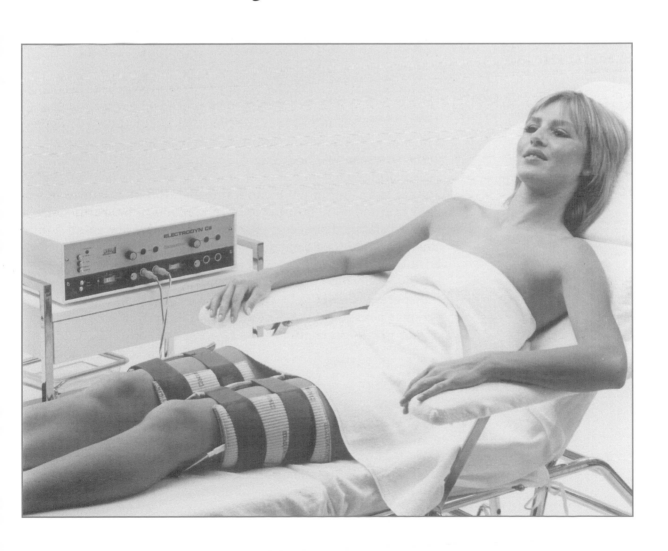

COMPONENTS

The endocrine system acts with the nervous system to control and co-ordinate the body's activities. It consists of the endocrine glands and the hormones or chemical messengers they secrete and/or store. Because the endocrine glands have no ducts and their hormones are transported by the blood, they are known as ductless glands. The secretory cells of the endocrine gland cluster round blood capillaries inside the gland, so the hormones can readily pass into the blood. In the blood, the hormones become attached to plasma proteins and are transported round the body to the target organs in which they produce a response. A hormone may affect a number of target organs which can be widely separated in the body.

RESPONSES

Hormonal responses in the target organs are usually less rapid than nervous responses and frequently continue over long periods of time. Many hormonal responses are related to growth and development which are slow and prolonged processes. Although only small amounts of hormones are present in the blood, their effects on the target organs are considerable.

What is a hormone? In what type of organs are hormones produced? What is their main function?

NERVOUS CONTROL

The activity of most endocrine glands is ultimately controlled by the nervous system. The hypothalamus links the functioning of the central nervous and endocrine systems by releasing regulating factors that affect hormone secretion by the endocrine glands. The hormone adrenalin is almost identical to the transmitter substance noradrenalin, produced at the synapses at the ends of sympathetic nerves. Both chemicals produce the same responses in the body.

FUNCTIONS

The main function of hormones is to maintain homeostasis by regulating the composition of the internal environment to keep it relatively constant. Some hormones produce cyclic patterns of activity (e.g. the sex hormones) and others control the rate of growth.

DISTRIBUTION

The endocrine glands are distributed throughout the body. They consist of the pituitary and pineal glands in the head, the thyroid and four parathyroid glands in the neck, the thymus gland in the thorax, and the two adrenal glands and the pancreas in the abdomen. In addition, the reproductive organs (ovary or testis) are endocrine glands.

THYROID GLAND

Structure

The thyroid gland occurs in the neck close to the larynx. It is composed of hollow spherical sacs called follicles, held together

Figure 13.1   *Positions of the endocrine glands*

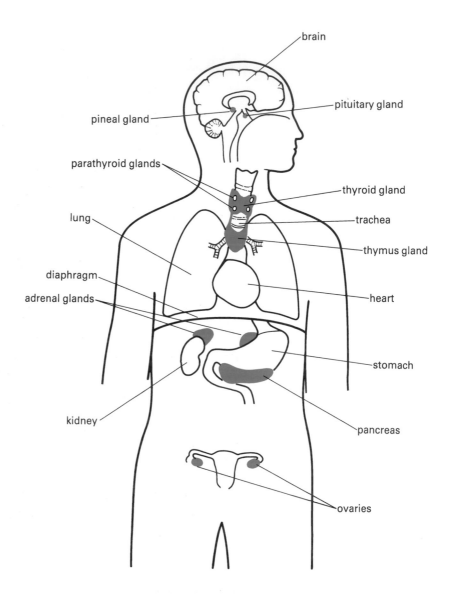

by connective tissue containing many blood capillaries. The follicle walls are composed of a simple cubical epithelium. The epithelial cells secrete hormone into the cavity of the follicle, where it is stored and later passed into the blood for transport to the target organs.

Thyroxin

The thyroid gland removes iodine from the blood, the iodine being provided by food and water in the diet. In the cells of the

Figure 13.2   *Section through part of the thyroid gland*

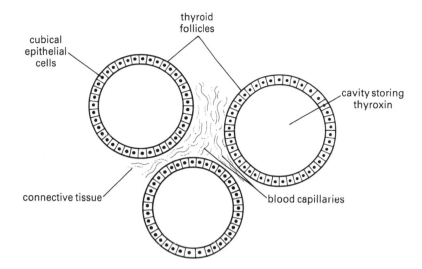

follicles, iodine is combined with the amino acid tyrosine to form the hormone thyroxin. Thyroxin affects all the body tissues and has two main functions. It controls the basal metabolic rate (BMR), adjusting it to a low level just adequate for survival when the body is at rest. Its other main function is to regulate the growth and development of the body, especially the growth of nervous tissue. Thyroxin increases the rate at which carbohydrates are oxidised in the tissue cells to produce energy, and it stimulates cells to break down proteins for energy instead of using them to build new tissues.

 Name the two materials which the body needs to synthesise thyroxin. Which activities of the body are controlled by this hormone?

Abnormal activity

HYPERSECRETION

Hypersecretion (overactivity) of the thyroid gland may be caused by a tumour in the gland, or it may be due to malfunction of the pituitary gland which controls thyroid activity. Too much thyroxin in the blood increases the BMR and the heart rate and results in considerable weight loss by using protein as an energy source. It also makes the person very excitable.

A side effect of overactivity of the thyroid gland is that the eyes bulge due to the accumulation of fluid behind the eyeball. The thyroid gland may increase in size to form a goitre or neck swelling. Because of its effect on the eyes and on the size of the thyroid gland, this disorder is called exophthalmic goitre or Graves' disease.

HYPOSECRETION

Hyposecretion (underactivity) of the thyroid gland may be due to a deficiency of iodine in the diet, and also results in the formation of a goitre. In adults the effect of too little thyroxin is to cause a condition called myxoedema. The BMR is slow and the body weight increases. Mental activity also slows down so the person is less alert. The skin becomes dry and puffy and the hair becomes thinned and brittle.

In children too little thyroxin results in cretinism, a condition in which mental, physical and sexual development are retarded. Thyroid hyposecretion is now treated by giving thyroxin in carefully controlled amounts.

Control of the thyroxin level in the blood

THYROID STIMULATING HORMONE (TSH)

The release of the thyroxin from the thyroid gland into the blood is stimulated by the presence of thyroid stimulating hormone (TSH) in the blood. TSH is secreted by the pituitary gland. An increase in the amount of thyroxin in the blood inhibits (suppresses) the secretion of TSH by the pituitary gland, a situation described as negative feedback control.

THYROXIN RELEASING FACTOR (TRF)

The pituitary gland is stimulated to produce TSH by a thyroxin releasing factor (TRF) formed in the hypothalamus of the brain, which is close to the pituitary gland. TRF passes into small blood vessels leading from the hypothalamus directly to the pituitary gland.

HOMEOSTASIS

A high level of TSH in the blood will inhibit TRF secretion, while a low level of TSH will stimulate TRF secretion. As information about the hormone level is fed back to the endocrine gland, this is negative feedback control. It prevents overproduction or underproduction of the hormone, and is an example of homeostasis.

Figure 13.3   *Homeostatic control of thyroxin level in the blood*

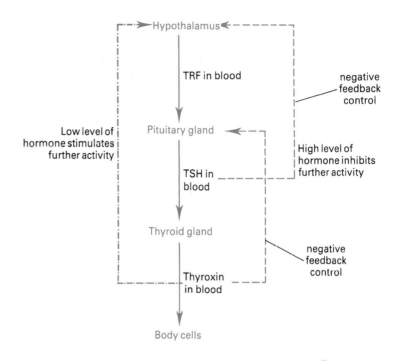

PARATHYROID GLANDS

There are four small parathyroid glands embedded on the posterior surface of the thyroid gland.

Parathyrin

They produce a hormone parathyrin, which is a protein. Parathyrin affects the level of calcium ions in the blood and other body fluids. By releasing calcium ions from bone, increasing calcium reabsorption in the kidney tubules and increasing calcium absorption from food in the intestine, parathyrin raises the calcium level of the blood. A high level of calcium in the blood has a direct effect on the parathyroid glands, inhibiting the secretion of parathyrin. This is an example of negative feedback control.

Abnormal activity

HYPERSECRETION

Hypersecretion of the parathyroid glands increases the level of calcium in the blood by breaking down bone structure. This activity of parathyrin increases after the menopause, when parathyrin is no longer inhibited by oestrogen hormone from the ovaries. The fragile bones of older women, a condition called osteoporosis, are due to the parathyroid overactivity resulting from oestrogen deficiency.

HYPOSECRETION

Hyposecretion of the parathyroid glands results in a low level of calcium ions reaching the skeletal muscles. This affects muscle contraction resulting in tetany, when muscles go into spasm producing involuntary convulsive contractions.

PANCREAS

The pancreas occurs in the abdominal cavity just below the stomach. It is both an endocrine and an exocrine gland.

Islets of Langerhans

Its endocrine portion consists of clusters of hormone-secreting cells called islets of Langerhans. These islets contain two types of hormone-secreting cells: α-cells which produce glucagon, and β-cells which produce insulin.

Insulin and glucagon

Both these hormones are proteins, and both affect the level of glucose in the blood. Glucagon raises the blood glucose level while insulin lowers it. Insulin also increases the rate of entry of glucose into living cells from the blood. Insulin is dominant immediately after meals to store glucose. Glucagon acts between meals to top up blood glucose as fast as it is used up by the tissues (see chapters 10 and 7).

 Explain the effects of insulin and glucagon on:
(a) the level of blood glucose
(b) the use of glucose in the tissue cells to produce energy

Abnormal activity

HYPOSECRETION

Hyposecretion of the islets of Langerhans results in diabetes mellitus (sugar diabetes) due to a shortage of insulin. The glucose level in the blood rises causing hyperglycaemia, and glucose is excreted in the urine (glycosuria). The presence of glucose in urine disturbs the body's fluid balance, as it reduces water reabsorption from the kidney tubules by increasing the osmotic pressure of the glomerular filtrate. Feeling thirsty is therefore one of the symptoms of diabetes mellitus.

The stores of glycogen in the liver are broken down rapidly where the insulin level is low, and glucose enters the tissue cells much more slowly. Fats are therefore broken down in the tissue cells to provide enough energy, which results in ketosis (see chapter 7). Weight loss occurs as proteins are also used to supply energy.

Diabetes mellitus is treated by regular doses of insulin and/or a low carbohydrate diet. In the elderly, diabetes mellitus is often not insulin-dependent. It can be due to raised levels of other hormones (e.g. cortisol, aldosterone, adrenalin, somatotropin), while insulin secretion is normal.

ADRENAL GLANDS

Structure

There are two adrenal glands, one above each kidney. Each gland is divided into an outer adrenal cortex and an inner adrenal medulla. The cortex has a firm texture and is deep yellow in colour, while the medulla is soft and dark brown in colour. The two parts of the gland secrete different hormones.

Adrenal cortex

The adrenal cortex secretes the steroid hormones cortisol and aldosterone.

CORTISOL

Cortisol affects normal metabolism and resistance to stress. It ensures that the body cells have sufficient glucose for energy and stimulates the use of fats and proteins as energy foods if necessary. It depresses the action of lysosomes in breaking down damaged cells and causes wounds to heal more slowly. Cortisol also controls the body rhythms, providing an 'internal clock' determined by the body's cortisol level. Around midnight the level of cortisol drops, reaching its lowest level between 2 and 4 a.m. The cortisol level then starts to rise again until there is enough to trigger waking from sleep between 6 and 9 a.m. Just after lunch the cortisol level falls slightly again, inducing sleepiness, but then rises towards the evening.

ALDOSTERONE

Aldosterone regulates the level of sodium and potassium ions in the body and affects the osmotic pressure of the body fluids and fluid balance. Aldosterone increases the reabsorption of sodium ions in the kidney tubules, thus increasing the sodium level of the blood. A high sodium level in the blood inhibits further secretion of aldosterone, providing negative feedback control.

SEX HORMONES

The adrenal cortex also secretes both the male and female sex hormones, androgen and oestrogen.

 Using aldosterone as an example, explain the meaning of negative feedback control in homeostasis.

ABNORMAL ACTIVITY

- **Hypersecretion** of

  (a) cortisol results in Cushing's syndrome. It can be due to an adrenal tumour. In this disorder the patient gains weight and the body fat is redistributed in a characteristic way. It results in very thin legs, a large 'moon face', a shoulder hump and an enlarged abdomen. The blood pressure is raised and the skin of the face appears flushed. Bruising of the tissues occurs readily. There is an increased growth of hair (hirsutism) in women, and the bones become soft and fragile due to osteoporosis. Beauty therapy treatments are contra-indicated where Cushing's syndrome is present.

  (b) aldosterone decreases the level of potassium in the body, which affects nerve transmission resulting in muscular paralysis. It also causes retention of sodium and water by the blood, resulting in high blood pressure and oedema in the tissues.

(c) the adrenal sex hormones may be due to a tumour in the gland. In most cases it is the male androgens which are increased, causing virilism in females, who develop male sexual characteristics such as the growth of a beard and deepening of the voice.

An adrenal tumour will result in an abnormal increase in the number of cells in the gland, a condition known as adrenal hyperplasia.

- **Hyposecretion** of androgen, cortisol and aldosterone results in Addison's disease. The symptoms of this disease are muscular weakness, weight loss and mental lethargy, as there is insufficient glucose in the blood for tissue cell respiration, particularly in skeletal muscle. Increased potassium and decreased sodium in the blood lead to reduced blood pressure and dehydration through water loss. Bronzing of the skin occurs and women may lose their axillary hair.

Adrenal medulla

ADRENALIN

The adrenal medulla secretes the hormone adrenalin. Larger quantities of adrenalin are secreted when the body is very active or under stress. The hormone prepares the body to use more energy during the 'flight-or-fight' response to stress or danger. It affects a large number of target organs and has the same effects as stimulation by the sympathetic nervous system.

Adrenalin increases the depth and frequency of contraction of the heart muscle, increasing the heart rate and blood pressure. It dilates the bronchi so that more air enters the lungs, increasing the oxygen supply. It causes the arterioles in the skin and alimentary canal to contract and those supplying the skeletal muscles to relax, to bring more food and oxygen for greater muscular effort. Glycogen in the liver and muscles is converted into glucose to provide additional energy, so the blood glucose level is raised.

Adrenalin increases the sensitivity of the nervous system so that the body responds more rapidly to external stimuli. The smooth muscle of the wall of the alimentary canal relaxes, slowing peristalsis. In addition, the pupil of the eye is dilated and the arrector pili muscles contract, making the hairs stand on end.

ABNORMAL ACTIVITY

Hypersecretion of adrenalin causes high blood pressure and an increase in the BMR. There are high levels of glucose in the blood and urine. Nervousness and sweating increase. Hypersecretion can be the result of a tumour, but can also occur where there is a continuously high stress level in an individual's lifestyle. It may be one factor in causing coronary thrombosis and early death by heart failure.

 What effect do the following hormones have on the basal metabolic rate (BMR)?
(a) thyroxin
(b) adrenalin

PITUITARY GLAND

The pituitary gland projects downwards from the hypothalamus of the brain, and is surrounded by the sphenoid bone which lies below.

Structure

It consists of two parts: the anterior and posterior lobes, which secrete different hormones. Some of the pituitary hormones regulate the activity of the other endocrine glands, so the pituitary has been described as the 'master gland'.

Anterior lobe

HORMONES

This region produces a number of hormones which act on other endocrine glands. One of these is TSH, which acts on the thyroid gland to control the secretion of thyroxin. Another is ACTH (corticotropin), which controls the secretion of cortisol by the adrenal cortex. The gonadotropins (FSH and LH), which control the secretion of ovarian hormones, and prolactin, which controls the milk secretion of the mammary glands, are also produced by the anterior pituitary (see chapter 14).

Figure 13.4 *Structure of the pituitary gland*

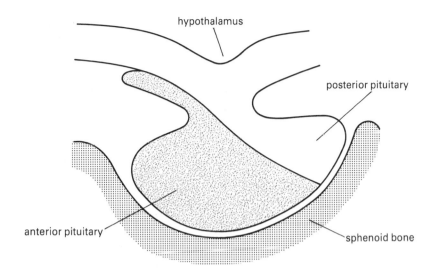

The growth hormone somatotropin, from the anterior pituitary, affects the body tissues directly, increasing protein synthesis in the cells which causes tissue growth. Although secretion of somatotropin occurs throughout life, the amount secreted falls once growth is completed at maturity. The anterior pituitary secretes a melanocyte stimulating hormone, which increases skin pigmentation.

ABNORMAL ACTIVITY

- **Hypersecretion** of
  (a) ACTH causes Cushing's syndrome by its effect on cortisol secretion.

  (b) the growth hormone somatotropin in childhood leads to giantism, as the limb bones increase in length enormously. If hypersecretion starts in adults it causes acromegaly, resulting in enlargement of the hands, feet, nose, jaws and ears.

- **Hyposecretion** of somatotropin in childhood leads to dwarfism.

  What is the effect of the following hormones on the external appearance of the body?
(a) cortisol
(b) somatotropin

Posterior lobe

HORMONES

This region stores two hormones which are secreted by the hypothalamus of the brain and pass into blood capillaries supplying the posterior pituitary. The two hormones are oxytocin and ADH (antidiuretic hormone) and both are proteins.

Oxytocin affects smooth muscle and causes the contractions of the uterine wall during childbirth. It also controls the flow of milk from the mammary glands. ADH increases the reabsorption of water into the blood by the kidney tubules and reduces the volume of urine formed, preventing excessive water loss.

ABNORMAL ACTIVITY

Hyposecretion of ADH is usually caused by damage to either the hypothalamus or the posterior pituitary lobe and causes diabetes insipidus. The kidney tubules reabsorb very little water due to the low level of ADH, so large volumes of very dilute urine are produced. Alcohol inhibits the secretion of ADH, increasing the volume of urine produced, so it has a dehydrating effect on the body.

THYMUS GLAND

The thymus gland lies in the thorax beneath the sternum. It is a bilobed gland composed of lymphoid tissue, and it forms part of the lymphatic system. It produces the hormone thymosin, which stimulates antibody production by the lymphocytes.

PINEAL GLAND

The pineal gland, which is shaped like a small pine cone, projects from the roof of the diencephalon of the brain. It is well developed in young children, but starts to degenerate from the age of seven. It secretes the hormone melatonin, which affects secretion of hormones by the ovaries. The hormone also controls body rhythms. Recent research shows that light entering the eyes makes the gland inactive; secretion of melatonin occurs in darkness.

Jet lag is thought to be due to changes in melatonin secretion, because of the altered day and night periods in other parts of the world experienced after long flights. Between Britain and the USA, jet lag is noticeable for about ten days following the return flight from the USA (after travelling east). It is less noticeable after the flight out, having travelled west.

 Q Which hormone may be associated with jet lag? Explain why the hormone is believed to produce this condition.

TESTES

In the male, the testes are two oval organs lying outside the body cavity in the scrotum. They produce the male sex hormones or androgens (e.g. testosterone) that stimulate the development of the male organs and maintain the male secondary sexual characteristics, such as body hair patterns, a deeper voice, and skeletal and muscular development.

OVARIES

In the female the two ovaries, which lie in the pelvic cavity, secrete two hormones, oestrogen and progesterone (see chapter 14).

Table 13.1   *Summary of the endocrine system*

Name of gland	Hormones	Effects	Associated disorders
Thyroid	Thyroxin	Controls BMR, growth and development	Exophthalmic goitre Simple goitre Myxoedema Cretinism
Parathyroid	Parathyrin	Raises blood calcium level	Osteoporosis Tetany
Pancreas islets of Langerhans	Glucagon	Raises blood glucose level	Hyperglycaemia
	Insulin	Lowers blood glucose level Increase entry of glucose into the cells	Diabetes mellitus

Table 13.1   *continued*

Name of gland	Hormones	Effects	Associated disorders
Adrenal cortex	Cortisol	Makes energy available for cell metabolism; resists stress; controls body rhythms	Cushing's syndrome Addison's disease
	Aldosterone	Controls potassium and sodium levels in the blood; affects fluid balance	Addison's disease
	Androgens	Cause male sexual characteristics to develop	Addison's disease Virilism in women
Adrenal medulla	Adrenalin	Increases BMR; prepares the body for the flight-or-fight response	High blood pressure
Anterior pituitary	TSH	Stimulates the release of thyroxin	
	ACTH	Increases the output of cortisol from the adrenal cortex	Cushing's syndrome
	Gonadotropins (FSH, LH)	Control the menstrual cycle and reproduction	Infertility
	Prolactin	Initiates and maintains lactation	
	Somatotropin	Controls growth	Giantism Acromegaly Dwarfism
Posterior pituitary	Stores and releases Oxytocin	Uterine contractions at childbirth; milk flow	
	ADH	Reduces urine volume	Diabetes insipidus
Thymus	Thymosin	Stimulates antibody production	
Pineal	Melatonin	Affects body rhythms and reproductive cycle	Jet lag
Testes	Testosterone	Male sexual characteristics	Infertility
Ovaries	Oestrogen Progesterone	Control the menstrual cycle and pregnancy	Breast cancer Premenstrual tension

Name the hormone which is concerned in the following disorders:
(a) osteoporosis
(b) diabetes mellitus
(c) Graves' disease
(d) female virilism
(e) diabetes insipidus

THE INFLUENCE OF HORMONE BALANCE ON EXTERNAL APPEARANCE

Hormones affect the size, masculinity or femininity of the body shape, the distribution of terminal hair, and the amount and distribution of subcutaneous fat. All these factors are involved in the external appearance of an individual.

As different hormones may affect one of these factors in opposite ways, the balance between the hormones can, to some extent, determine an individual's appearance. The situation is very complex, however, as genetic factors and diet also have marked effects on external appearance.

Height

An individual's height is affected by somatotropin, the anterior pituitary growth hormone, and by thyroxin. A childhood deficiency in either of these hormones retards growth, resulting in small stature in the adult. Hypersecretion of somatotropin in childhood will result in very tall stature as the limb bones are likely to grow longer than average. Hypersecretion of somatotropin, which begins in adult life, will have a marked effect on the appearance of the face, as the nose, jaws and ears enlarge. The hands and feet also increase in size. These changes are due to the deposition of extra bone. The lips thicken and the skin coarsens at the onset of the acromegaly.

Body shape

The masculinity or femininity of the body shape in women is influenced by the balance between the ovarian hormones and the adrenal sex hormones. Hypersecretion of adrenal androgens

322 THE SCIENCE OF BEAUTY THERAPY

and/or reduced secretion of ovarian hormones will result in the development of a more masculine body shape. Ovarian hormones will promote the increased width of the pelvis and the development of the breasts. Reduced secretion of thyroxin in children prevents the maturation of the body normally promoted by the ovarian sex hormones.

Hair distribution

The masculine type of distribution of terminal hair in women (hirsuties), with hair growth in the moustache and beard region, may result from hypersecretion of adrenal androgens or cortisol counteracting the feminising effect of ovarian hormones. After the menopause, when the level of ovarian hormones falls, the adrenal sex hormones become dominant and facial hair may develop. A deficiency of thyroxin causes thinning and loss of terminal hair, including that of the eyebrows.

Fat distribution

The typical female subcutaneous fat distribution on thighs, hips, shoulders and breasts is an effect of the ovarian hormones. Hypersecretion of cortisol results in a change in the distribution of fat from the legs and thighs to the face and abdomen, with increased deposition on the shoulders. Thyroxin imbalance affects the amount of fat deposited. Hypersecretion results in loss of subcutaneous fat and therefore in weight loss. Hyposecretion of thyroxin causes increased deposition of fat and weight gain.

 Describe the effects of the following hormones on the hair distribution in women:
(a) androgen
(b) oestrogen
(c) thyroxin

CHAPTER 14

The Reproductive System

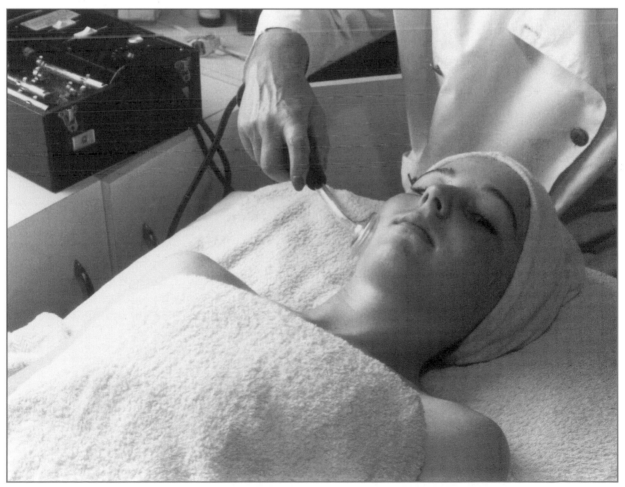

High frequency therapy – direct method

SEXUAL REPRODUCTION

Gametes

Sexual reproduction occurs in humans. The reproductive cells or gametes are produced separately in males and females, in the sex organs or gonads. The testes are the male gonads and the ovaries are the female gonads. The reproductive cells or gametes are the sperms in the male and the ova or eggs in the female.

Fertilisation

The sperms gain access to the ova through sexual intercourse so that fertilisation, the fusion of egg and sperm, can occur within the female reproductive system. This ensures that any resulting embryo can be protected and nourished. Sexual reproduction allows considerable genetic variation to occur among the offspring.

THE FEMALE REPRODUCTIVE SYSTEM

Organs

The female organs of reproduction occur in the pelvic cavity, except the mammary glands (breasts) which are on the anterior wall of the chest. The ovaries are two organs, 3 cm long and 1.5 cm wide, which produce the ova and secrete sex hormones. They occur, one on each side, in a depression on the lateral wall of the pelvis, attached to it by a suspensory ligament. An ovarian ligament anchors each ovary to the uterus also. Two fallopian tubes, which are lined with ciliated epithelium and have a funnel-shaped opening close to the ovary, carry the ova to the uterus (womb) following ovulation (the extrusion of a ripe ovum from an ovary). It is accompanied by a small rise in body temperature.

An ovum is fertilised in the fallopian tube, and the embryo becomes attached to the lining of the uterus. The foetus then continues to develop in the uterus during pregnancy. The uterus connects with the vagina by a narrowed cervix. The external genital organs, known as the vulva, occur at the entrance to the vagina. The urinary opening is just anterior to that of the vagina. The vagina serves as a passageway for the menstrual flow and acts as the birth canal. It also holds the male penis during sexual intercourse so that the sperms can enter the uterus and reach the fallopian tubes. At the lower end of the vagina is a thin fold of mucous membrane called the hymen, which initially partly closes the vaginal opening. The vaginal opening is enlarged during the first experience of sexual intercourse.

Figure 14.1   *Female reproductive organs (anterior view)*

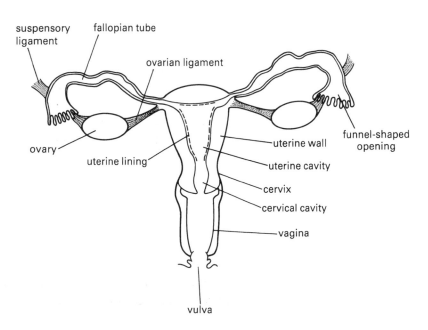

Where in the body could you expect to find the following?
(a) a newly fertilised ovum
(b) female gamete
(c) a foetus

PUBERTY IN THE FEMALE

Puberty is the period in life at which the reproductive organs become functional. It usually occurs between 10 and 14 years of age.

Hormones

At puberty the ovary responds to pituitary gonadotropic (gonadotrophic) hormones which appear in the blood, and ova are produced. The ovary then begins to produce the two hormones, oestrogen and progesterone, which travel in the blood to the body tissues. Under the influence of these hormones bones begin to grow, so that the body height increases and the pelvis becomes broader. Extra fat is deposited in the subcutaneous layer on the thighs, hips and shoulders.

Menstruation

The ovaries and uterus enlarge and change shape. As the menstrual cycle becomes established, the uterus lining undergoes a cycle of thickening, followed by the sloughing off of the extra tissue at menstruation.

Secondary sexual characters

Terminal hair grows on the axillae and in the pubic region, and the mammary glands develop. These are known as the secondary sexual characters. Psychological and personality changes occur of the type associated with adolescence.

Precocious puberty

Precocious puberty occurs when females become fertile at a very young age, even as young as five years. This may be due to an ovarian tumour which is secreting oestrogen. Surgical removal of the tumour is necessary.

THE MENSTRUAL CYCLE

The 28-day (average) menstrual cycle involves changes in the ovaries and uterus controlled by interacting hormones. If pregnancy occurs, the cycle is interrupted. Each cycle starts at the onset of menstruation and ovulation from one of the ovaries occurs at the midpoint of the cycle.

Stages

During the first 14 days, an ovum develops inside a follicle in the ovary. During the second 14 days, following ovulation, the empty follicle in the ovary develops into a corpus luteum (yellow body) as yellow pigment accumulates there. If the released ovum is not fertilised, the corpus luteum degenerates at the end of the cycle.

From the end of menstruation, around the fifth day of the menstrual cycle, the uterus lining thickens and becomes very vascular. This tissue is separated from the uterus at the end of the cycle and forms the menstrual flow. If the ovum is fertilised, the thick uterus lining remains intact and the embryo becomes attached to it, to begin pregnancy.

Figure 14.2   *Stages in the menstrual cycle*

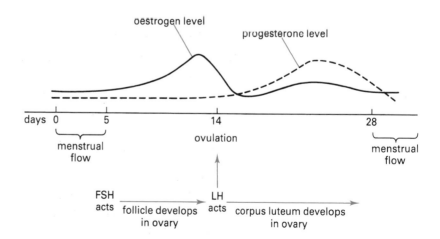

Regulating hormones

The stages in the menstrual cycle are regulated by four hormones which interact. Two are gonadotropins, formed by the anterior lobe of the pituitary gland and known as FSH (follicle stimulating hormone) and LH (luteinising hormone). The other two are the ovarian hormones oestrogen and progesterone.

 Q Name two gonadotropins and state where they are produced in the body.

At the end of menstruation, FSH causes a follicle to develop in the ovary and stimulates the secretion of oestrogen. Oestrogen initiates the repair and thickening of the uterus lining. The level of oestrogen in the blood steadily increases towards the midpoint of the cycle. At its peak, oestrogen stimulates the pituitary gland to produce LH, while inhibiting the production of FSH so that no further follicles start to develop. LH induces ovulation followed by the conversion of the empty follicle into a corpus luteum, which then secretes progesterone. The oestrogen level in the blood then falls, while the progesterone level rises and continues to promote the thickening of the uterus lining. Progesterone inhibits the production of LH so the corpus

Figure 14.3   *Hormonal control of the menstrual cycle*

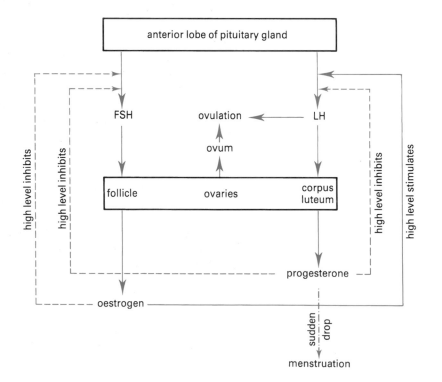

luteum degenerates. Progesterone also inhibits the production of FSH so that new follicles do not start to develop in the ovary. Degeneration of the corpus luteum occurs if fertilisation has not taken place and this causes a sudden drop in progesterone level which triggers menstruation thus starting the next menstrual cycle.

Premenstrual tension syndrome (PMT or PMS) commonly occurs just before the onset of menstruation. It causes mood changes, depression, headache and pain in the breasts and abdomen. It appears to be triggered by changes which occur in the levels of oestrogen and progesterone at the end of the menstrual cycle.

Homeostasis

The interaction between the four hormones controlling the menstrual cycle is a negative feedback mechanism which stabilises the reproductive cycle and is therefore an example of homeostasis.

SUMMARY

The cycle of changes in the ovary and uterus, occurring on average over a 28-day period, is a menstrual cycle. These cycles start at puberty in females and end at the menopause, being interrupted during pregnancy.

During the first half of the cycle, an ovum matures within a follicle in the ovary. It is released at ovulation at the mid-point of the cycle. During the second half of the cycle the empty follicle forms a corpus luteum (yellow body) inside the ovary.

From the fifth day of the cycle, the uterus wall thickens and becomes very vascular. If pregnancy does not occur, the extra tissue separates from the uterus wall as the menstrual flow at the end of the cycle.

The cycle is regulated by four hormones, two produced by the pituitary gland (FSH and LH) and two produced by the ovaries (oestrogen and progesterone).

Q   What are the effects of progesterone on the body?

FEMALE REPRODUCTIVE DISORDERS

These may be abnormalities of the menstrual cycle, ovarian cysts, or infectious diseases of the reproductive ducts.

Amenorrhoea

Amenorrhoea is the absence of menstruation and is usually due to hormone imbalance. In cases where menstruation usually occurs but then stops for two or three months, a sudden weight change may be the cause. Both obesity and extreme weight loss due to anorexia nervosa may stop menstruation.

Dysmenorrhoea

Dysmenorrhoea is painful menstruation accompanied by vomiting, diarrhoea and headache. It can be due to over-production of tissue hormones (prostaglandins) by the uterus, or the presence of ovarian or uterine tumours.

Ovarian cysts

Ovarian cysts are tumours in the ovary which may become cancerous and must be surgically removed. The cysts are filled with a thick jelly-like material and are usually painless until their increasing size causes pressure on other organs. This may result in abdominal swelling, frequent urination, vomiting and constipation. Pressure on leg veins may cause varicose veins and swelling ankles.

If the cyst becomes inflamed, sudden severe pain may occur in the pelvic region. Some ovarian cysts produce oestrogen, causing irregular menstrual bleeding or precocious puberty. Their presence may be suspected by the beauty therapist where abdominal swelling occurs, when the client should be directed to seek medical advice.

Sexually transmitted diseases

Sexually transmitted diseases are a group of infectious diseases spread primarily through sexual intercourse.

GONORRHOEA
Gonorrhoea affects the mucous membrane of the urinogenital

ducts and rectum and is caused by a Neisseria bacterium. If untreated it causes sterility.

SYPHILIS

Syphilis causes lesions in the vagina. If untreated it leads to stillbirths and finally to degenerative conditions of most of the body systems. It is caused by a spirochaete Treponema bacterium.

GENITAL HERPES

Genital herpes is caused by the Herpes simplex II virus and is uncurable. It causes painful blisters on the vulva or vagina and may be associated with the later development of cervical cancer.

TRICHOMONIASIS

Trichomoniasis is an inflammation of the vaginal lining by a protozoan pathogen called Trichomonas. It causes itching and vaginal discharge.

AIDS

AIDS (acquired immune deficiency syndrome) is caused by the HIV virus, which attacks the body's defence system so that it becomes unable to fight off other diseases from which the person eventually dies. The virus can be present in semen, vaginal fluid and blood, and may be passed on by intimate contact with any of these infected fluids.

Give the causal agents of the following diseases:
(a) gonorrhoea
(b) genital herpes
(c) AIDS

THE FEMALE MENOPAUSE

The menopause marks the end of the reproductive phase of life. It occurs between the ages of 39 and 59, with 47 being the average age of onset.

Effects

• The ovaries stop responding to gonadotropic hormones.

- Menstrual cycles become less frequent until they cease altogether.

- The ovaries shrink and no longer produce ova.

- Production of the hormones oestrogen and progesterone is reduced.

- Atrophy of the fallopian tubes, uterus, vagina and vulva occur.

- The vaginal epithelium becomes thinner and the secretion less acid, so the protection against vaginal infections is reduced.

- The breasts shrink as the glands and ducts atrophy and the amount of adipose tissue is reduced.

- The mammary blood vessels narrow so blood flow to the breast is reduced.

- The nipples become smaller and less erectile.

- The bones become structurally weaker due to the loss of calcium, resulting in some degree of osteoporosis.

- The cholesterol level in the blood rises and atherosclerosis results from fatty deposits in the arteries. This leads to an increased risk of coronary thrombosis in post-menopausal women.

- Vascular disorders such as hot flushes, headache and excessive sweating may occur.

- Muscular pains and cramps commonly occur.

- There may be emotional disturbances severe enough in a few cases to cause clinical depression.

HRT

In some cases hormone replacement therapy (HRT) may be a possible treatment for the symptoms of reduced oestrogen levels in post-menopausal women.

THE BREASTS

The two breasts or mammary glands are involved in milk secretion or lactation and are modified apocrine sweat glands.

Position

They occur on the anterior surface of the thorax over the pectoralis major muscles, to which they are attached by a layer of connective tissue. Each breast extends from the second to the sixth rib, and from the edge of the sternum to the axilla.

 Q Define the position of a mammary gland on the body surface.

External structure

Just below the mid-line of the hemispherical breast is a small projection, or nipple, onto which about 15 milk ducts open. A circular pigmented area of skin called the areola surrounds the nipple. The surface of the areola appears rough, because it contains modified sebaceous glands which secrete a fatty material to protect the skin of the nipple. The skin of the areola and nipple is hairless and very thin.

Internal structure

The mammary glands are branched tubuloacinar glands, and the layer of connective tissue which attaches them to the underlying muscle is the deep fascia. Each mammary gland consists of 15 to 20 lobes, arranged radially round the nipple and separated by an amount of adipose tissue which determines the size of the breast. Thus the amount of milk secreted by a mammary gland is not related to the size of the breast. Excessive milk production is known as Galactorrhoea.

In each lobe are many smaller lobules, 1 to 8 mm in diameter and composed of connective tissue in which the milk-secreting cells occur. Between the lobules are strands of fibrous connective tissue called Cooper's ligaments. These suspensory ligaments run between the skin and the deep fascia and support the breasts. They are better developed over the upper part of the breast. The tubuloacinar glands form grape-like clusters in the lobules. The milk they secrete passes into secondary tubules which drain into larger mammary ducts. Where these ducts converge on the nipple, each widens to form an ampulla where the milk may be stored. From each ampulla a lactiferous duct continues and opens on the nipple.

Figure 14.4 *Vertical section through a mammary gland (breast)*

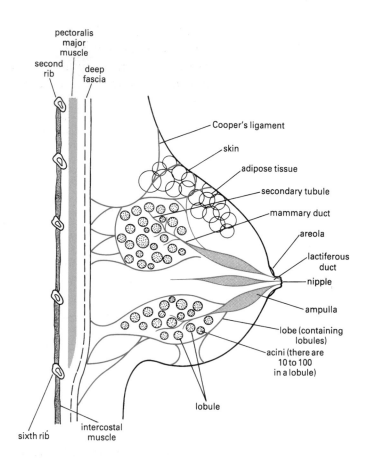

> **Q** List the ducts that a milk drop will pass through on its way from an acini gland cell to a baby's mouth.

The blood supply

The subclavian and axillary arteries supply blood to the breast. The subclavian artery has an internal mammary branch which passes downwards alongside the sternum and supplies the medial half of the breast. The axillary artery is a continuation of the subclavian artery and has lateral thoracic and subscapular branches which supply the lateral half of the breast. From the arteries, the blood passes into an extensive capillary network and is collected from the breast by veins. Surrounding the nipple is a network of small veins called the circulus venosus, which drain into an internal mammary vein. This opens into a large innominate vein at the base of the neck.

Figure 14.5   *Arterial blood supply to mammary gland (breast)*

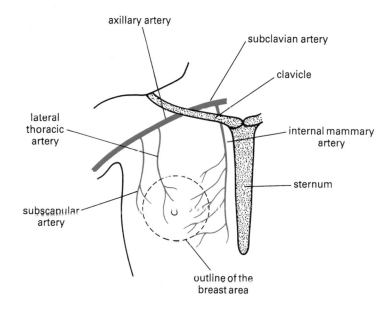

Lymphatic drainage

The axillary lymph nodes receive 75% of the lymph draining from the breast, and the internal mammary (parasternal) nodes

Figure 14.6   *Lymphatic drainage of mammary gland (breast)*

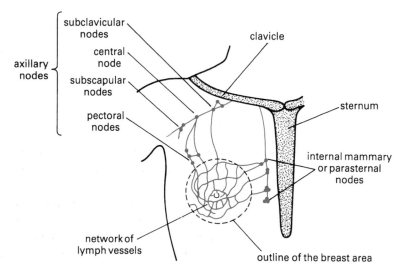

receive the rest. The axillary nodes include four groups, the subclavicular, central, subscapular and pectoral nodes. The internal mammary nodes are a linear group following the edge of the sternum. The extensive lymph drainage allows metastasis (spread) of cancerous cells to other parts of the body if breast cancer develops.

 List the groups of nodes involved in lymph drainage from the breast.

Changes in the breast

BIRTH

At birth the mammary glands in both male and female babies appear as slight elevations on the anterior chest wall.

PUBERTY

At puberty in the female the breasts begin to develop, stimulated by the female sex hormones. The mammary glands enlarge and the ducts elongate. Additional adipose tissue is laid down, and the areola and nipple grow.

ADOLESCENCE

In adolescence, sexual maturity is attained and continues until the menopause. As the menstrual cycle becomes established and ovulation occurs, the increased production of oestrogen causes the ducts of the mammary glands to lengthen and branch. More adipose tissue is laid down in the breast as sexual maturity is reached. During this phase the volume of the breast is at its minimum between the fifth and seventh day of the menstrual cycle. The hormone progesterone, which causes increased blood flow through the mammary vessels and retention of tissue fluid, will increase breast size in the second half of the menstrual cycle and may cause discomfort. Progesterone also stimulates the acini of the mammary glands to develop.

PREGNANCY

In pregnancy the increased production of the hormones oestrogen and progesterone stimulate further growth of the mammary glands, and the blood vessels dilate to increase blood flow. The areola and nipple enlarge and become darker in colour. The breasts enlarge further during the second month of pregnancy and their upper surface becomes more rounded. In late pregnancy the milk ducts contain colostrum, a yellowish milk-like fluid rich in antibody proteins.

CHILDBIRTH

After childbirth, when the levels of oestrogen and progesterone fall, the anterior pituitary lobe releases extra prolactin hormone which stimulates the glandular acini to secrete true milk. The constituents of the milk are obtained from the blood flowing through the mammary glands. When the baby suckles, nerve impulses to the posterior pituitary lobe cause it to release the hormone oxytocin. This is carried in the blood to the breast where it stimulates milk flow to the baby. Suckling is also the principle stimulus in releasing prolactin, which stimulates milk secretion. This is an example of positive feedback, since the harder the baby sucks, the greater the volume of milk produced.

LACTATION

Lactation often prevents menstrual cycles for the first few months after childbirth by inhibiting FSH and LH release. When the menstrual cycle becomes re-established, oestrogen and progesterone are again produced and prolactin secretion is suppressed. When lactation stops the ducts and glandular tissue of the breast are reduced, but the breast still remains slightly larger than it was before pregnancy. The lower surface of the breast is more pendant, and the nipple appears to be placed at a lower level.

MENOPAUSE

At the menopause there is a shrinkage of breast tissue as the acini and ducts atrophy and are replaced by connective tissue. The lobular structure of the mammary glands therefore disappears. The amount of adipose tissue in the breast also decreases and the blood vessels become narrow, reducing blood flow. With the decrease in size the breasts become more pendant. The nipples become smaller and less erectile.

Q   List three changes in the female breast which occur at menopause.

Figure 14.7   *Successive changes in the shape of the breast*

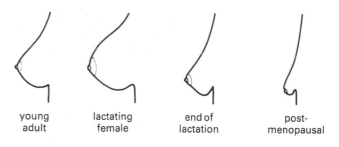

young adult   lactating female   end of lactation   post-menopausal

Table 14.1   *Summary of the effects of the reproductive hormones on the body*

Hormone	Origin	Effects on the body
Oestrogen	Ovarian follicles	Regulates the development of the sex organs and secondary sexual characters; stimulates LH and inhibits FSH production in the control of the menstrual cycle; initiates the thickening of the uterine wall; causes growth of the ducts in the mammary glands
Progesterone	Corpus luteum in the ovary	Inhibits LH and FSH production in the control of the menstrual cycle; causes further thickening of the uterine wall; causes tissues to retain fluid; stimulates acini of the mammary glands to develop
FSH	Anterior lobe of the pituitary gland	Stimulates follicle development in the ovary; causes the ovary to secrete oestrogen; interacts with ovarian hormones to control the menstrual cycle
LH	Anterior lobe of the pituitary gland	Causes ovulation; stimulates the development of a corpus luteum in the ovary; causes the ovary to secrete progesterone; interacts with ovarian hormones to control the menstrual cycle
Prolactin	Anterior lobe of the pituitary gland	Causes the mammary glands to secrete milk after childbirth
Oxytocin	Posterior lobe of the pituitary gland	Causes contraction of the uterus during childbirth; causes the release of milk from the breast

ABNORMALITIES OF THE BREAST

Breast size

The size of the breast in different individuals can vary considerably, mainly due to variations in the amount of fat present. Its size is determined by two genetic factors: (a) the level of ovarian hormones in the blood, and (b) the sensitivity of breast tissue to these hormones.

SMALL BREASTS

Small breasts can be enlarged by cosmetic surgery, in which breast augmentation by implants is carried out. An incision is made in the breast and the implant is inserted underneath the breast tissue against the muscle. The implant consists of a sac containing silicone gel.

There is recent controversy over the use of silicone gel implants. Occasional leakage of silicone from the implant does occur and this may cause an allergic reaction in sensitive individuals. In the USA, silicone gel implants are no longer allowed for cosmetic reasons.

ATROPHY

Atrophy of the breast due to loss of adipose and glandular tissue occurs in all post-menopausal women. It may also be associated with general weight loss.

HYPERTROPHY

Hypertrophy of the breast is its excessive enlargement, which can be counteracted by cosmetic surgery to remove some of the surplus tissue. In breast reduction an incision is made round the areola and down the front underside of the breast. Skin, fat and glandular tissue are then removed. Some hypertrophy of the breast is normal during pregnancy and lactation, due to the enlargement of the mammary lobules.

Tumours

The female breast is highly susceptible to the development of tumours, which are often visible externally or can be felt under the skin.

CYSTS

A cyst is a hollow tumour containing fluid or soft material, which forms a rounded lump in the breast. It may appear at any age, and though it is benign and does not invade the tissue, it is usually removed by minor surgery. Retention cysts are due to blockage in milk ducts caused by inflammation.

FIBROADENOMA

A fibroadenoma is a benign tumour, composed of glandular and fibrous tissue which feels firm and rubbery and is easily moved about under the skin. It occurs most frequently in young women taking the oral-contraceptive pill, and in childless menopausal women. It is usually removed by minor surgery.

CANCER

Breast cancer is due to malignant tumours which are not enclosed in a capsule and which invade and destroy the breast tissues. The symptoms of breast cancer are the presence of lumps, discharges from the nipple, or a nipple which becomes pulled in on one side. Puckering of the skin of the breast may also occur, but the tumour is seldom painful. Breast cancer is more likely to develop in post-menopausal women. It can be treated effectively if it is noticed in the early stages. The beauty therapist may detect its presence in a client, who should then seek immediate medical advice.

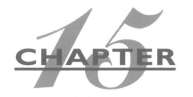

CHAPTER 15

Electrical Equipment

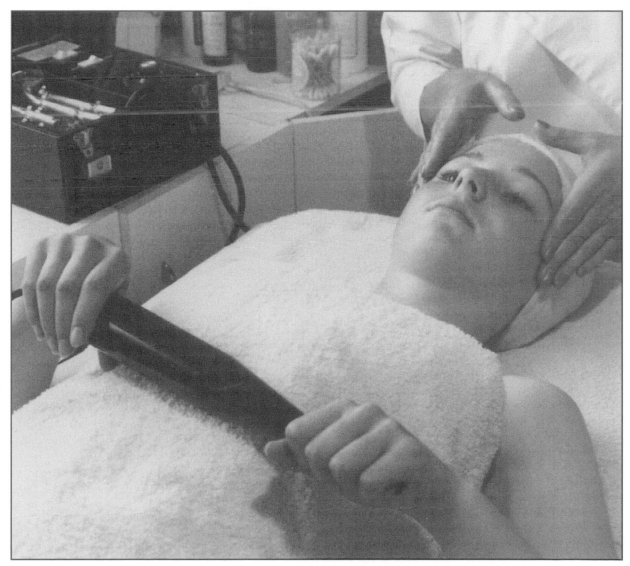

High frequency therapy – indirect method

The electrical equipment used in beauty therapy treatments contains a number of electrical devices whose actions are described below.

ELECTRICAL DEVICES

Electromagnet

When an electric current flows through a copper wire coil, known as a solenoid, it acts as a magnet. The magnetic field is stronger when the coil is wound round a soft iron core. The south pole of the electromagnet is at the end of the wire coil where the current flows clockwise, and the north pole is at the other end where it flows anticlockwise. An electromagnet loses its magnetic effect when the electric current is switched off.

Figure 15.1   *Simple electromagnet*

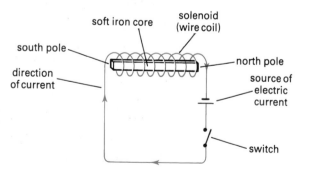

Electric motor

An electric motor is a device to convert electrical energy into mechanical energy. It contains a solenoid, the rotor, through which an electric current passes to produce an electromagnet.

The rotor is placed between the two opposite poles of a permanent magnet. When the north pole of the electromagnet is close to the north pole of the permanent magnet it is repelled, causing the rotor to rotate. To keep turning always in the same direction, the electric current passing through it must change direction every half-turn of the rotor. A split-ring commutator is used for this purpose. The two free ends of the wire in the rotor arc connected to one of the semi-circular plates of the split ring. These plates rotate with the coil and while doing so press against carbon brushes, which pass the electric current to them. Every half-turn the commutator halves interchange brushes, and the current flows through the rotor in the opposite direction. The rotor is attached to a shaft, which is made to rotate continuously in the same direction as long as the motor is in operation.

Figure 15.2   *Electric motor*

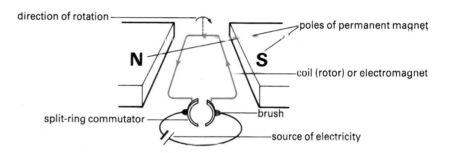

Changing the mains supply electric current

Many of the machines used in beauty therapy treatments require a different type of electric current to that supplied by the salon mains power circuit. Mains current has certain properties. It is an alternating current (AC), with a frequency of 50 cycles/second or 50 hertz (Hz). Mains current has a particular electrical pressure, or voltage, usually 240 volts (V).

There are a number of devices, described below, which will alter one or more of these properties of the mains current.

TRANSFORMER

A transformer is a device to change the voltage of an alternating current without changing its frequency. A changing magnetic field induces an alternating electric current in a copper wire coil. A changing magnetic field can be obtained by passing the mains alternating current through the coil of an electromagnet. The coil of the electromagnet carrying the mains current is called the primary coil. The coil from which the induced current of altered voltage is obtained is the secondary coil. The two coils are wound round a soft iron core and insulated from one another.

A transformer which converts the mains voltage of 240 V to higher values is a step-up transformer. If the conversion is to a lower voltage, it is a step-down transformer. In a step-up transformer the secondary coil has more turns than the primary coil. In a step-down transformer the secondary coil has the smaller number of turns.

RECTIFIER

A rectifier changes the mains alternating current into a direct current (DC) by acting as a 'valve', allowing electrons to pass through it in one direction only.

Electric heating and lighting are unaffected by the direction of flow of a current, but galvanism and electrical muscle stimulation (faradism) require direct current or the effect on the body would be counteracted each time an alternating current changed direction.

Although a rectified mains current only flows in one direction, the rate of flow still varies continuously. This variation is smoothed out to a steady value by the use of a capacitor.

CAPACITOR

A capacitor is a device which stores electric charge. It consists of two conducting metal plates with a thin layer of insulating material sandwiched between them. There is a build-up of charge on the two plates, as electricity cannot readily pass through the insulating layer. A capacitor can smooth out a rectified mains current by storing charge when the current passing is high, thereby reducing it. By releasing charge when the current passing is low, the capacitor boosts it. The direct current then becomes an almost constant flow of electrons.

High frequency devices

In addition to requiring an alternating current of high voltage, beauty therapy equipment may need to produce a current of very high frequency, e.g. 20,000 Hz or higher. This must be generated from the mains current which has a frequency of only 50 Hz.

OSCILLATOR

The basic principle of generating a current that changes direction at a frequency of very high value is to use an electronic switch called an oscillator, which can switch on and off several million times a second. Unfortunately, the rapid switching also generates harmonics of the required frequency. These harmonics must be filtered out by a circuit like that used to select a programme on a radio, that is a tuning circuit. A tuning circuit is usually made up of an inductor (coil) and a capacitor. In this way it is possible to choose the frequency of the alternating current produced.

Figure 15.3   *Oscillator and tuning circuit*

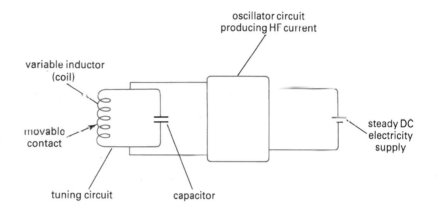

SPARK GAP AND TRANSISTOR

The repeated rapid switching on and off by the oscillator is commonly produced by using either a spark gap or a transistor. A spark gap is a break in the circuit where there are two pieces of metal placed close together but separated by a small air gap. Once the voltage has built up sufficiently in the circuit, it can pass current in the form of a spark across the air gap, so the voltage is suddenly reduced. The voltage then starts to build up again. A transistor is an electronic device that is fast enough for this switching on and off operation.

 State the purpose of each of the following electrical devices:
(a) rectifier
(b) electronic oscillator
(c) step-up transformer
(d) capacitor

INDUCTION COIL

In the past, high frequency current of up to 20,000 Hz were produced from mains current by means of an induction coil containing a spark gap. An induction coil forms part of the traditional high frequency apparatus. Where very high frequencies of several million hertz are required, as in high frequency epilation equipment, an electronic oscillator must be used.

Figure 15.4   *Induction coil*

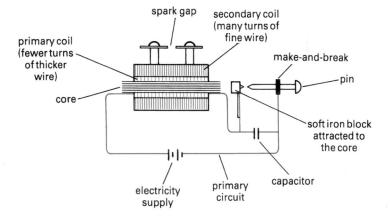

Potentiometer

A potentiometer is a variable resistance used as a volume control for radio, but in electrical stimulation machines it can be used to control the size (intensity) of the current. It consists of a coil acting as a resistance to the flow of current, over which a contact is moved. The movable contact is attached via a shaft to the control knob.

Figure 15.5   *Potentiometer intensity control*

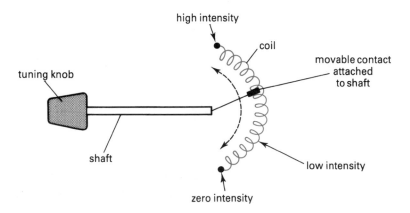

ELECTRICAL STIMULATION THERAPY

A number of different machines are available to increase the blood and lymph flow in the skin, and to stimulate motor nerves and muscles, causing muscle contractions.

Vacuum suction machine

- **Purpose**
  It is used on the face to aid the movement of lymph through the superficial lymph vessels. It is used on the body for stubborn fat conditions, as it is thought to aid the softening of subcutaneous fat cells.

- **Effect**
  The partial vacuum produced beneath the suction cup causes the skin to arch upwards into the cup. This stimulation brings an increased blood supply to the treated area of skin. Moving the suction cup along the path of a lymph vessel increases the rate of lymph flow.

- **Apparatus**
  It consists of an electric motor which drives a vacuum pump. The pump sucks out some of the air from below the cup and forces it through an outlet into the salon air.

- **Safety precautions**
  The cup should be disinfected before use with an alcohol wipe. The skin should be previously lubricated with massage cream so that the suction cup will slide easily over the skin. Suction should not be applied over lymph glands, but only over lymph vessels.

- **Hazards**
  If the machine dial is turned up too rapidly, suction increases so strongly that bruising of the tissues due to capillary breakage may occur. It can also tear the skin.

A photograph of the machine in use will be found on page 295.

Brush cleanser

- **Purpose**
  It is used on the face and body for desquamation.

- **Effect**

  Brushing loosens dead scales from the skin surface. It causes erythema due to the increased blood flow to the skin.

- **Apparatus**

  It contains an electric motor which rotates the brush, driven by dry batteries. The brush is moistened with a detergent solution.

- **Safety precautions**

  The entire brush surface should be in contact with the skin to give uniform pressure. The brush size and texture should be suitable for the area of skin being treated. If too much liquid is applied to the brush, spraying will occur. The brush should be disinfected with a 70% ethanol solution.

- **Hazards**

  If the brush attachment is not firmly in place, the brush could fly off during use.

A photograph of the machine in use will be found on page 189.

Belt massager (heavy vibrator)

- **Purpose**

  It is used to stimulate the muscles of the thighs and hips.

- **Effect**

  It improves the drainage of tissue fluid, reducing oedema which swells the tissues. It creates some erythema by increasing the blood flow due to frictional heating of the skin. The muscles are shaken and stimulated by the movements of the canvas belt.

- **Apparatus**

  An electric motor rotates a disc, causing the end of the canvas belt attached to the disc to rotate as well. This produces vibratory movements along the length of the belt.

- **Safety precautions**

  The belt should be placed in a steriliser before use, to ensure that pathogens are not transferred from one client to the next.

- **Hazards**

  It should not be used by clients with rheumatic conditions who are likely to bruise easily, or by anyone with a back problem.

A photograph of the machine in use will be found on page 52.

Gyratory vibrator

- **Purpose**
  It is used on the body to increase the rate of blood flow to the skin and muscles.

- **Effect**
  The friction between the vibrator and the skin produces heat, resulting in erythema.

- **Apparatus**
  It contains an electric motor, which rotates a shaft to which the applicator is attached.

- **Safety precautions**
  The applicator heads must be parallel with the skin surface during the treatment to give uniform pressure. A powder lubricant should be applied to the skin before starting the treatment. After use, applicators should be washed with hot water and detergent and dried with a paper towel. Alternatively an ethanol or ethanol/chlorhexidine wipe may be used for disinfection.

- **Hazards**
  Bruising can occur if the treatment is prolonged or an unsuitable applicator is used.

Percussion vibrator

- **Purpose**
  It is used to massage localised areas of the body, using different types of applicator for different body regions. A sponge applicator is used for facial work, an ebonite one for the shoulders and back.

- **Effect**
  The tapping movements of the applicators have their main effects on the skin surface. The frictional heat causes vasodilation in the skin blood vessels, which increases the rate of blood flow and the activity of the sebaceous glands. Superficial dead skin scales are loosened and removed.

- **Apparatus**
  An electric motor produces rotation, which is then converted into an up-and-down tapping motion of the applicator.

- **Safety precautions**
  The applicator heads must be parallel with the skin surface during the treatment. Powder should be used as a lubricant. All applicators should be disinfected after use. Some therapists believe that a percussion vibrator should not be used on the face.

- **Hazards**
  Bruising can occur if the treatment is prolonged or an unsuitable applicator is used.

 List three machines used in electrical stimulation therapy which contain an electric motor.

Audiosonic vibrator

- **Purpose**
  It is used on facial muscles to increase the rate of blood and lymph flow through the skin. It may be used to treat fibrositis nodules in the muscles of the neck and shoulders.

- **Effect**
  The vibrations produced can penetrate the skin to reach the underlying muscles, where they produce heat for treating fibrositis and increasing blood flow. As there is no surface banging from the audiosonic vibrator, it can be used on the face and for mature sensitive skins.

- **Apparatus**
  A coil is placed between the poles of a magnet, and an alternating current passes through the coil. The coil moves forward when the current is passing one way through the coil, and backwards when the direction of the current reverses. This is known as the electromotive effect, as a conductor moves in a magnetic field. The coil vibrates, moving to and fro, and the movement of the coil is transferred to the applicator placed on the skin. The vibrations alternately compress and decompress (rarefy) the molecules in the surrounding air, as well as in the body tissues. The waves produced have particular frequencies (the number of compressions and decompressions produced per second, expressed in hertz). The frequencies to which the human ear responds are in the range of 20 Hz to 1,500 Hz in the average

person. Vibrations within this frequency range are described as audiosonic because they can be heard and are produced by this type of vibrator.

- **Safety precautions**
Powder should be used as a lubricant when plastic applicators are used. Spongy applicators should be used where gentler stimulation is necessary, for example over bony areas of the face. Applicators should be disinfected before use.

Electrical muscle stimulation (faradic) machine

- **Purpose**
It is used on the body as a passive muscle exerciser for toning very specific areas, and on the face to improve facial contour. It is used in cases where taking active exercise may not be possible for medical reasons.

- **Effect**
The muscles which are stimulated contract and relax involuntarily, which improves muscle tone and prevents atrophy. The muscular movements increase the rate of flow of blood and lymph.

- **Apparatus**
(a) In one type the machine supplies an interrupted direct current, where the size (intensity) of the current rises and falls rapidly so that the current pulsates. The pulses last for such a short time that chemical effects will be too small to cause discomfort. Each brief pulse is followed by a longer interval when no current is flowing. The pulses of current pass through the body between two electrodes applied at different points on the skin over the muscle being treated. The interrupted direct current is produced by an electronic oscillator with a make-and-break circuit. A photograph of the machine in use will be found on page 127.
(b) Micro-current facial toning uses a low frequency micro current, that is an alternating current at a frequency of 0.6 Hz and a pressure of 50 V. The two electrodes from the machine producing the current each have cotton covered applicators wetted with saline solution, which are pressed onto the skin to conduct the current. The electrodes are placed a short

distance apart, and the micro current flows through the tissue separating the two electrodes for a few seconds. The micro current acts as a triggering force whose effects continue for around 24 hours. Muscles are tightened and toned, and lines and wrinkles in the skin are said to be smoothed out, thus improving facial contours.

- **Safety precautions**
  The current must not change in intensity too rapidly or the pain receptors of the skin may be stimulated in addition to the muscle.

- **Hazards**
  The treatment is ineffective in the case of very obese clients as the electrical pulses cannot penetrate the thick layer of subcutaneous fat to reach the muscle.

 In each case, name a machine used in beauty therapy which features the following:
(a) desquamation
(b) an electromotive effect
(c) frictional heat
(d) a partial vacuum

Galvanic machine

- **Purpose**
  It is used on the face to introduce chemicals into the intact skin during iontophoresis, and for skin cleansing during desincrustation. It is used on the body to treat areas of hard fat.

- **Effect**
  The direct (galvanic) current produces a chemical effect within the skin. Around the negative electrode (cathode) there will be an excess of hydroxyl ions, resulting in increased pH. The effect of this increased alkalinity is to reduce the oiliness of the skin and to break down the keratin of the dead skin scales. These effects are used in desincrustation.

  When used for iontophoresis, positive or negative ions thought to have therapeutic effects may be driven into the skin. This will occur if positive ions in solution are placed on the skin below the positive electrode (anode), while negative ions are placed below the cathode. The similarly charged electrode will repel the ions so that they are driven below the skin surface.

- **Apparatus**
  The galvanic machine produces a direct current by means of a rectifier which converts the mains AC into DC. A smoothing capacitor produces a steady DC from the rectified current. Two metal electrodes, connected by leads to the machine, are placed on the skin. The current travels through the skin from one electrode to the other. The active electrode is placed over a pad soaked in electrolyte solution. This is the cathode when used for desincrustation. When used for iontophoresis, the active electrode may be either the anode or the cathode. The other electrode is wrapped in damp lint and held by the client. The damp pads improve the electrical contact between the electrodes and the skin.

- **Safety precautions**
  The client's skin should be washed immediately after the treatment to dilute and remove the alkaline solution produced by electrolysis, which will soften the skin and cause redness. The size of the current should be changed gradually, and electrodes must not be suddenly lifted from the skin while the machine is operating. Sudden changes in current may cause muscles to contract violently. The pad should be evenly soaked with the electrolyte solution to prevent galvanic burns. The size of the current should be reduced where bony regions of the face are being treated. The absence of softer tissues causes reduced resistance to the current and galvanic burns may occur.

- **Hazards**
  If the current size is too great, a galvanic burn may be produced in the skin due to high alkalinity. If the two electrodes are allowed to touch while the machine is operating, short circuiting may occur and damage the machine.

A photograph of the machine in use will be found on page 167.

 Distinguish between iontophoresis and desincrustation. Which type of machine is used in both of these processes?

Interferential machine

- **Purpose**
  It is used on the body, but not on the face, to stimulate muscle contraction.

- **Effect**
  It causes muscles to contract and speeds up the rate of blood and lymph flow. It causes little skin heating and affects motor nerves, but not sensory nerves, so there is little skin discomfort during treatment.

- **Apparatus**
  The machine contains two oscillators which produce two high frequency alternating currents of slightly different frequencies. As these two currents flow through the same region of tissue, they mix to produce an interferential current whose frequency is the difference between the frequencies of the currents actually supplied. The difference between the frequencies of the two currents is usually between 0 and 100 Hz, so the interferential current is of low frequency. Interferential currents with frequencies at the lower end of the range (0 to 10 Hz) will cause muscle contractions. Currents with the higher frequencies (close to 100 Hz) do not cause muscle contraction, but increase the rate of blood and lymph flow and have an analgesic effect.

- **Safety precautions and hazards**
  The low current intensity makes interferential therapy a completely safe method of treatment.

A photograph of the machine in use will be found on page 305.

High frequency machine

- **Purpose**
  On the face, the direct method is used to treat seborrhoea (greasy skin), while the indirect method increases the rate of blood and lymph flow through the skin and is beneficial for dry skins.

- **Effects**
  It warms the skin, as the high frequency current produces resistance heating which causes vasodilation. The ozone produced by the machine when using the direct method has an antiseptic action on the skin and may improve acne. These

high frequency currents do not stimulate motor nerves to cause muscle contraction.

- **Apparatus**
  The machine contains an oscillator which changes the frequency of the current from the 50 Hz of the mains supply to above 100,000 Hz. The voltage of the current is also increased to 2,000 V by a transformer, but the current is small and remains in the skin – it does not penetrate into the deeper tissues. A rectifier and capacitor convert the AC mains supply to the steady DC current required by the oscillator.

  In the direct method of treatment, frequent very short pulses of current flash across a spark gap inside the glass electrode which is placed on the skin. In the indirect method, the client holds the metal rod electrode (saturator), from which the current passes through the client's skin to the therapist who is carrying out manual massage on the face of the client. In both methods the current returns to the machine through the air and salon furniture to complete the circuit.

- **Safety precautions**
  Metal objects, such as jewellery, should be removed as through resistance heating they can become hot enough to cause a burn. Electrodes should be disinfected with ethanol (surgical spirit) before and after use. The intensity should be reduced to zero and the current switched off before the electrode, or therapist's hand, is lifted from the skin. Sudden breaks in the circuit cause the client to feel discomfort. Shorter treatment times are required for dry mature skins.

- **Hazards**
  The ozone produced during the sparking which occurs in the direct method is poisonous at high concentrations. The sparking itself may cause alarm in some clients.

A photograph of the machine in use applying the direct method will be found on page 323. A photograph showing the indirect method will be found on page 341.

Contra-indications

A number of disorders of the cardio-vascular system contra-indicate electrical stimulation therapy, for example heart disorders (angina), abnormal pulse rates, high or low blood pressure, varicose veins and highly vascular skin conditions. Skin lesions such as bruises, scar tissue, inflammation or pustules, and excessively loose, fragile or hypersensitive skins also contra-indicate treatment.

Facial treatments are contra-indicated where the client suffers from asthma, migraine or sinus disorders. Neuritis, neuralgia or the presence of much metalwork in teeth or dentures may also contra-indicate treatment.

Electrical stimulation treatments should not be applied to the abdomen during menstruation or pregnancy.

> **Q** | List six contra-indications for facial electrical stimulation therapy.

EPILATION

This process results in the permanent removal of unwanted terminal hair by destroying the hair roots. Destruction of the hair root may be due to heat or chemical burning caused by an electric current. Epilation is principally used on facial hair.

Diathermy machine

- **Purpose**
  It is used for the removal of unwanted facial hair.

- **Effect**
  The hair root is destroyed by heat within the hair follicle. The hair can then be removed and no further hairs will grow in the follicle.

- **Apparatus**
  It resembles the high frequency machine described above. It produces an alternating current with a very high frequency. In the USA, by law this frequency must be 13.16 million hertz. While there is as yet no set frequency in the EU, most machines operate at the lower frequency of 7 million hertz.

This current is directed to the hair root from the tip of a needle electrode inserted down the hair follicle. Intense heat develops at the tip of the needle which destroys the matrix of the hair root.

- **Safety precautions**
  It is essential when placing the needle that its tip should be in contact with the hair root. Regrowth of the hair will occur if the root is not destroyed.

- **Hazards**
  Infection and scarring of the skin can occur if the upper part of the hair follicle is damaged by an incorrectly placed needle, or by moving the needle in or out of the follicle while the current is still flowing through it.

A photograph of the machine in use will be found on page 70.

Galvanic electrolysis

- **Purpose**
  It is used for the removal of unwanted facial hairs, but is a slower method than diathermy.

- **Effect**
  The region round the tip of the needle electrode inserted down the hair follicle becomes very alkaline. The hair root is therefore destroyed by a chemical (galvanic) burn and can be removed from the follicle.

- **Apparatus**
  A steady direct electric current is applied to the skin from a galvanic machine. It passes from an anode, consisting of a sponge pad soaked in salt solution, to a cathode which is the electrolysis needle inserted into the hair follicle. The tissue fluid acts as the electrolyte, conducting the current from anode to cathode.

- **Safety precautions**
  The needle electrode must be placed correctly so that its tip is in contact with the hair root.

- **Hazards**
  Galvanic burns may occur through over-treating a small area of skin. The positions of the sponge anode and needle cathode must not be too close together.

Blend machine

This method of epilation combines the galvanic current (DC) with the diathermy current (AC). This combines the chemical effect of the direct current with the heating effect of the high frequency current. The galvanic current produces alkaline sodium hydroxide at the hair root which is then heated by the diathermy current. The hair root is thus destroyed very rapidly by a combination of galvanic burn and resistance heating. It is the most effective method of epilation and is widely used in the UK and abroad.

Contra-indications

The skin conditions which contra-indicate epilation are psoriasis, eczema and infectious skin diseases. Acne, moles, warts, bruises or inflammation, as well as hypersensitive, very vascular or fragile skin, are contra-indications. In clients suffering from diabetes, epilepsy, asthma or hayfever, epilation is contra-indicated. The use of a sunbed immediately before or after epilation treatment is inadvisable.

HEAT THERAPY

A number of appliances used in beauty therapy treatments involve the heating effect of an electric current as it flows through a high resistance wire which is present in the heating element. In some appliances, the heating element produces steam by heating water.

Facial steamer

- **Purpose**
  It is used for preheating the skin, to aid the absorption of materials applied subsequently as masks or face packs. It is also used for deep cleansing of the skin of the face.

- **Effect**
  It has a diaphoretic effect, that is it increases sweating. It also causes vasodilation, increasing the rate of flow of blood and lymph. If the steamer also produces ozone, its antiseptic action on the skin may improve acne.

- **Apparatus**
  An electric heating element, containing a nichrome high resistance wire, is present in a kettle in which distilled water is boiled. Distilled water is used to prevent scaling in the kettle. The steam produced passes into a pipe where it is mixed with air and condenses, forming a fine spray which is directed onto the client's face. The steamer may contain a high-pressure mercury vapour lamp, producing ultra-violet radiation which converts molecular oxygen in the air to ozone.

- **Safety precautions**
  The client's eyes can be protected by damp cotton wool pads.

- **Hazards**
  The steamer should be isolated from other electrical equipment as the presence of water makes the occurrence of electric shocks from faulty equipment more likely. The steam treatment may make the client's pulse rate rise and lower the blood pressure, which could cause a client who already had abnormally low blood pressure to faint.

A photograph of the steamer in use will be found on page 226.

Steam bath

- **Purpose**
  It is used for preheating the body prior to massage and deep cleansing the skin.

- **Effect**
  The heat has a diaphoretic effect and increases the rate of flow of blood and lymph due to vasodilation. Activity of the sebaceous glands increases and muscular relaxation is promoted.

- **Apparatus**
  An electric heating element in a water tank heats water to 50–55 °C. The temperature is regulated by a thermostat and there is a thermal cut-out device in case the water level in the tank falls below the level of the heating element. The tank is contained in a thermally insulated cabinet from which the client's head will project. Warm air with a relative humidity of 95% surrounds the rest of the client's body.

- **Safety precautions**
  A towel soaked in cold water should be placed round the

client's neck to keep steam away from the head. The slatted seat over the water tank should be covered with a towel to protect the skin of the buttocks. The therapist should make regular temperature and pulse checks throughout the treatment. There should be an internal door handle to allow the client to come out of the cabinet immediately if she feels any discomfort during the treatment. A cooling down period of at least half an hour should elapse before a client is allowed to leave after treatment.

- **Hazards**
  Clients with low blood pressure, or who are on a low calorie slimming diet, could faint during the treatment.

Sauna

- **Purpose**
  It is used to induce a feeling of relaxation followed by vigour.

- **Effect**
  The heat increases the rate of flow of blood and lymph due to vasodilation. There is a fall in blood pressure and the pulse rate rises. Sweating is increased.

- **Apparatus**
  The sauna is a heated wooden cabin where steam is made. The cabin walls are both thermally insulating and water absorbing. The cabin contains a stove, inside which a thermostatically controlled electric element heats rocks. Water is poured onto the hot rocks to create steam. An air inlet is present just above floor level and there is an outlet near the top of the cabin. Warm air circulates by convection. The relative humidity of the air remains low at around 10%. An air temperature between 80 and 100 °C is usual for a ten minute treatment. Wooden benches on which the clients lie are provided in the cabin.

- **Safety precautions**
  Clients should be watched for symptoms of faintness during the treatment. It should be followed by a cool shower or a cooling down period of at least half an hour.

- **Hazards**
  Heating elements can cause fires and burns and must be heavily guarded. Clients often overestimate their ability to tolerate heat.

A photograph of a sauna will be found on page 256.

 Describe the safety precautions you would carry out for a client having a sauna treatment:
(a) before starting treatment
(b) during treatment
(c) after treatment

Far infra-red lamp

- **Purpose**
  It can be used for preheating the skin,

- **Effect**
  The heat rays produced do not penetrate below the epidermis of the skin, but the heat absorbed at the surface will spread downwards by conduction. The heat increases the rate of blood and lymph flow in the skin, and erythema results from vasodilation in the skin capillaries. Far infra-red rays are non-irritant and treatments of up to 30 minutes' duration can be tolerated.

- **Apparatus**
  A coil of high resistance wire is embedded in fireclay to form the heating element. When an electric current passes through the wire, it heats up and passes on the heat to the fireclay by conduction. The heating element produces only invisible far infra-red rays, which have a wavelength of around 4,000 nm (or 40,000 Angstrom units (Å) where 10 Å = 1 nanometre). Far infra-red rays thus have a long wavelength. The rays are reflected and focused by a polished metal concave reflector behind the element. The front of the lamp is covered by a wire guard. The lamp takes between 5 and 15 minutes to heat up.

- **Safety precautions**
  The client's skin must be clean and free from greasy preparations. Goggles should be worn to protect the eyes when the lamp is used on the face. The principle of the inverse square law must be applied. Treatment should never be continued for longer than 30 minutes or burning of the skin may occur.

- **Hazards**

  As the far infra-red radiation is invisible, it is impossible to tell by its appearance whether the lamp is switched on or off. There is thus the danger of burns due to touching the hot lamp. Too frequent use of these lamps can cause cataract by damaging the eye lens, and mottling of the skin with a network of dark brown lines.

These far infra-red lamps have been largely replaced in beauty salons by radiant heat lamps which produce mainly near infra-red radiation.

Radiant heat lamp

- **Purpose**

  It is used to relieve muscle tension.

- **Effects**

  The heat rays produced penetrate more deeply into the body, reaching the muscles. As the skin is warmed, the rate of blood and lymph flow increases and erythema occurs as a result of vasodilation. Sweating increases and muscles relax, relieving tension at the joints.

- **Apparatus**

  It consists of a glass bulb containing a tungsten filament which becomes hot when an electric current passes through it. The radiation emitted by the filament contains near infra-red of around 1,000 nm (10,000 Å) wavelength, some white (visible) light, and a small amount of ultra-violet. The bulb has a red glass filter which allows only the infra-red and visible red light to pass through it. The ultra-violet rays and the other colours in the visible white light are stopped by the filter. The bulb is filled with an inert gas at low pressure, and the top half of the bulb is coated with polished metal to reflect the radiation downwards. The lamp has an electric power rating of 200 to 250 watts, and heats up immediately it is switched on.

- **Safety precautions**

  The client's skin must be clean and free from greasy preparations. The principle of the inverse square law must be applied. The distance of the client from the lamp should be such that erythema does not occur until 10 minutes after the treatment starts. The application time should be short or the skin will burn. The lamp face should be parallel to the skin surface being irradiated so that a uniform heating effect is produced. The client's eyes should be protected by goggles to prevent cataract.

- **Hazards**
  The glass bulb becomes very hot in use and will burn the skin if it is touched. The bulb must not be dropped, knocked or splashed with water when hot or the glass will break. The bulb will then implode due to the partial vacuum inside it.

 What are the effects of a radiant heat lamp on the skin?

Figure 15.6   *Infra-red bulb*

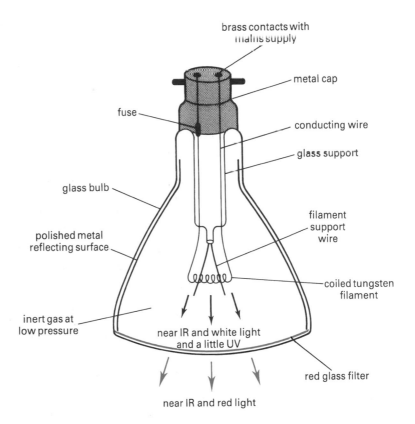

Contra-indications

Cardio-vascular disorders (angina and high or low blood pressure), epilepsy, asthma and migraine are all contra-indicated. Diabetics, who have a reduced sensitivity to heat and could be unaware that skin burning was taking place, should not receive heat therapy. Other contra-indications are the recent consumption of alcohol or a heavy meal, being on a low calorie slimming diet, and menstruation or pregnancy.

ULTRA-VIOLET THERAPY

Ultra-violet (UV) is electromagnetic radiation used in beauty therapy for its property of producing a 'suntan'. It is invisible, with a wavelength range shorter than that of visible light. It is divided into three regions, UVA (wavelength 400–320 nm), UVB (wavelength 320–290 nm) and UVC (wavelength 290–100 nm). UVC radiation with a wavelength shorter than 250 nm will convert molecular oxygen into ozone.

The UVA radiation will pass through ordinary glass, but UVB and UVC will not. UVA and UVB both pass through Perspex (plastic). All three types of UV radiation will pass through quartz glass. UVA rays penetrate the skin most deeply, reaching to the lower levels of the dermis. UVB rays penetrate only as far as the stratum basale of the epidermis. UVC rays only reach the outermost layers of the epidermis.

Lamps

Some ultra-violet lamps produce UVC rays as well as UVA and UVB rays, while others produce mainly UVA radiation.

- **Low-pressure mercury vapour** (LPMV) tubes produce mainly UVA radiation, not more than 1% being UVB. The electric current passing through the mercury vapour inside these tubes produces some UVC, but this is absorbed by the special coating of phosphors on the inside of the tube and is converted into UVA radiation which can pass out through the glass tube. R-UVA tubes have an internal reflector to boost the amount of UVA. The amount of UVB is reduced to 0.1%.

- **High-pressure mercury vapour** (HPMV or solarium) lamps produce all three types of ultra-violet radiation. These lamps are often bulb-shaped and contain a quartz tube of mercury vapour at high pressure which produces the ultra-violet radiation when an electric current passes through it. The lamp

Figure 15.7 *Low-pressure mercury vapour tube*

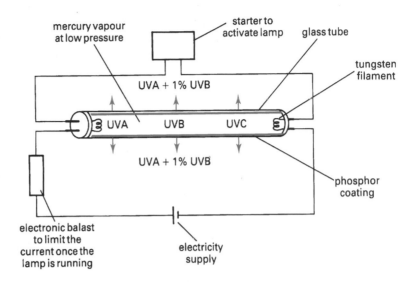

is fitted with a filter to stop UVC rays and to reduce the amount of UVB radiation to below 1% of the total.

 Compare the type of radiation emitted from a low-pressure mercury vapour tube and a high-pressure mercury vapour lamp.

Sunbeds and canopies

- **Purpose**
  They are used to produce a whole body tan.

- **Effects**
  These are entirely cosmetic. The tanning effect is due to increased activity of the melanocytes in the epidermis of the skin. Slight erythema may precede tanning. The skin is not protected against the UVB radiation in sunlight.

- **Apparatus**
  The sunbed and canopy contain LPMV tubes so almost all the radiation emitted is UVA. The tubes in the sunbed are covered by a Perspex sheet, over which the client lies. The canopy is supported from the ceiling at an adjustable height above the sunbed. A timer switch is incorporated, the safest type switching off the radiation automatically at the end of the selected treatment period.

- **Safety precautions**
The length of the treatment should be related to the amount of previous exposure to ultra-violet radiation and to the client's skin type. The inverse square law applies, so the distance of the canopy from the client's body must be carefully controlled. Goggles should be worn by both the client and the therapist to protect the eyes (see p. 245). Cotton wool pads or sunglasses provide insufficient protection from reflected radiation. Creams or perfume, which can increase the skin's sensitivity to ultra-violet radiation, should not be applied to the skin before the treatment.

- **Hazards**
Sunburn and conjunctivitis will result from overexposure to ultra-violet radiation. Premature ageing of the skin due to loss of elasticity can be caused by UVA. The development of skin cancers and thickening of the epidermis can result from overexposure to UVB radiation.

Individual tanning units

- **Purpose**
These units are used for tanning the face.

- **Apparatus**
They contain HPMV lamps which produce all three types of ultra-violet radiation.

- **Safety precautions**
Goggles must be worn to protect the eyes as UV rays cause conjunctivitis. The inverse square law applies.

- **Effects and hazards**
As for sunbeds.

Contra-indications

Pregnancy, a hypersensitive skin prone to sunburn, and a susceptibility to cold sores (Herpes simplex) are all contra-indications for ultra-violet therapy. It is also inadvisable for clients taking drugs which cause photosensitivity, e.g. tetracycline.

 List the beauty therapy treatments which necessitate protecting the client's eyes.

CHAPTER 16

Cosmetic Preparations

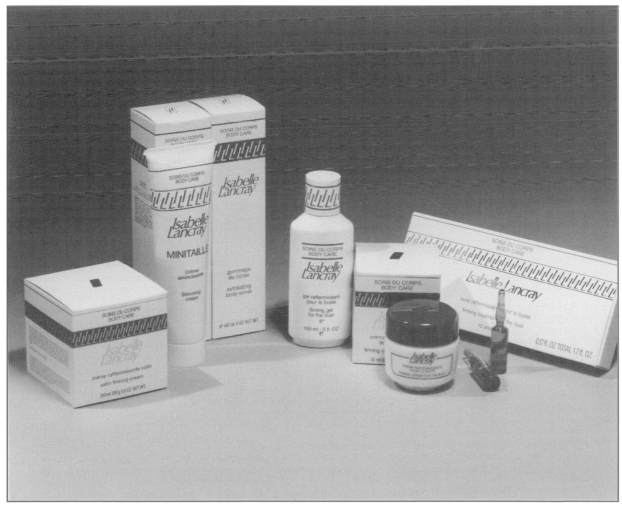

Beauty therapy preparations

EFFECTS

Cosmetic preparations are intended to improve the appearance, or to alter it to promote attractiveness. The main effects of cosmetics on the skin are to remove dirt; alter the colouring; retain water in the epidermis and delay wrinkling; and protect the skin from the harmful effects of ultra-violet radiation.

EU REGULATIONS

The wide variety of chemical substances used in cosmetic preparations have different effects on the skin, and in the past some of these substances have proved to be hazardous to the health of the users. There is now an EU directive regulating the use of substances in cosmetics. The hormones oestrogen and progesterone, for example, may not be included in any cosmetic preparation. Certain other substances are only permitted in quantities below a specified maximum, for example hydroquinone must not exceed 2% of a skin bleaching cream, and para-dye must not exceed 1.7% in a hair tint.

Many of the chemicals used in cosmetics are listed in the EU Code, and have E numbers like the food additives. The E numbers are given for just a few of the cosmetic ingredients listed in later sections of the chapter. In the case of lipstick, some of each application will inevitably reach the alimentary canal, being swallowed with food and drink. The same restrictions must therefore apply to its ingredients as apply to the food additives. As eye cosmetics come into contact with the delicate eye membrane (conjunctiva), stringent regulations apply here, particularly to the pigments permitted to colour the cosmetics.

A number of terms are used to describe the action of cosmetic preparations on the skin. These terms, with examples of the chemicals involved, are listed in the following section.

DESCRIPTIVE TERMS APPLIED TO COSMETIC INGREDIENTS

Emulsions

A cosmetic emulsion, or cream, is a suspension of droplets of one liquid in another (see chapter 1), where the two liquid phases are oil and water. The chemicals used to form the oil phase are either esters (produced from organic acids neutralised by alcohols) or hydrocarbons (mineral oils and paraffin wax).

ESTERS

The esters employed are oils, fats and waxes of vegetable and animal origin.

- The non-volatile or 'fixed' vegetable oils which are used include almond, olive, coconut and castor oils. Because they are unsaturated (see chapter 7), they are liable to go rancid. They are insoluble in ethanol (alcohol) with the exception of castor oil.

- The vegetable fat cocoa butter, which comes from crushed cacao seeds, is often included in cosmetic emulsions as it melts at body temperature and, being a saturated fat, does not go rancid.

- Carnauba wax, which is scraped from the leaf surfaces of the plant, makes cosmetic creams firmer in consistency.

- Waxes of animal origin, such as beeswax, lanolin and spermaceti, are also used. Lanolin comes from sheep's wool, and is a sensitiser, so it may cause dermatitis in some people. Spermaceti is obtained from the mixed oils of the sperm whale and consists mainly of cetyl palmitate and cetyl myristate, which are esters formed from cetyl alcohol and fatty acids.

- Synthetic waxes (e.g. Lanette wax), derived from cetyl alcohol, are also used as components of cosmetic creams.

HYDROCARBONS

Hydrocarbons are not true oils and waxes, but are also used in the preparation of some emulsions. The mineral oils and waxes used are obtained from petroleum. They are liquid paraffin, petroleum jelly and hard paraffin wax.

EMULSIFYING AGENTS

The emulsifying agents (emulsifiers) used in making cosmetic creams include soaps, cetrimide (a cationic soapless detergent), lecithin (E322 from egg yolk and soya beans) and synthetic emulsifying waxes (lanette). The emulsifying agent helps the droplets of one liquid to disperse in the other liquid by coating the surface of each tiny droplet. One end of each emulsifier molecule is attracted to the droplets of the disperse phase, and the other end is attracted to the molecules of the continuous phase.

STABILISERS

Emulsions can be stabilised (so that the oil and water phases do not separate out on storage) by adding gums, protein, starch or synthetic resin (e.g. PVP resin). When a cosmetic cream is applied to the skin, the two phases of the emulsion, which were homogeneously mixed, separate out. The water evaporates while the oil remains as a surface coating.

Humectants

A humectant is a substance which attracts water vapour from the atmosphere, that is it is hygroscopic. It will prevent a cream from drying out when exposed to air and thus becoming difficult to apply. Glycerol (E422), sorbitol and propylene glycol are added to creams as humectants. Glycerol must not be placed neat on dry skin or it removes water from the epidermis causing severe dehydration. It must always be applied with water.

Emollients

An emollient is a substance which reduces water loss from the dead stratum corneum forming the skin surface, thus preventing it from drying and cracking. By maintaining the water content of the epidermis it produces the emollient (softening) effect on the skin. Fats, oils and waxes are emollients as they form a waterproof film over the skin surface and greatly reduce evaporation from it. The skin's natural emollient is the wax sebum.

 Distinguish between an emulsion and an emollient.

Astringents

An astringent is a substance which has a tightening effect on the skin, making it look less flaccid. Some astringents (e.g. ethanol) are volatile liquids which cool the skin as they evaporate. Fruit and vegetable juices (lemon, carrot, cucumber) and orange flower water contain mild astringents. Stronger astringent effects are obtained from witch-hazel, lactic acid, menthol and potassium aluminium sulphate (alum). Stronger astringents should not be used on hypersensitive or dry mature skins as they are dehydrating.

Cleansers

A cleanser removes the skin's surface film of sebum, sweat and scales, together with soluble and particulate dirt and its associated bacteria and fungi.

DETERGENTS

Water alone removes soluble dirt, but oily dirt must be emulsified by using a detergent with water. Sodium stearate, potassium palmitate (soft soap) and lauryl sulphates (soapless) are suitable detergents for use on skin.

CREAMS

Cream cleansers consist of w/o emulsions, where oily dirt on the skin mixes readily with the oily continuous phase and particulate dirt adheres to the emulsion. Where the dirt to be removed is largely stale heavy make-up with a high wax content, the mineral oil liquid paraffin is an effective cleanser.

CLAYS

Natural clays or earths mixed into a paste and applied as a face mask can act as a cleanser. Surface dirt adheres to the inside of the paste mask and is removed with the hardened mask at the end of the treatment. Kaolin (china clay from decayed granite), bentonite (a volcanic clay) and fuller's earth (aluminium silicate clay) used in these pastes must be steam-sterilised to destroy any spores of the Bacillus tetani bacterium which causes tetanus (lockjaw).

 State the source of the following components of cosmetic preparations:
(a) spermaceti
(b) lanette wax
(c) kaolin
(d) liquid paraffin

Desquamators (exfoliators)

A desquamator removes some of the outermost layers of the stratum corneum from the skin epidermis. Comedones (blackheads) and milia (whiteheads) are removed, and deeper cleansing occurs. Soap solutions applied with a facial brush, or skin massage with an abrasive (e.g. oatmeal granules or crushed nuts), are used for facial desquamation. Pumice, which is a stronger abrasive, can be used on the thick skin of the soles of the feet where callosities occur.

Lubricants

A lubricant allows other surfaces to slide easily over the skin, providing slip. Many of the machines used in beauty therapy treatments have applicators which are moved over the skin, and during manual massage the therapist's hands must slide freely and painlessly on the client's skin. There are three main types of lubricant.

POWDER

Talc (magnesium silicate), the metallic soaps (magnesium and zinc stearates) and rice starch are powder lubricants. These fine powders should not be shaken into the air as they damage the lungs when breathed in. Talc, like other minerals, must be steam-sterilised to destroy tetanus spores.

CREAM

Cream lubricants contain a high proportion of petroleum jelly in their oil phase, and silicones (derived from sand) are added for extra slip.

MINERAL OIL

Unscented mineral oil (liquid paraffin) is an excellent lubricant for massage.

Barriers

BARRIER CREAM

One type of barrier forms an impervious layer over the skin surface, which protects the skin against dirt and some harmful chemicals and is resistant to water. Mineral oil is the major component of protective barrier creams. An effective barrier cream should have a pH between 5.6 and 6.5. It should also be non-sticky and stable to avoid the need for frequent re-application. Its protection against detergent solutions is short-lived however, as mineral oils in the cream, as well as other oils and waxes, will be emulsified.

SUNSCREENS

Another type of barrier, called a sunscreen, is used on the skin to protect it against ultra-violet radiation.

- Talc, chalk, kaolin, magnesium oxide and zinc oxide, in a cream or lotion base, act as a sun block to prevent all types of ultra-violet radiation reaching the skin, so tanning cannot occur. The sun-protection factor (SPF) indicates its sun-blocking ability.

- Barriers are available which filter out the more damaging UVB radiation of shorter wavelength, but allow UVA radiation to reach the skin and cause tanning. Para-aminobenzoic acid acts as this type of barrier, but it can be a sensitiser and cause dermatitis in some people.

Opacifiers

An opacifier is a substance used to make a transparent or translucent cosmetic preparation opaque, so that visible light cannot pass through it and be reflected from the skin surface. Opacifiers are used in preparations formulated to cover skin blemishes such as scars, naevi or acne pustules. Kaolin, titanium dioxide (E171) and zinc oxide are all white mineral powders which are good opacifiers.

What is meant by the following terms?
(a) a desquamator
(b) a humectant
(c) a fixed oil
(d) an opacifier

Colourants

Colourants are used in cosmetics to provide an overall skin-coloured tint, or to highlight particular features such as cheeks, eyes, lips and nails.

PIGMENTS AND LAKES

Pigments occur as solid coloured particles which are insoluble in water, ethanol or oil.

Lakes are solid coloured particles, obtained synthetically by adsorbing dyes onto the surface of insoluble metal oxides or hydroxides. For example, the dye cochineal adsorbed onto aluminium hydroxide forms the lake called carmine.

The insoluble pigments and lakes are usually used in cosmetic preparations as they neither 'run' by dissolving in sweat, tears or rain, nor permanently colour the skin by being adsorbed onto keratin molecules or dissolving in tissue fluid.

Natural pigments are inorganic materials and are non-sensitising, although lead- and mercury-containing pigments are highly toxic and not permitted in cosmetics. Examples of natural pigments that are used are carbon black (charcoal from burnt wood) and the mineral ores chrome green, ultramarine and yellow iron oxide (ochre).

SOLUBLE DYES

Soluble dyes form coloured solutions with one of the liquids present in cosmetics – water, ethanol or oil.

Dyes used in cosmetics are mainly synthetic materials, although cochineal obtained from the Mexican cochinellid beetle is of animal origin. Azo dyes are synthetic dyes derived from the coal tar product aniline. Azo dyes are sensitisers and cross-sensitisers, but are commonly used to form lakes as they provide a wide colour range. Cochineal (E120) is also a sensitiser.

Diaphoretics

Diaphoretics are substances that increase sweating by providing a waterproof and thermally insulating layer over the skin. A layer of wax, latex (rubber) or polyvinyl acetate (PVA) resin, applied as a face mask, has this effect.

Antiperspirants

An antiperspirant reduces the flow of sweat to the skin surface from the sweat glands, so it has the opposite effect to a diaphoretic. Antiperspirants may function by increasing the permeability of the sweat duct wall, so that less of the sweat secreted reaches the surface pore. Aluminium chlorhydrate is the compound usually used as an antiperspirant, but it can cause contact dermatitis in some people, particularly if the skin has been damaged by removing unwanted hair.

Deodorants

A deodorant removes unpleasant smells (body odour) from the skin. The odour is caused by the breakdown of the sweat and sebum of the skin's 'acid mantle' and the fatty materials in stale make-up. When triglycerides are broken down by bacteria, free fatty acids are produced which are largely responsible for the unpleasant smell. Apocrine sweat produced in the axillae contains small amounts of protein and sugars which are also broken down by bacteria. Unpleasant ammonia-related compounds are produced from the proteins.

The bacterial activity on the skin can be reduced by antiseptics which prevent the bacteria multiplying. Hexachlorophene which used to be used as a deodorant is no longer thought to be non-toxic, and hexamine has replaced it. The amount of antiseptic allowed in a skin deodorant is controlled by EU regulations.

Depilatories

A depilatory removes unwanted hair from the upper lip, chin, axillae and legs in women. The condition of terminal hair growth on the upper lip in women is hirsuties. The temporary removal of unwanted hair is known as depilation. It removes only the part of the hair shaft which projects from the skin and does not destroy the hair root, so the hair regrows.

CHEMICAL

Chemical depilatories break down the keratin forming the hair shaft by destroying its peptide and disulphide bonds. This weakens the hair sufficiently for it to break at skin surface level. Because of their action on keratin, chemical depilatories also damage the stratum corneum of the skin epidermis.

- Calcium thioglycollate is the active compound in most chemical depilatories. The preparation is made alkaline by calcium hydroxide to give a pH between 10 and 12.5. Both these chemicals attack disulphide bonds, and the alkaline calcium hydroxide destroys the peptide bonds in the polypeptide chains of the keratin. As thioglycollate is the active chemical in hair perming lotions as well, these depilatories have the same characteristic smell.

- Strontium sulphide is used in another type of faster acting chemical depilatory. It too breaks the disulphide bonds of hair keratin, but in contact with water forms hydrogen sulphide gas which has a 'bad egg' smell, making the preparation unpleasant to use.

WAX

Depilatory waxes are used to remove hair from the legs. The melted paraffin wax applied to the skin solidifies and the hairs become embedded in it. When the solidified wax is stripped off, the hairs break at skin surface level.

SUGAR

Sugar can be used as a depilatory and, unlike wax, it does not stick to the skin and can be applied at a lower temperature. This makes the process less painful than salon waxing. A paste of sugar is made with warm water and formed into a ball. It is massaged onto the skin area from which hair is to be removed, then pulled away against the direction of hair growth.

 In each case, state the effect on the skin of a cosmetic preparation containing:
(a) calcium thioglycollate
(b) hexamine
(c) aluminium chlorhydrate
(d) para-aminobenzoic acid

Perfumes

Perfumes add fragrance because they are absorbed by the outer layers of the skin. They are also used to cover the less pleasant smell of the oily components of skin cosmetics. A perfume consists of a blend of pleasantly smelling volatile plant products dissolved in methanol. A perfume is described in 'notes'. On first applying perfume to the skin, the most volatile ingredients give the 'top note'. Once the perfume has dried on the skin, the less volatile 'middle notes' are registered. The 'base note' remains after some time has passed. This persistent impression of the perfume is due to the least volatile oils.

ESSENTIAL OILS

The volatile plant products used in perfumes are essential oils (bergamot, rose, citrus, lavender, jasmine, etc.), resins such as pine terpenes, and balsams such as myrrh, which are mixtures of resins and essential oils. Unlike fixed plant oils, essential oils are soluble in the alcohols ethanol and methanol.

FIXATIVES

Fixatives are added to cause the scented molecules to evaporate at equal rates, so that the balance of the perfume does not change as it is used. The fixatives are usually animal products (ambergris, musk, civet and castor), but synthetic fixatives, such as benzyl benzoate and phthalates, may also be used.

SENSITISATION

Some balsams and essential oils, particularly bergamot and citrus oils, are sensitisers and photosensitisers. Perfume should never be placed on the skin before sunbathing or ultra-violet treatment because of the photosensitisation risk.

AROMATHERAPY

Aromatherapy is a branch of alternative medicine that uses essential oils from a variety of plants to treat the mind and body. The essential oils are usually applied to the skin during massage, but must always be diluted first. Up to 1 ml of the essential oil is dissolved in 50 ml of a fixed oil such as almond or wheatgerm oil. A few drops of an essential oil can also be added to bath water, or to a bowl of hot water from which it can be inhaled. Essential oils are absorbed by the skin and enter the blood.

Aromatherapy is said to alleviate disorders such as asthma, PMT

(PMS), anorexia, migraine and arthritis. Certain essential oils may affect a person's mood, for example jasmine and lavender oils are said to relieve depression, inducing a feeling of well-being. Tea-tree (Cajuput) oil is said to be effective in treating acne.

Aromatherapy treatment is contra-indicated in some cases as described below.

- Essential oils should not be taken internally or applied in concentrated form to the skin, as they can cause inflammation and allergic reactions.

- Some oils should not be used on pregnant clients as they are said to carry a slight risk of causing miscarriage (e.g. basil, rosemary, sage and thyme).

- Some essential oils induce a photosensitive response to UV radiation (e.g. bergamot and citrus oils).

- Varicose veins, scar tissue and inflamed skin areas contra-indicate aromatherapy by massage.

- Epilepsy, very high blood pressure and heart disease are also contra-indications.

Preservatives

A preservative is added to a cosmetic preparation to prevent large numbers of micro-organisms becoming established in it and being transferred to the skin when it is applied. The vegetable oils, starches and proteins in cosmetics are a source of food for bacteria and fungal spores present in the air. Mineral oils cannot be used as a food source by micro-organisms and do not require preservatives. The preservatives added to cosmetic preparations include para- and ethyl-hydroxybenzoates (parabens and nipagin respectively) at a concentration of 0.2%, benzoic acid (E210), cetrimide and essential oils. All of these compounds may act as sensitisers, causing dermatitis in some people. People with asthma may be particularly sensitive to benzoic acid.

Antioxidants

An antioxidant will prevent the unsaturated oils in a cosmetic preparation becoming rancid. This occurs when the double bonds ($C=C$) in their molecules are attacked by atmospheric oxygen to release unpleasant smelling fatty acids. Ascorbic acid (Vitamin C E300) and lecithin are used as antioxidants in most cosmetic creams. Sodium sulphite is used as an antioxidant in para dye base to prevent it darkening in the tube due to premature oxidation.

Bleaches

Hydroquinone is a skin bleach which acts by reducing the activity of the skin melanocytes so that less dark melanin pigment is produced. Hydroquinone is applied at a maximum strength of 2%, but it acts as a severe skin irritant on a number of people even at this low concentration, and these preparations may be a health hazard.

Palliatives

A palliative is used to treat incurable diseases and disorders as it will reduce the symptoms and alleviate pain, but it cannot effect a cure. Calamine lotion is a palliative used to treat sunburn.

COSMETIC PREPARATIONS FOR THE FACE

Emollient cream (skin conditioner)

These creams are used on the face overnight and have a softening effect on the skin. They may be o/w or w/o emulsions containing spermaceti and lanolin, together with vegetable oils for their emollient action.

Moisturising cream

These creams are used on the face overnight or as a make-up base for dry mature skins. They are o/w emulsions containing a mixture of natural and synthetic waxes which will coat the skin to reduce water loss from the epidermis. Added silicone helps the cream to spread rapidly and evenly over the skin. The cream contains a preservative (paraben or nipagin), and a humectant to maintain its water content. Alpha hydroxy acids (AHAs) are often included.

Moisturising creams are particularly valuable for all black skins and for ageing white skins. The older the skin becomes, the less

A suitable formula for vanishing cream would be:

Distilled water	73%
Lanette wax	15%
Glycerol	6%
Stearic acid	5%
Triethanolamine	1%
+ preservative and perfume	

Figure 16.1
Removing eye make-up

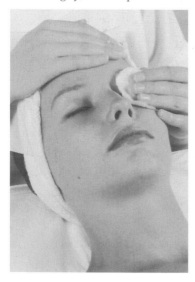

A suitable formula for a cold cream would be:

Liquid paraffin	50.0%
Distilled water	32.0%
Beeswax	16.0%
Sodium borate	1.0%
Perfume	0.8%
Nipagin	0.2%

efficient it is at retaining water. Moisturising creams do not nourish the skin as only the blood can supply nutrients. Adding collagen, elastin, lecithin or Vitamin E to the moisturising cream is ineffective as an anti-ageing aid.

Vanishing cream

This is an o/w emulsion used as a day cream and as a foundation for light make-up. Stearic acid and lanette wax or spermaceti are used for the disperse phase and are emulsified by an in situ soap formed from triethanolamine and stearic acid. A humectant, such as glycerol, may be included. A preservative (nipagin) and perfume are added.

Coloured foundation cream

A foundation cream must have good holding properties so that powder will cling to it. Adding lanolin to the blend of oils and waxes in the o/w emulsion achieves this. Pigments and lakes are added to give a uniform coloration to the skin of the face when the cream is applied. Titanium dioxide or zinc oxide are included to give opacity, and silicone is added to make the cream spread quickly and evenly. A preservative is required and perfume may be added.

Cold cream

This is a w/o emulsion which is used as a skin cleanser. When applied to the skin, the water in it quickly evaporates, and this has a cooling effect due to the removal of latent heat. Cold cream contains a high percentage of liquid paraffin which is effectively emulsified by an in situ soap, produced from beeswax and sodium borate.

Acid cream (pH balanced cream)

These creams are used to counteract the effects of alkaline soap solutions on the skin by maintaining a slightly acid pH of 5.6 to 5.8. An acid cream is an o/w emulsion of the vanishing cream type which contains a weak acid, such as citric acid, and a buffer to maintain the slightly acid pH.

Face packs and masks

The effects on the skin produced by using the various types of face pack or mask may be cleansing, stimulating, astringent, diaphoretic or emollient.

Certain precautions are necessary when applying face masks. The eyes must be protected by dampened cotton wool pads, and the preparation kept away from the nostrils, mouth and eyes. Clay-based masks must be made from sterilised materials because of the danger from tetanus spores.

CLAY BASE

Clay-based face packs are cleansing and stimulating in their action. They consist of a paste of clays and water which dries rapidly by evaporation of the water when it is applied to the face and neck. The pack is cleansing as surface dirt from the skin adheres to the clay. The warmth retained by the clay covering causes dilation of the skin blood capillaries, producing the stimulatory effect. The clay base is either kaolin or bentonite. By the addition of a humectant such as glycerol, enough water is retained to keep the face pack flexible and easier to apply. Titanium dioxide is added to the clay base as a whitener to improve its colour. Perfume and a preservative (paraben) are added. These face packs are most suitable for naturally greasy skins.

ASTRINGENT

Astringent masks are clay based and contract as they dry, producing the sensation of skin tightening. The clay base contains the more astringent fuller's earth and kaolin, instead of bentonite. Lactic acid, witch-hazel or orange flower water are added to increase the astringent effect. These masks should not be used on mature or hypersensitive skins, but they may help in treating acne on a greasy skin.

WARM OIL

Warm-oil masks are diaphoretic and emollient in their effect. A gauze mask is fitted over the face and neck, leaving holes for the eyes, nostrils and lips. The gauze is then soaked in warm almond oil. An infra-red lamp is directed onto the mask, the additional warmth increasing the diaphoretic effect. This type of mask is very suitable for mature dry skins.

A suitable formula for a clay-based face pack would be:

Distilled water	75%
Bentonite	15%
Glycerol	4%
Sulphonated castor oil	3%
Titanium dioxide	2%
Perfume and preservative	1%

WAX

Wax masks are diaphoretic and stimulating in their action. Paraffin wax, blended with petroleum jelly or cetyl alcohol, is melted and brushed onto the face and neck at a temperature very slightly above body temperature. It rapidly solidifies on the skin, forming a waterproof layer which is thermally insulating. The blood capillaries of the skin therefore dilate and the sweat glands become more active.

LATEX

Latex masks are similarly diaphoretic and stimulating in their action. They are applied as an emulsion of latex and water. The water evaporates, leaving a rubber film over the skin which is waterproof and thermally insulating. Emulsions of synthetic resins, such as polyvinyl acetate, can replace latex in this type of mask. Wax and latex or resin masks are all suitable for dry mature skins.

HYDROCOLLOID

Hydrocolloid (biological) masks consist of a sol or gel which is a colloidal suspension of gums, starches, or the proteins gelatin and casein. Polyvinyl synthetic resins may be used instead of the natural colloidal materials. Fruit or vegetable juices can be added to the colloids for particular effects, otherwise the masks are stimulating in their action.

Figure 16.2   *Application of face powder*

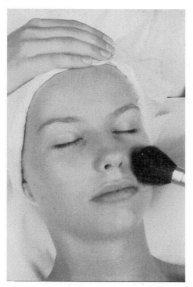

The sol or melted gel is applied over the face and dries quickly to form a plastic film which does not tighten. The fruit or vegetable juices can be selected to produce a slight astringency (e.g. cucumber), or to adjust the pH of the skin's surface film. Lemon juice will increase its acidity while carrot juice will reduce it. These hydrocolloid masks are suitable for mature, hypersensitive or dehydrated skins. They are useful for clients who dislike the greater tightening effect of other types of mask, or who prefer to have natural products used on their skin.

Q For a mature dry skin, name a suitable type of
(a) overnight cream
(b) face mask
(c) cleanser

Face powder

A face powder is a mixture of inert white powders to which pigment is added for a flesh tint. Titanium dioxide and zinc oxide are included to provide opacity, while talc and rice starch give slip. The absorption of sweat and sebum is performed well by magnesium carbonate and precipitated chalk, although chalk has a tendency to cake. Silicon dioxide (silica or sand) is anti-caking, but harmful to the lungs when breathed in. The metallic soaps (magnesium and zinc stearates) provide good skin adhesion, and rice starch gives a smooth matt surface. Lakes are the usual colourants. By the addition of a gum (karaya or tragacanth) to bind it, the powder can be marketed as a cake.

A suitable formula for a face powder would be:

Sterilised talc	70%
Rice starch	10%
Precipitated chalk	10%
Magnesium stearate	5%
Titanium dioxide	5%
+ colour and perfume	

Rouge and blushers

Red lakes or pigments are added to a variety of bases and applied to the skin of the cheeks as rouge or blusher. The ingredients used in face powder form one type of base, but cream or wax bases may hold the colourants. Silicone is added to cream and wax bases to aid smooth application of the blusher.

Lipstick

The base for a lipstick consists of a blend of oils and waxes which allows easy application and good adhesion. Castor oil (to hold the colourant), carnauba wax (to harden the base), beeswax, spermaceti, cetyl alcohol, petroleum jelly and lanolin (emollient) are commonly included in lipsticks. Silicone increases their ease of application and gives improved staying power. Pigments and lakes are used as colourants, and adding titanium dioxide produces paler shades. Lanolin in lipstick may act as a sensitiser.

A suitable formula for a lipstick would be:

Beeswax	30%
Petroleum jelly	25%
Carnauba wax	15%
Cetyl alcohol	15%
Castor oil	10%
Lanolin	5%
+ colourants, preservative and silicone	

Mascara

The base for mascara is either a blend of waxes similar to those used in lipsticks, or a w/o emulsion as in cream mascara. Inorganic pigments, which do not irritate the conjunctiva, are used as colourants, e.g. carbon, ultramarine, chrome green and iron oxides. Silicone is added for easier application and improved staying power.

A suitable formula for mascara would be:

Petroleum jelly	63%
Carbon black	20%
Cocoa butter	6%
Beeswax	4%
Spermaceti	4%
Cetyl alcohol	2%
Silicone + preservative	1%

Figure 16.3   *Application of eye liner*

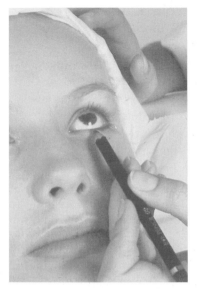

Eye shadow and eye liner

The base for these preparations consists of an o/w emulsion similar to vanishing cream, or a mixture of waxes. Inorganic pigments are used as colourants.

Eyebrow pencils

These pencils have a hard wax base which holds the inorganic pigments used as colourants.

Eyelash dye

Paratoluene diamine hair dyes, oxidised by hydrogen peroxide, are usually used to permanently colour eyelashes. As there is a high frequency of contact dermatitis due to these dyes, patch tests for sensitivity should be given 48 hours before the treatment and great care exercised when applying the dye.

 State the possible hazards associated with the following ingredients of cosmetic preparations:
(a) bentonite
(b) lanolin
(c) witch-hazel
(d) paratoluene diamine

COSMETIC PREPARATIONS FOR THE NAILS

Nail cream

Like the rest of the skin keratin, nails lose water and become brittle, resulting in the disorder Fragilitas unguium. This is particularly likely to occur in older people, or where a person spends a lot of time with their hands in hot detergent solutions.

A cream for treating degreased dehydrated brittle nails is:

2% Salicyclic acid ointment	50%
Glycerin of starch	50%

 Distinguish between dyes, pigments and lakes. Which of these colourants would be most suitable for:
(a) mascara
(b) blusher
(c) lipstick

Nail lacquer

Nail lacquer is a solution which, when painted onto the nails, leaves a film of varnish (enamel) when the solvent has evaporated. The film-former used in nail lacquer is nitrocellulose (produced from plant celluloses) which holds colourants well. As a nitrocellulose film does not adhere to the nail plate very firmly, and chips easily, an adhesive is added to the lacquer. Formaldehyde resin improves film adhesion and hardens the varnish, but can cause contact dermatitis in some people. Adding silicone will also toughen the varnish. Phthalates or isopropyl myristate are added as plasticisers to give the varnish elasticity and prevent flaking.

All these materials are dissolved in a mixture of volatile solvents which evaporate at slightly different rates. Toluene and ethyl, butyl and amyl acetates may be included in the solvent blend. These solvents are highly flammable so nail lacquer should be kept away from heat and flames, including lighted cigarettes. If inhaled, the solvents can damage the lungs. If the solvent evaporates too rapidly, the lacquer will not flow well and brush marks will show in the varnish.

COLOURED

Coloured nail lacquer contains inorganic pigments or lakes, and titanium dioxide can be added to obtain paler shades. Adding bentonite helps to keep the pigments and lakes in suspension. Pearl nail lacquers commonly contain Timicas (mica flakes coated with titanium dioxide) or bismuth oxychloride. Guanine from fish scales may be used as a pearliser but is expensive.

BASE COAT

This is a clear lacquer which is applied to the nail and allowed to dry before brushing on coloured nail lacquer. Base coat contains a lower percentage of nitrocellulose and an increased percentage of formaldehyde resin to improve adhesion to the nail. It forms a harder varnish as less plasticiser is added. The coloured lacquer adheres more readily to this base coat of varnish than it does to the nail.

 List four components of nail lacquer and explain the role of each component in the preparation.

Cuticle remover

A 2% solution of the alkalis sodium or potassium hydroxide is caustic and will soften the keratin of the cuticle by attacking its disulphide bonds. The cuticle can then be pushed back from the nail plate to expose the lunula of the nail more fully. Alkalis also remove sebum, so the skin round the base of the nail may become brittle and crack after using this preparation. A humectant, such as glycerol, is usually added to counteract its degreasing and dehydrating effect.

Less alkaline cuticle removers are available which contain sodium phosphate instead of sodium hydroxide. Sodium phosphate is the salt of a strong base and a weaker acid. It ionises to form an alkaline solution, but the presence of the weak acid lowers the pH.

Liquid nail varnish remover

This preparation consists of a mixture of solvents which dissolve nail varnish readily, such as ethyl, butyl and amyl acetates. The mixture of solvents is not identical to that present in nail lacquer, so the preparation cannot be used successfully to dilute thickened nail lacquer. These acetates are also fat solvents and remove sebum from the skin round the nail plate, so lanolin or castor oil are added to the preparation to counteract the degreasing effect. Nail varnish remover is flammable and can damage the lungs if much is inhaled.

Nail hardener

This is a lacquer containing formaldehyde resin as the film-former so that the varnish adheres very firmly to the nail plate. This varnish helps to prevent soft nails chipping or peeling. Formaldehyde resin may cause contact dermatitis round the edges of the nail. It is therefore helpful if the cuticle and skin round the nails are protected by a film of oil before the nail hardener is applied.

Nail repairer

This preparation contains nitrocellulose and formaldehyde resin film-formers, together with fine suspended fibres of rayon or nylon which will reinforce the varnish. A phthalate plasticiser is added to keep the varnish flexible. The solvent is a blend of toluene and ethyl acetate. Several coats of this preparation are required to repair torn or damaged finger nails.

Nail white

Special pencils, containing a wax core in which titanium dioxide and zinc oxide are dispersed, are used to apply a film of white material below the translucent free edge of the nail.

Nail polish

To give shine to the nail and remove small irregularities, an abrasive powder or paste is applied and rubbed over the nail with a buffing pad. The frictional heat causes dilation of the blood capillaries below the nail. The best abrasive for this purpose is stannic oxide, which is mixed with talc to give slip. As stannic oxide is expensive, the cheaper precipitated chalk may be the abrasive ingredient.

COSMETIC PREPARATIONS FOR BLACK SKIN

Skin bleach

A skin bleach may be used by black women to lighten the complexion, so that its coloration is both paler and more even and make-up has a greater impact. Skin bleaches containing hydroquinone are available, but only about 60% of treatments appear to give satisfactory results. A course of treatment requires two applications of the bleach daily for up to four months. The skin must not be exposed to sunlight over the treatment period.

Concentrations of hydroquinone above 2% are illegal in skin bleaches, but even at this low level hydroquinone can be a health hazard. It has been found to cause skin cancers or irreversible skin damage in some women. The permanent destruction of small groups of melanocytes commonly causes small white patches (vitiligo) on black skin.

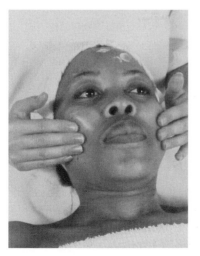

Figure 16.4 *Moisturising black skin*

Desquamators

These preparations are used on black skin to leave leave a smoother, less ashy surface for the application of make-up. The most suitable desquamators contain plant products, e.g. oatmeal granules. The AHA glycolic acid is a mild desquamator used in night creams.

Moisturising cream

As black skin, though shiny, is not oily, moisturising cream should be applied during the day as well as overnight, in preference to other types of cosmetic creams. The oil phase of the cream should consist of plant waxes and oils and fats such as cocoa butter, rather than mineral oils and glycerol which form a heavier film on the skin surface.

Cleansers

Highly degreasing cleansing lotions containing ethanol should not be used on black skins. Cleansing clay-based face packs are effective and they also have a desquamating effect.

Foundation

White creams should not be used on black skins. A colourless gel base which will hold powder is a more a suitable make-up foundation.

Face powder

Face powder should be composed of very fine particles of the usual inert powders with suitable colourants. Titanium dioxide or zinc oxide should not be present as these substances produce a greyish appearance on black skin.

COSMETIC PREPARATIONS FOR THE BODY

Massage cream

An emollient cream can be used to lubricate the skin during massage as an alternative to unscented mineral oil or talcum powder. The cream is usually a w/o emulsion with a high mineral oil content.

A suitable formula for talcum powder would be:	
Sterilised talc	80%
Precipitated chalk	15%
Magnesium stearate	5%
+ perfume	

Talcum powder

This preparation is an absorbent powder which removes traces of water left on the skin after towel drying and absorbs sweat and sebum from the skin surface. Talcum powder also has lubricating properties, preventing skin surfaces from sticking together and allowing clothing to slide over the skin easily. It also provides lubrication for manual or electrical massage treatments. For absorbency, the powder contains precipitated chalk, magnesium carbonate, silicon dioxide or kaolin. Talc provides good lubrication, while magnesium and zinc stearates are necessary for skin adhesion. The talc used should be sterilised, and talcum powder should not be breathed in as it may cause lung damage.

 In each case, give the name of one ingredient which gives the following properties to talcum powder:
(a) skin adhesion
(b) lubrication
(c) sweat absorption

Foot powder

A foot powder has a talcum powder base containing kaolin for additional absorbency. Medicating agents may be added to protect against fungal attack between the toes which causes athlete's foot, and bacterial breakdown of sweat causing hyperidrosis or bromidrosis. Zinc undecenoate is added as a fungicide, and salicylic acid reduces the bacterial activity which causes unpleasant foot odour.

Antiperspirant and deodorant preparations

Chemicals having these two effects on the skin are usually combined in a single preparation. It may be applied from an aerosol spray, a roll-on stick or as a cream, and is mainly used on the underarm area. In addition to aluminium chlorhydrate as the antiperspirant and hexamine as the deodorant, the preparation contains silicone to make it flow smoothly and dry quickly. Silicone also reduces any stinging sensation when the preparation is applied. Zirconium salts can be used, but not in sprays as they are harmful if inhaled.

Artificial suntan lotion

Some of these lotions contain a brown pigment and, when applied, their effect on the skin is entirely cosmetic as they give no protection against sunburn. They are difficult to apply sufficiently evenly to get uniform coloration and the pigment is often unconvincing as a suntan.

Another type of artificial suntan lotion contains the colourless compound dihydroxyacetone as a 2.5% solution in an ethanol/water solvent. The dihydroxyacetone reacts with some of the keratin amino acids to form a brown compound, so the tanning effect occurs gradually. This preparation can be used to disguise areas of skin where vitiligo occurs. Dihydroxyacetone may cause severe contact dermatitis in some people.

Suntanning pills

Suntanning pills containing canthaxanthin and beta-carotein have been available. They produce a tanning effect by colouring the subcutaneous fat. Although both the active ingredients of these pills are permitted food colourings, the pills have been found to cause eye damage and are being withdrawn. In no case should clients be persuaded to take suntanning pills containing canthaxanthin.

Sunburn lotion

Sunburn is treated by applying calamine lotion which is a suspension of zinc carbonate. It has a palliative cooling effect on the skin. Lacto-calamine is a lotion containing 4% zinc carbonate, 5% witch-hazel and 0.2% phenol. The witch-hazel reduces skin inflammation. The phenol acts as an anaesthetic to reduce the pain from sunburn and prevents infection of the damaged skin.

 Explain the reason for applying:
(a) Base coat nail lacquer
(b) Calamine lotion
(c) 2% hydroquinone solution

Table 16.1   *Summary of the characteristics of the major cosmetic ingredients*

Name	Source or nature	Effect	Cosmetic use	Hazards
Acetone	Organic solvent	Degreaser	Nail varnish remover	Flammable
Almond oil	Fixed plant oil	Emollient	Warm oil mask	–
Aluminium chlorhydrate	Inorganic salt	Antiperspirant	Antiperspirant	Irritant
Amyl acetate	Organic solvent	-	Nail lacquer	Flammable
Ascorbic acid	Vitamin C	Antioxidant	Cosmetic creams	–
Azo dyes	From coal tar	Colourant	As lakes	Cross-sensitisers
Beeswax	Animal wax	Emollient	Creams, lipstick	–
Bentonite	Volcanic clay	Cleanser	Clay face pack	Tetanus spores
Calamine	Mineral salt	Palliative	Sunburn lotion	–
Calcium thioglycollate	Organic salt	Depilatory	Depilatories	Irritant
Carmine	Cochineal lake	Colourant	Rouge	Irritant
Carnauba wax	Plant wax	Emollient	Lipstick	–
Cetyl alcohol	Synthetic wax	Emollient	Emulsifier	–
Chalk	Mineral salt	Absorbent	Talcum powder	Dries the skin
Cocoa butter	Plant fat	Emollient	Creams	–
Dihydroxyacetone	Synthetic	Browns skin	Tanning lotion	Sensitiser
Essential oils	Volatile plant oil	Perfume	Perfumes, aromatherapy	Sensitisers
Ethanol	Organic solvent	Astringent	Toners	Hardens skin
Formaldehyde resin	Synthetic resin	Hardens nail	Base coats	Irritant
Fuller's earth	Mineral clay	Cleanser	Astringent mask	Tetanus spores
Glycerol	From triglyceride	Humectant	Moisturisers	Dehydrating
Hexamine	Organic base	Antiseptic	Deodorants	–
Hydroquinone	Phenol derivative	Bleaching	Skin bleach	Irritant, vitiligo
Inorganic pigments	Mineral ores	Colourant	Lipstick, mascara	–

Table 16.1   *continued*

Name	Source or nature	Effect	Cosmetic use	Hazards
Kaolin	Clay from quartz	Cleanser	Clay packs	Tetanus spores
Lactic acid	Sour milk	Astringent	Astringent mask	–
Lanolin	Sheep wool	Emollient	Hand cream	Sensitiser
Lauryl sulphates	Soapless detergent	Cleanser	Shampoo	Degreaser
Lecithin	Egg yolk lipid	Antioxidant	Creams	–
Liquid paraffin	Mineral oil	Emollient	Barrier cream	–
Magnesium stearate	Metallic soap	Lubricant Adhesion	Talcum powder	
Nitrocellulose	Plant celluloses	Varnish	Nail lacquer	–
Orange flower water	Essential oil	Astringent	Toners	–
Para-aminobenzoic acid	Organic acid	UVB filter	Sunscreens	Sensitiser
Paraffin wax	Mineral wax	Diaphoretic	Wax mask, depilatory	–
Paraben	Organic acid	Antiseptic	Preservative	Sensitiser
Phthalate	Ester	-	Plasticiser	Sensitiser
Polyvinyl acetate resin	Synthetic resin	Coating	Hydrocolloid mask	–
Propylene glycol	Organic alcohol	Humectant	Vanishing cream	
Rice starch	From rice grains	Lubricant	Face powder	–
Salicylic acid	From willow bark	Desquamator	Desquamators	Irritant
Silicone	From sand	Lubricant	Lipstick, rouge	–
Sodium stearate	Hard soap	Cleanser	Toilet soap	–
Spermaceti	Animal wax	Emollient	Creams	–
Talc	Mineral	Lubricant	Skin powders	Tetanus spores
Titanium dioxide	Mineral	Opacifier	Powders, lipstick	–
Witch-hazel	Plant extract	Astringent	Toners	–
Zinc oxide	Mineral	Opacifier	Face powder, sunscreen	–
Zinc stearate	Metal soap	Lubricant Adhesion	Talcum powder	–

Longer questions

1   (a)   By means of a diagram only, describe a ring main circuit.
    (b)   List three advantages of this type of circuit compared with older methods of wiring.
    (c)   State where you would find the following structures in a ring main circuit.
          (i)   a conductor
          (ii) a device to prevent electric shock
          (iii) a 30 amp circuit breaker
          (iv) a brown insulating cover

2   (a)   State the position, origin and insertion of the following muscles:
          (i)   brachialis
          (ii) brachioradialis
          (iii) triceps brachii.
    (b)   Give a labelled diagram of the joint where movement occurs due to the action of these three muscles.
    (c)   Name the type of movement each muscle produces at the joint.

3   (a)   Draw up a table to show the source, chemical nature and cosmetic use of the following cosmetic ingredients:
          (i)   bentonite
          (ii) lanolin
          (iii) glycerol
          (iv) ethyl acetate
          (v)   para-aminobenzoic acid
          (vi) hydroquinone
          (vii) aluminium chlorhydrate
    (b)   For each substance, explain the possible hazards of its use.

4   (a)   Draw a simple labelled diagram of a section through the female breast.
    (b)   Describe the influence of hormones on:
          (i)   the development of the breast
          (ii) lactation

5 (a) Compare the chemical structure of starch and protein molecules.
   (b) Explain why unrefined carbohydrates should be present in the diet in preference to refined ones. List six foods which would supply unrefined carbohydrates to a diet.
   (c) What are the main uses of dietary starch and protein in the body's metabolism?

6 (a) Describe one appliance producing infra-red radiation and one producing ultra-violet radiation which are used in a beauty therapy salon.
   (b) Indicate any precautions which should be taken when using these appliances to treat a client.
   (c) Name any contra-indications associated with the use of these appliances.

7 (a) By means of a fully labelled diagram only, describe the blood supply to the liver.
   (b) Draw up a table to indicate the differences in structure and function of an artery and a vein.
   (c) List the functions of each of the following blood components:
        (i)   erythrocytes
        (ii) leucocytes
        (iii) thrombocytes
        (iv) plasma proteins

8 Give a diagram and explain the action of each of the following components of the nervous system:
   (a) a synapse
   (b) a motor neuron
   (c) a reflex arc
   (d) the fifth cranial nerve

9 (a) Draw a simple labelled diagram of a longitudinal section through a finger nail.
   (b) Describe the effects on the nail of the following diseases or disorders:
        (i)   pterygium unguium
        (ii) onycholysis
        (iii) agnail
        (iv) paronychia
   (c) List the constituents of nail lacquer and explain the function of each in this cosmetic preparation.

10 (a) Describe each of the following bones in terms of its type, position and main role in the body:
        (i)   femur
        (ii) scapula
        (iii) thoracic vertebra
        (iv) patella
        (v)   calcaneum
   (b) Draw a clear labelled diagram of a thoracic vertebra.

Definitions of Terms

GENERAL TERMS

Acromegaly is an increase in growth of the extremities (hands, feet, chin, jaws, nose and ears) in adults who secrete an abnormally large amount of the growth hormone somatotropin.

Actin is the protein occurring in the thin contractile filaments of muscle tissue which slide towards each other as a muscle contracts.

Active transport is a process by which substances can cross a membrane from a region of lower concentration to one of higher concentration, using energy in order to do so.

Adrenal hyperplasia is an abnormal increase in size of the adrenal gland resulting from a tumour.

Aerobic describes the type of respiration which requires oxygen.

Allergen is a substance causing an allergic reaction in people who are hypersensitive to it. It may be present in the environment, in food or in drugs.

Allergy is a condition of hypersensitivity to a substance to which the majority of people do not react.

Alternating current is an electric current in which the direction of flow in a circuit reverses many times a second according to its frequency.

Amino acids are the units linked by peptide bonds to form proteins.

Anaerobic describes the type of respiration which occurs in the absence of oxygen.

Anagen is the growing phase of the hair-growth cycle.

Antagonistic pairs of muscles act on the same joint with opposite effects, as each muscle of the pair contracts alternately.

Antibody is a substance produced by some types of white blood cell, e.g. lymphocytes, which destroys pathogens.

Antigens are chemicals carried on a person's red blood cells which determine their blood group.

Antioxidants are chemicals which prevent the oxidation of fats and oils – a reaction which makes a cosmetic preparation become rancid.

Apocrine glands are the large sweat glands found in the armpits which secrete a milky fluid containing organic substances. Bacterial breakdown of this sweat causes 'body odour'.

Areola is the circular pigmented area surrounding a nipple.

Arteries are blood vessels taking blood from the heart.

Assimilation is the incorporation of nutrients into the living cells of the organism, where they are involved in cell metabolism.

Astringents are substances which tighten the skin.

Atoms are the smallest particles of an element which can be involved in a chemical change.

ATP is the molecule which stores the energy produced by the breakdown of nutrients. It can release this energy for use by the living body cells.

Atria are the two upper chambers of the heart into which blood enters from veins.

Autonomic nervous system controls the involuntary activities of glands, e.g. sweat glands, and of cardiac and smooth muscle. It involves sympathetic and parasympathetic nerves.

Balanced diets contain all six main nutrient groups in adequate amounts for energy, growth, reproduction and protection of the body.

Breathing is the process by which air enters and leaves the body during inspiration and expiration respectively.

Capacitors are devices which store electric charge. They are used to smooth out a direct current.

Capillaries are very narrow blood vessels which form networks in the body tissues linking arterioles to venules. They allow exchange of materials between the blood and the tissue cells.

Cardiac cycle is the inherent rhythm with which the heart muscle contracts and relaxes.

Cells are the units which make up the human body.

Cisterna chyli is a small widening of the thoracic duct in the abdomen. Lymph from the lower regions of the body drains into it.

Collagen is the protein fibre giving strength and flexibility to connective tissue.

Compounds can be split up into two or more simpler substances by a chemical change.

Cooper's ligaments occur in the breast to support the glandular tissue and fat. They run between the skin and deep fascia and are composed of fibrous connective tissue.

Cretinism is a condition of retarded mental, physical and sexual development found in children with insufficient thyroxin.

Cystitis is an inflammation of the wall of the bladder.

Deamination is the stage in protein breakdown where the nitrogen-containing amino group is removed and converted into urea.

Deep Further away from the surface, lying underneath other structures

Deodorants prevent an unpleasant body odour from the skin by reducing the activity of skin bacteria which break down sweat and sebum.

Depilatories remove unwanted hair by destroying the part of the hair shaft that projects from the skin surface.

Desincrustation is a skin cleansing process. A direct electric current produces a chemical effect by increasing the alkalinity of an area of the skin.

Desquamation occurs when skin scales flake off from the epidermal surface.

Desquamators remove some of the scaly cells of the outermost layer of the skin to produce a smoother surface.

Diabetes is a disease in which glucose is present in urine. It results from inadequate amounts of the hormone insulin being produced by the pancreas.

Diaphoretics are substances applied to the skin that increase sweating.

Diaphysis is the shaft of a long bone. It contains yellow bone marrow in the central cavity.

Diastole is the relaxation of the cardiac muscle.

Diffusion is a physical process by which a substance moves from a region of higher concentration to one of lower concentration.

Digestion is the conversion of complex food materials into simpler soluble substances.

Direct current is an electric current which flows in one direction only round a circuit.

Dispersion is the splitting up of light into its component coloured rays, producing a spectrum.

Distal Further from the mid-line. In the case of the limbs, those parts lying furthest away from the trunk

Diuretic is a substance which increases the volume of urine produced.

DNA is the chemical forming the genes (heritable material). It is present in the cell nucleus.

Earth wires are safety devices included in electric circuits to prevent electric shock.

Electrolytes are solutions containing ions. An electric current will flow through such a solution.

Elements are substances which cannot be split into two or more simpler substances by a chemical change.

Emollients are skin softeners. They reduce water loss from the skin surface, preventing it from drying and hardening.

Emulsions are suspensions of droplets of one liquid in another, forming a cream. The two liquids must be insoluble in one another.

Endocrine describes a gland whose secretion passes directly into the blood.

Endocrine glands are ductless glands which secrete hormones directly into the blood stream.

Enzymes are biological catalysts which speed up chemical reactions in the body. They are present in most digestive juices.

Epilation is a process where the destruction of a hair root results in the permanent removal of an unwanted terminal hair.

Erythrocytes are red blood cells.

Excretion is the removal of the waste products of metabolism.

Exocrine describes a gland whose secretion is passed into a duct.

External respiration is the gaseous exchange which occurs in the lungs between the blood and the alveolar air.

Fertilisation is the fusion of an ovum and a sperm to produce an embryo which develops into a new individual.

Fibrinogen is a plasma protein dissolved in blood and lymph which acts as a clotting agent.

Fuses are safety devices in an electric circuit to protect the wiring from damage when the circuit becomes overloaded.

Gametes are reproductive cells which fuse together to produce a new individual. Male gametes are sperms and female gametes are ova.

Glomerulus is a knot of blood capillaries lying in the capsule of each nephron.

Glycosuria is a condition where glucose is excreted in the urine. It is one of the symptoms of diabetes mellitus.

Goitres are anterior swellings at the base of the neck due to enlargement of the thyroid gland.

Gonads are the sex organs which produce gametes. The male gonad is the testis and the female gonad is the ovary.

Haemoglobin is the purple oxygen-carrying pigment in the blood. It is bright red in colour when saturated with oxygen and is then known as oxyhaemoglobin.

Haversian systems consist of concentric rings of bone cells round a central canal. They occur in compact bone tissue.

Homeostasis is the maintaining of stable conditions within the body.

Hormones are chemical messengers secreted by endocrine glands and carried round the body by the blood.

Humectants attract water vapour from the atmosphere as they are hygroscopic. They retain water in an emulsion, preventing it from drying out.

Humidity is the amount of water vapour in the air.

Hyaluronic acid is the natural skin moisturiser present in the dermal matrix.

Hyperaesthesia is over-sensitivity to touch and contra-indicates massage.

Hyperglycaemia is an abnormally high level of glucose in the blood.

Hypertension is high blood pressure, the most common disease affecting the cardio-vascular system.

Immunity is the ability to resist disease. It is conferred by the presence, in the person's blood, of the specific antibody to the pathogen involved.

Insertion is the point of attachment of a muscle to a bone which will move as the muscle contracts. The insertion is the pulling end of the muscle.

Internal respiration is the gaseous exchange which occurs in the tissues between the blood and living tissue cells.

Ions are particles carrying an electric charge formed from atoms or molecules which have lost or gained electrons.

Iontophoresis is the process whereby chemicals are introduced into the intact skin by a direct electric current.

Isometric describes muscle contractions where the muscle tenses but does not shorten.

Isotonic describes muscle contractions where the muscle shortens and bulges.

Keratinisation is the formation of horny keratin granules within a cell. It makes the cell waterproof, but kills it in the process.

Latent heat is the heat either given out or absorbed when a substance changes its state, for example heat absorbed from the skin when sweat evaporates.

Leucocytes are white blood cells. They are of several types found in the blood and infected tissues.

Ligaments are fibroelastic bands of connective tissue holding bones in position. They are usually found at joints.

Lymph nodules are blocks of lymphocytes in the outer cortex of lymph nodes.

Lymphocytes are white blood cells produced in the lymph nodes. They make antibodies to destroy bacteria and their toxins.

Lymphoid tissue is a specialised form of connective tissue found in lymph nodes, the spleen, tonsils, thymus gland and Peyer's patches.

Macrophages are cells in the outer cortex of lymph nodes which filter the lymph by ingesting bacteria, damaged cell material and unwanted proteins.

Meiosis is the type of cell division occurring only when eggs and sperms are produced. Each new cell contains only half the parental DNA and is therefore not identical to the parent cell.

Melanin is the pigment in skin and hair produced by melanocytes.

Meninges are the membranes surrounding the brain and spinal cord.

Menopause is the stage at which an individual's reproductive phase ends. In women this occurs in late middle age.

Menstrual cycles are periodic changes in the ovary and uterus in women, each cycle lasting around 28 days. During each cycle an egg is released from an ovary, and changes occur in the uterus wall terminating in menstruation.

Metabolism is the sum of all the living processes of the body which use and supply chemicals and energy, and remove waste materials.

Micturition is the emptying of the bladder so that urine is passed out of the body.

Minute volume is the volume of air taken in with each normal quiet breath, multiplied by the number of breaths per minute, e.g. $0.5 \times 16 = 8$ litres.

Mitosis is the type of cell division where the daughter cells are identical to the parent cell, containing the full amount of parental DNA.

Molecules are the smallest particles of an element or compound that can exist alone.

Motor point is the place where a motor nerve enters a muscle to stimulate contraction.

Myelin is a fatty, non-conducting material which surrounds some nerve fibres to prevent loss of the nerve impulse.

Myoglobin is a red oxygen-storing pigment in red skeletal muscle.
Myosin is the protein occurring in the thicker contractile filaments of muscle tissue.
Myxoedema is the slowing down of the metabolic rate due to a shortage of the hormone thyroxin.
Nephrons are the functional units of the kidney which separate waste products from the blood and maintain the body's osmotic balance.
Neurons are cells which conduct nerve impulses.
Nutrients are components of food needed for energy and warmth, growth and repair, and protection against disease.
Oedema is the accumulation of fluid in the tissues causing puffy local swellings.
Opacifiers make a cosmetic preparation opaque so that light does not pass through it. Such preparations are used to cover skin blemishes and as sun blocks.
Organelles are characteristic structures occurring within cells.
Organs are structures within the body which carry out one or more particular functions. They may contain several different types of tissue.
Origin is the point of attachment of a muscle to a bone remaining stationary as the muscle contracts.
Oscillators are electronic switches used to produce an alternating current of very high frequency.
Osmoregulation is the process maintaining the normal salt/water balance in the body.
Osmosis is a physical process by which water passes from a dilute solution into a more concentrated solution through a semi-permeable membrane.
Osteoporosis is a decrease in bone mass causing softening and shortening of the bones.
Ovulation is the release of a ripe ovum from an ovary. It occurs at the mid-point of the menstrual cycle.
Pathogens are disease-causing organisms.
Periosteum is the membrane that covers a bone.
Peristalsis consists of squeezing movements of the walls of the alimentary canal which push the food along.
pH is the scale from 0 to 14 on which the degree of acidity or basicity is measured.
Phagocytosis is one form of active transport by which a cell can engulf solid particles.
Pheromones are sexual attractants present in apocrine sweat.
Plexus is a nerve network comprising branches (rami) from several spinal nerves.
Potentiometers are variable resistances used as an intensity control in electrical equipment.
Proprioceptors provide the kinesthetic sense. They occur in muscles, joints, tendons and ears and are the receptors defining the body's position and movements.
Puberty is the stage at which an individual's reproductive organs become functional. It normally occurs between 10 and 14 years of age.
Pulmonary circulation is the stream of blood going from the heart to the lungs and back.
Rectifiers change an alternating current into a direct current.
Red pulp is a type of lymphoid tissue present in the spleen around the splenic venules. It destroys worn out red blood cells.
Reflex action is a rapid automatic response to a particular stimulus and is usually involuntary.
Respiration is the process by which the living cells of the body obtain energy by breaking down food.
Respiratory centre is a region of the brain stem where reflex breathing movements are controlled.
Saprophytes are organisms which feed on dead organic material.
Selectively permeable describes a membrane which allows only some substances to pass through it.
Sesamoid describes a type of bone which develops in a tendon.
Sinu-auricular node (SAN) is a patch of tissue in the wall of the right atrium where contraction of cardiac muscle starts. It is known as the 'pacemaker', as it causes the heart to beat automatically at a regular rate.

Sutures are interlocking joints between two flat bones.

Synapse is a junction between two neurons, allowing a nerve impulse to pass in one direction by means of a chemical transmitter.

Systemic circulation is the stream of blood going from the heart to the body organs, except the lungs, and then returning to the heart.

Systole is the contraction of the cardiac muscle.

Target organs are the particular organs in which a hormone produces a response.

Telogen is the resting phase of the hair-growth cycle.

Tendons are pieces of tough, fibrous, non-elastic connective tissue attaching a muscle to a bone.

Thermostats regulate temperature by cutting off the fuel supply to a heater once it reaches a selected temperature.

Thrombocytes are cell fragments in the blood which aid clotting.

Tissues are composed of specialised cells which carry out particular functions in the body.

Transformers are devices to change the voltage of an alternating current by either increasing or decreasing it.

Triglycerides are a type of lipid occurring in fats and oils. They consist of three fatty acid molecules combined with glycerol to form an ester.

Ultra-filtration is the process occurring in the capsule of each nephron whereby a fluid (glomerular filtrate) is absorbed from the blood in the glomerulus.

Ureter is a duct carrying urine from a kidney to the bladder.

Vasomotor control affects the diameter of the arteries, arterioles and capillaries. It is carried out by the sympathetic nerves of the autonomic nervous system.

Veins are blood vessels taking blood to the heart.

Ventricles are the two lower chambers of the heart from which blood leaves via arteries.

Vitamins are chemicals present in foods which are essential for metabolism but which the body cannot synthesise.

White pulp is a form of lymphoid tissue present in the spleen surrounding the splenic arterioles. It produces lymphocytes.

ANATOMICAL TERMS

Anterior or **Ventral** Front side of the body. Palms of the hands are anterior.

Posterior or **Dorsal** Back or rear side of the body.

Medial Near the mid-line (a line running from the centre of the forehead to between the feet).

Lateral Further from the mid-line – at the sides.

External On the outside.

Internal On the inside.

Superficial Close to the external body surface but not actually on it.

Deep Further away from the surface, lying underneath other structures.

Proximal Closest to the mid-line. In the case of the limbs, those parts nearest the trunk.

Distal Further from the mid-line. In the case of the limbs, those parts lying furthest away from the trunk.

Superior Closer to the head.

Inferior Further away from the head.

Terms Used in the Description of Bones

Condyle A large projection, either convex or concave, at the end of a bone at the joint, for example the occipital condyles on the occipital bone at the base of the skull.

Foramen A round opening in a bone through which blood vessels, nerves, or ligaments can pass, for example a foramen occurs in each transverse process of a cervical vertebra for the vertebral artery and vein.

Head A rounded projection at the end of a bone, for example the head of the femur where it articulates with the pelvis.

Process A projection from a bone, for example the transverse processes project laterally from the centrum of a vertebra.

Spine A sharp slender process projecting from a bone, for example the neural spine is a posterior projection from the centrum of a vertebra, and the scapula has a ridge-like posterior spine.

Sulcus A groove along a bone in which a blood vessel, nerve or tendon lies, for example the sulcus on the head of the humerus called the bicipital groove carries the tendon of the long head of the biceps muscle.

Tubercle A small rounded process, for example the tubercle on each rib which articulates with a transverse process of a vertebra.

Tuberosity A large rounded roughened area on a bone, for example the ischial tuberosity on the posterior region of the pelvis where the quadratus femoris muscle has its origin.

Bibliography

Baum, G., *Aquarobics*, Arrow Books, 1991

Bembridge, R.A., *Beauty Therapy Science*, Longman, 1985

Harvard, C.W.H. (ed.), *Black's Medical Dictionary*, 35th edn., A&C Black, 1987

Gersh, S. & Gersh, I.G., *The Biology of Women*, Junction Books, 1981

Gibney, M.J., *Nutrition, Diet and Health*, Cambridge University Press, 1986

Gray, H., *Gray's Anatomy*, 36th edn., R. Warwick & P.L. Williams (eds.), Churchill Livingstone, 1980

Hibbott, H.W., *Handbook of Cosmetic Science*, Pergamon Press, 1963

Hodgson, G., 'The hazards of beauty culture', *The Practitioner*, vol. 189, 1962, pp. 667–673 and pp. 778–787

Martindale, W., *The Extra Pharmacopoeia*, 28th edn., The Pharmaceutical Press, 1982

Pierantoni, H., 'Essential notions about black skin', *Les Nouvelles Esthetiques*, Paris, 1977

Reuben, C. & Priestley, J., *Essential Supplements for Women*, Thorsons, 1991

Rogers, A.W., *Cells and Tissues*, Academic Press, 1983

Rounce, J., *Science for the Beauty Therapist*, Stanley Thornes, 1983

Rowett, H.G.Q., *Basic Anatomy and Physiology*, 2nd edn., John Murray, 1973

Samman, P.D. & Fenton, D.A., *The Nails in Disease*, 4th edn., Heinemann, 1986

Simpkins, J. & Williams, J.I., *Biology of the Cell, Mammal, and Flowering Plant*, Mills & Boon, 1980

Stoppard, M., *Everywoman's Life Guide*, Macdonald & Co., 1982

Tortora, G.J. & Anagnostakos, N.P., *Principles of Anatomy and Physiology*, 3rd edn., Harper & Row, 1981

Thompson, C.W., *Manual of Structural Kinesiology*, 11th edn., C.V. Mosby Co., 1989

Young, A., *Practical Cosmetic Science*, Mills & Boon, 1972

Wing, T.W., 'Star Trek Therapy here today', *The Digest of Chiropractic Economics*, 1979/1983

INDEX